Thyroid Disease and Reproduction

Jennifer L. Eaton
Editor

Thyroid Disease and Reproduction

A Clinical Guide to Diagnosis and Management

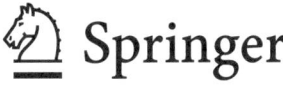 Springer

Editor
Jennifer L. Eaton, MD, MSCI
Division of Reproductive Endocrinology and Infertility
Department of Obstetrics and Gynecology
Duke University Medical Center
Durham, NC
USA

ISBN 978-3-030-07563-7   ISBN 978-3-319-99079-8   (eBook)
https://doi.org/10.1007/978-3-319-99079-8

© Springer Nature Switzerland AG 2019
Softcover re-print of the Hardcover 1st edition 2019
This work is subject to copyright. All rights are reserved by the Publisher, whether the whole or part of the material is concerned, specifically the rights of translation, reprinting, reuse of illustrations, recitation, broadcasting, reproduction on microfilms or in any other physical way, and transmission or information storage and retrieval, electronic adaptation, computer software, or by similar or dissimilar methodology now known or hereafter developed.
The use of general descriptive names, registered names, trademarks, service marks, etc. in this publication does not imply, even in the absence of a specific statement, that such names are exempt from the relevant protective laws and regulations and therefore free for general use.
The publisher, the authors, and the editors are safe to assume that the advice and information in this book are believed to be true and accurate at the date of publication. Neither the publisher nor the authors or the editors give a warranty, express or implied, with respect to the material contained herein or for any errors or omissions that may have been made. The publisher remains neutral with regard to jurisdictional claims in published maps and institutional affiliations.

This Springer imprint is published by the registered company Springer Nature Switzerland AG
The registered company address is: Gewerbestrasse 11, 6330 Cham, Switzerland

This book is dedicated to the students, residents, and fellows who challenge me to excel as a teacher and physician. You are the future of reproductive medicine.

To Sam: thank you for being the best husband and father. I appreciate the countless hours you spent at the pool with our children while I was working on this project. It would not have been possible without you.

Preface

The link between overt thyroid disease and obstetrical outcomes is well-established. The potential impact of subtle thyroid dysfunction on reproduction, however, is still being investigated. As a fellow in Reproductive Endocrinology and Infertility, I frequently debated this topic with my attending physicians. At that time, it was difficult to obtain clear, evidence-based guidance. Five years later, the body of evidence had grown substantially, but there was still no central source of information on this subject. After speaking on thyroid and reproduction at the Annual Meeting of the American Society for Reproductive Medicine, I was inspired to fill this gap in the existing literature.

This book may be subdivided into five basic sections: (1) thyroid physiology and pathophysiology, (2) thyroid function during pregnancy and fetal development, (3) thyroid pathophysiology in pregnancy, (4) the role of thyroid disease in infertility and miscarriage, and (5) postpartum thyroid disease. The first three chapters give a basic introduction to thyroid physiology and pathophysiology. These chapters will serve as a basis for understanding Chap. 4, which discusses the changes in thyroid physiology that occur during pregnancy. In turn, fetal thyroid development is discussed in Chap. 5. Chapters 6, 7, and 8 focus on thyroid dysfunction, nodules, and cancer during pregnancy. The most hotly debated topics are subsequently discussed in Chap. 9 on "Thyroid Dysfunction and Infertility" and in Chap. 10 on "Thyroid Autoimmunity and Miscarriage." Finally, in Chap. 11, the focus turns to postpartum thyroiditis, a common condition that may be missed due to mild symptomatology and overlap with normal postpartum stress.

This evidence-based text was written to serve as a straightforward reference for students, house staff, obstetrician-gynecologists, and endocrinologists. I hope that providers will find this book useful to inform their clinical decisions when providing patient care. Each chapter is written by an expert in the field, and I feel truly honored to have had the opportunity to work with these outstanding authors. Given that the existing knowledge on this topic is rapidly expanding, I look forward to working with them to update this resource in the future.

Durham, NC, USA   Jennifer L. Eaton

Contents

1 **Thyroid Hormone Biosynthesis and Physiology** 1
  Malini Soundarrajan and Peter A. Kopp

2 **Hypothyroidism**... 19
  Vishnu Vardhan Garla, Licy L. Yanes Cardozo,
  and Lillian Frances Lien

3 **Thyrotoxicosis** 45
  Adva Eisenberg, Rebecca Herbst, and Tracy L. Setji

4 **Thyroid Function and Pregnancy** 69
  Nathan King and Lia A. Bernardi

5 **Fetal and Neonatal Thyroid Physiology** 79
  Laura C. Page and Robert W. Benjamin

6 **Hypothyroidism in Pregnancy**................................. 101
  Elizabeth N. Pearce

7 **Thyrotoxicosis in Pregnancy** 117
  Wilburn D. Bolton III and Jennifer M. Perkins

8 **Thyroid Nodules and Cancer in Pregnancy** 137
  Sarah E. Mayson and Linda A. Barbour

9 **Thyroid Dysfunction and Infertility** 157
  Shweta J. Bhatt, Emily C. Holden, and Aimee Seungdamrong

10 **Thyroid Autoimmunity and Miscarriage** 169
   Kelly S. Acharya and Jennifer L. Eaton

11 **Postpartum Thyroiditis**..................................... 183
   Benjamin S. Harris and Jennifer L. Eaton

Index.. 189

Contributors

Kelly S. Acharya, MD Duke University Medical Center, Division of Reproductive Endocrinology and Infertility, Department of Obstetrics and Gynecology, Durham, NC, USA

Linda A. Barbour, MD, MSPH University of Colorado School of Medicine, Divisions of Endocrinology, Metabolism, and Diabetes; and Maternal-Fetal Medicine, Aurora, CO, USA

Robert W. Benjamin, MD Duke University Medical Center, Department of Pediatrics, Durham, NC, USA

Lia A. Bernardi, MD, MSCI Northwestern University, Feinberg School of Medicine, Division of Reproductive Endocrinology and Infertility, Department of Obstetrics and Gynecology, Chicago, IL, USA

Shweta J. Bhatt, MD Rutgers New Jersey Medical School, Department of Obstetrics, Gynecology, and Women's Health, Newark, NJ, USA

Wilburn D. Bolton III, MD Duke University Medical Center, Division of Endocrinology, Metabolism, and Nutrition, Department of Medicine, Durham, NC, USA

Jennifer L. Eaton, MD, MSCI Medical Director of Assisted Reproductive Technologies, Director of Oocyte Donation, Duke University Medical Center, Division of Reproductive Endocrinology and Infertility, Department of Obstetrics and Gynecology, Durham, NC, USA

Adva Eisenberg, MD Duke University Medical Center, Division of Endocrinology, Metabolism, and Nutrition, Department of Medicine, Durham, NC, USA

Vishnu Vardhan Garla, MD University of Mississippi Medical Center, Department of Internal Medicine, Jackson, MS, USA

Benjamin S. Harris, MD, MPH Duke University Medical Center, Division of Reproductive Endocrinology and Infertility, Department of Obstetrics and Gynecology, Durham, NC, USA

Rebecca Herbst, MD Duke University Medical Center, Division of Endocrinology, Metabolism, and Nutrition, Department of Medicine, Durham, NC, USA

Emily C. Holden, MD Rutgers New Jersey Medical School, Department of Obstetrics, Gynecology, and Women's Health, Newark, NJ, USA

Nathan King, MD Northwestern University, Feinberg School of Medicine, Department of Obstetrics and Gynecology, Chicago, IL, USA

Peter A. Kopp, MD Northwestern University, Feinberg School of Medicine, Division of Endocrinology, Metabolism, and Molecular Medicine, Chicago, IL, USA

Lillian Frances Lien, MD, FACP University of Mississippi Medical Center, Division Chief of Endocrinology, Metabolism, and Diabetes, Department of Medicine, Jackson, MS, USA

Sarah E. Mayson, MD University of Colorado School of Medicine, Division of Endocrinology, Metabolism, and Diabetes, Aurora, CO, USA

Laura C. Page, MD Duke University Medical Center, Department of Pediatrics, Durham, NC, USA

Elizabeth N. Pearce, MD, MSc Boston Medical Center, Boston University School of Medicine, Section of Endocrinology, Diabetes, and Nutrition, Boston, MA, USA

Jennifer M. Perkins, MD, MBA Duke University Medical Center, Division of Endocrinology, Metabolism, and Nutrition, Department of Medicine, Durham, NC, USA

Tracy L. Setji, MD, MHS Duke University Medical Center, Division of Endocrinology, Metabolism, and Nutrition, Department of Medicine, Durham, NC, USA

Aimee Seungdamrong, MD Rutgers New Jersey Medical School, Department of Obstetrics, Gynecology, and Women's Health, Newark, NJ, USA

Damien Fertility Partners, Shrewsbury, NJ, USA

Malini Soundarrajan, MD Northwestern University, Feinberg School of Medicine, Division of Endocrinology, Metabolism, and Molecular Medicine, Chicago, IL, USA

Licy L. Yanes Cardozo, MD University of Mississippi Medical Center, Departments of Cellular and Molecular Biology, and Internal Medicine, Jackson, MS, USA

Chapter 1
Thyroid Hormone Biosynthesis and Physiology

Malini Soundarrajan and Peter A. Kopp

> **Clinical Case**
> A 6-year-old girl is referred for evaluation of resting tachycardia and abnormal thyroid function tests. On systematic questioning, she reports frequent bowel movements, and she has difficulties concentrating. On physical examination, her heart rate is 110 bpm, and her thyroid is diffusely enlarged. She has no signs of endocrine ophthalmopathy. Her height is at the 50th percentile, and her weight is at the 20th percentile. Her TSH is mildly elevated at 7.2 mU/l (0.5–4.5), the T4 is 31 mcg/dl (6.0–12.0), and the T3 is 1915 ng/dl (80–178). TSH receptor-stimulating antibodies (TSAB) and anti-thyroperoxidase antibodies (TPO-Ab) are negative. What is your differential diagnosis? What type of medical treatment do you recommend?

Thyroid Hormone Physiology

Thyroid hormones play a key role in development, growth, and metabolic regulation. A normally developed thyroid gland, an intact hypothalamic-pituitary-thyroid axis, adequate nutritional iodine intake, and a sequence of regulated biochemical steps within thyroid follicular cells are all essential for appropriate thyroid hormone synthesis. Thyroid hormones act largely by regulating nuclear transcription factors, the thyroid hormone receptors α and β (TRα, TRβ), to alter gene expression. Transcriptional regulation is either positive or negative, depending on the target

---

M. Soundarrajan · P. A. Kopp (✉)
Northwestern University, Feinberg School of Medicine, Division of Endocrinology, Metabolism, and Molecular Medicine, Chicago, IL, USA
e-mail: p-kopp@northwestern.edu

gene. In addition to transcriptional regulation, thyroid hormones can also exert non-genomic effects, which are not well characterized.

The estimated prevalence of hypothyroidism and hyperthyroidism are 3.7% and 0.5%, respectively, in the United States (Chaps. 2 and 3). Overall, thyroid disease is more prevalent among females than males [1]. Thus, these entities are of significant clinical relevance. Importantly, the hypothalamic-pituitary-thyroid axis and thyroid hormone-binding proteins undergo significant changes during pregnancy (Chap. 4) [2]. Alterations in thyroid function or the presence of thyroid autoimmunity can impact conception rates and pregnancy outcomes (Chaps. 4, 6, 7, 9, and 10) [3]. While it is well accepted that significant alterations in thyroid function also impact fetal outcomes, the consequences of subclinical thyroid dysfunction (subclinical hypo- and hyperthyroidism) remain controversial [4].

Overview of the Hypothalamic-Pituitary-Thyroid Axis

The thyroid gland, like many endocrine organs, is regulated by positive and negative feedback pathways via the hypothalamic-pituitary-thyroid (HPT) axis (Fig. 1.1) [5]. Thyrotropin-releasing hormone (TRH) secreted from the hypothalamus stimulates production and release of TSH, a glycoprotein hormone, in the anterior pituitary gland. TSH is comprised of an α and a β subunit. The α subunit of TSH is common to several other glycoproteins including follicle-stimulating hormone (FSH), luteinizing hormone (LH), and human chorionic gonadotropin (hCG), while the β subunit is unique. TSH binds to the TSH receptor, a G protein-coupled transmembrane receptor, at the basolateral membrane of the follicular cells in the thyroid gland resulting in stimulation of cell growth, differentiation, and thyroid hormone synthesis (Fig. 1.2) [6]. TSH receptor activation leads to coupling with G protein Gsα and activation of adenylyl cyclase with a resulting increase in intracellular cyclic AMP (cAMP) concentrations, phosphorylation of protein kinase A, and activation of various cytosolic and nuclear target proteins. At high concentrations of TSH, the TSH receptor also couples to $G_{q/11}$, activating the phospholipase C-dependent inositol phosphate Ca^{2+}/diacylglycerol pathway resulting in increased production of hydrogen peroxide (H_2O_2) and iodination. In Graves' disease, thyroid-stimulating immunoglobulins (TSI) bind the TSH receptor resulting in overproduction of thyroid hormones (Chap. 3) [6].

In the thyroid, the follicles form the functional units that are necessary for the synthesis of thyroid hormone (Fig. 1.3). In a series of biochemical steps, which are discussed in more detail below, the thyroid hormones thyroxine (T4) and triiodothyronine (T3) are synthesized and then released into the blood stream. In the serum, T4 and T3 are largely bound to proteins including thyroxine-binding globulin (TBG), transthyretin (TTR), and albumin. Only a small fraction of T4 and T3 are present as free hormone [7]. T3 in the circulation exerts a negative feedback on TRH and TSH secretion thereby regulating the HPT axis.

1 Thyroid Hormone Biosynthesis and Physiology

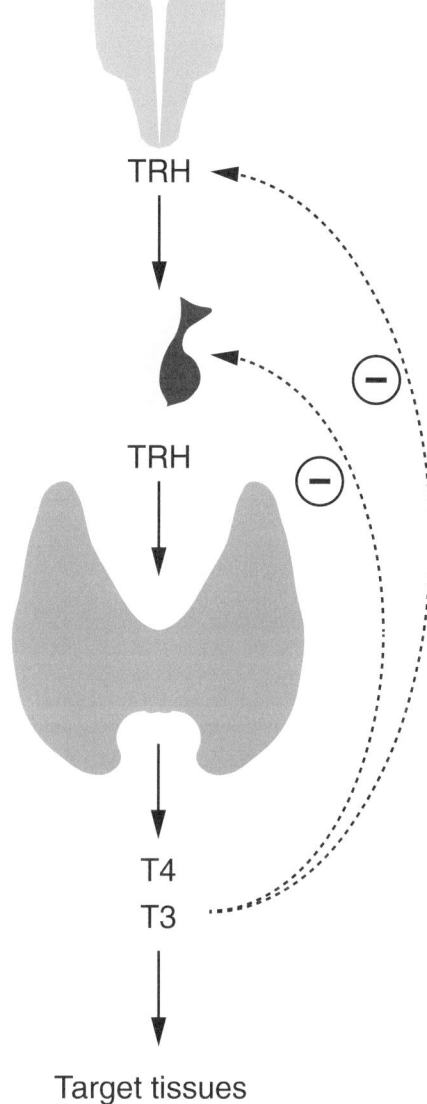

Fig. 1.1 The hypothalamic-pituitary-thyroid axis. TRH TSH-releasing hormone, TSH Thyroid-stimulating hormone, T4 Thyroxine, T3 Triiodothyronine

Entry of thyroid hormones into target peripheral cells is mediated by several thyroid transporters [8]. Within the cells, T4 either undergoes 5′-deiodination by deiodinase type I or II to form the more active T3 or undergoes deiodination of the inner ring to form reverse T3 (rT3), the inactive thyroid hormone (Fig. 1.4) [9]. Thyroid hormone action is predominantly mediated by two ligand-regulated nuclear receptors, TRα and TRβ, which regulate gene expression [10]. Thyroid hormones also have several non-genomic actions, which are less well understood.

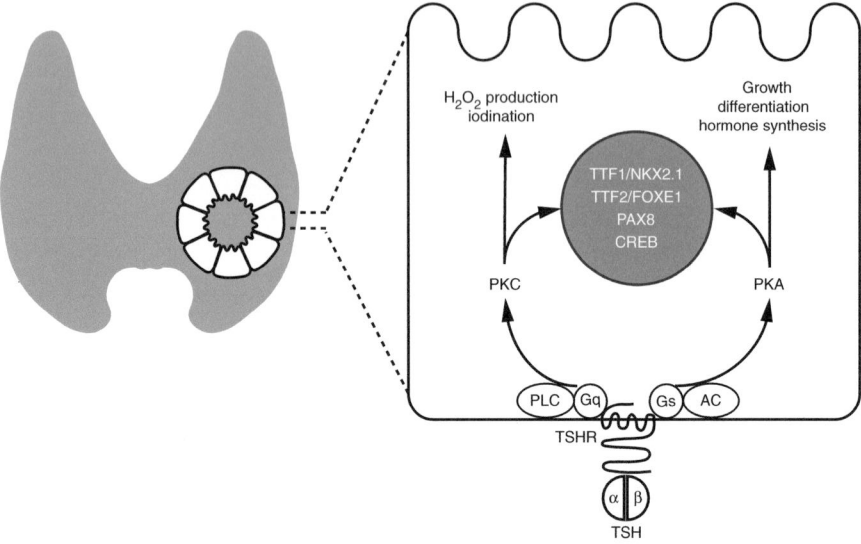

Fig. 1.2 Signaling pathways in thyroid follicular cells. The functional unit in the thyroid is the thyroid follicle, which is formed by a monolayer of thyroid cells and a colloid-filled lumen. TSH, thyroid-stimulating hormone consisting of an α and a β subunit. TSHR TSH receptor, AC Adenylyl cyclase, cAMP Cyclic adenosine monophosphate, PKA Protein kinase A, DAG Diacylglycerol, PKC Protein kinase C, PLC Phospholipase C, IP3 Inositol triphosphate, PAX8 Transcription factor PAX8, TTF1/NKX2.1 Thyroid transcription factor 1, TTF2/FOXE2 Thyroid transcription factor 2, CREB cAMP response element-binding protein

Thyroid Hormone Synthesis

Thyroid hormone synthesis occurs within the spherical thyroid follicles, which are formed by a monolayer of thyroid cells and the follicular lumen [11]. A sequence of biochemical steps within the follicle results in the synthesis of T4 and T3 (Fig. 1.3). The sodium-iodide symporter (NIS) at the basolateral membrane of the thyroid follicular cell actively transports iodide into the cells [12, 13]. The sodium-potassium (Na^+/K^+) ATPase generates the electrochemical gradient needed for the iodide transport. Iodide then reaches the apical membrane and is released into the follicular lumen through pendrin, an anion exchanger, and possibly anoctamin [14]. In the follicular lumen, iodide is oxidized by the enzyme thyroperoxidase (TPO) in the presence of H_2O_2 [15]. Dual oxidase 2 (DUOX2) is an enzyme that catalyzes the production of H_2O_2; this enzyme requires the DUOX2 maturation factor (DUOXA2) to reach the apical membrane [16, 17]. The colloid within the follicular lumen is predominantly formed by thyroglobulin (TG). TG is the matrix upon which synthesis of T4 and T3 occurs [18]. First, an organification reaction occurs whereby specific tyrosyl residues on TG are iodinated by TPO, forming mono-and diiodotyrosines (MIT, DIT). Subsequently, via a coupling reaction, the iodotyrosines are coupled by TPO to form T4 and T3. TG is internalized from the follicular lumen into the

1 Thyroid Hormone Biosynthesis and Physiology

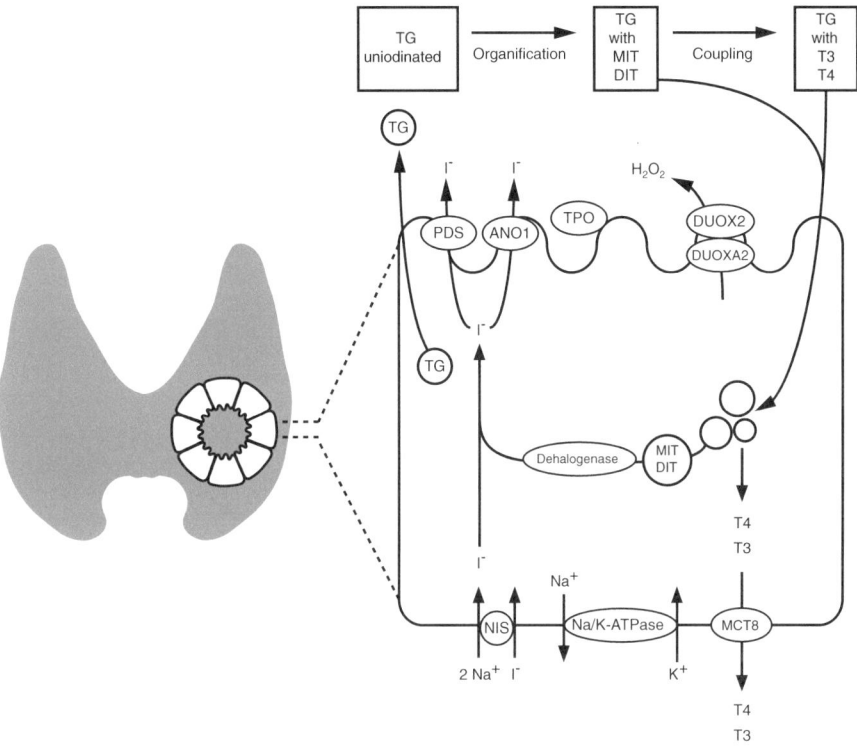

Fig. 1.3 Thyroid hormone synthesis. Thyroid hormone synthesis occurs in thyroid follicles. NIS Sodium-iodide symporter, PDS Pendrin, ANO1 Anoctamin, TPO Thyroperoxidase, TG Thyroglobulin, DUOX2 Dual oxidase 2, DUOXA2 DUOX2 maturation factor, MIT Monoiodotyrosine, DIT Diiodotyrosine, T4 Thyroxine, T3 Triiodothyronine, MCT8 Monocarboxylate transporter 8

follicular cell by pinocytosis and the thyroid hormones are released into the circulation, at least in part via the thyroid hormone-transporting channel MCT8 [17]. About 80% of the released hormone consists of T4 and 20% of T3. Remarkably, MIT and DIT are retained in the cell and deiodinated by the iodotyrosine dehalogenase DEHAL1/IYD, and the released iodide is recycled back into follicular lumen for thyroid hormone synthesis [19].

Parafollicular (C) cells of the thyroid gland secrete calcitonin. While calcitonin is not necessary for calcium homeostasis, at supraphysiological doses, it has a hypocalcemic effect. Further, evidence from mice studies suggests it may inhibit bone resorption during growth, pregnancy, and lactation [20]. Whether this has relevance in human physiology remains uncertain [20]. Similarly to thyroglobulin, which serves as tumor marker for thyroid carcinomas originating from thyroid follicular cells (papillary and follicular thyroid carcinomas), calcitonin is used as a tumor marker in the surveillance of patients with medullary thyroid cancer [21].

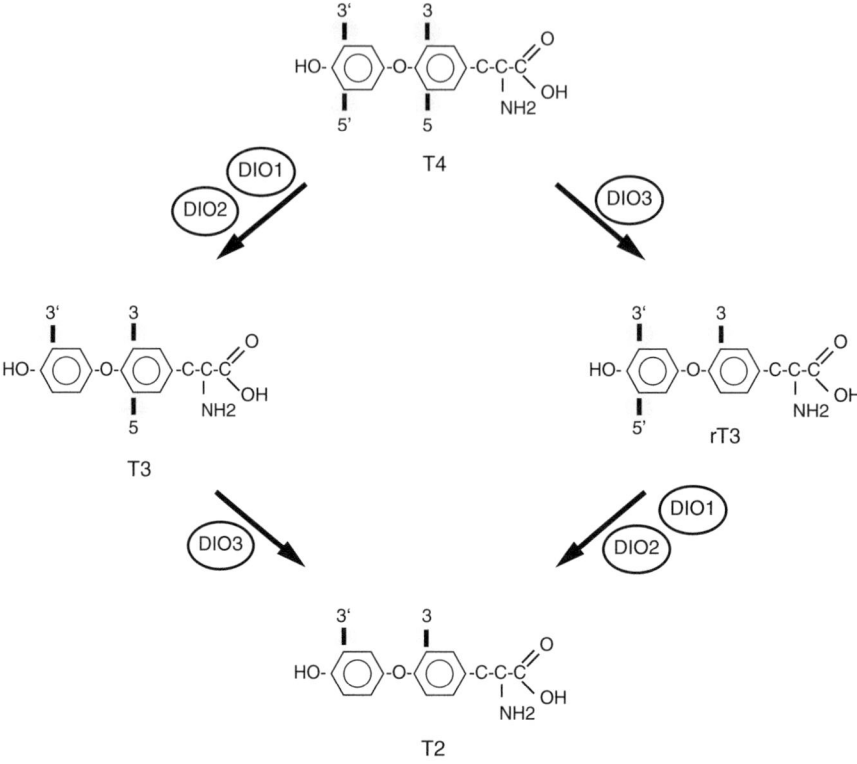

Fig. 1.4 Structure of thyroid hormones and modification by deiodinases. Structure of thyroxine (T4), triiodothyronine (T3) and reverse T3 (rT3), and diiodothyronine (T2). T4 undergoes 5′-monodeionation by deiodinase 1 and 2 (DIO1, DIO2), which are differentially expressed. T3 is more active, and T4 is in general considered a prohormone. T4 can be inactivated to rT3 by deiodinase 3

Iodide Uptake by the Sodium-Iodide Symporter (NIS)

The iodide concentration is significantly higher within thyroid cells compared to serum due to the active uptake by the sodium-iodide symporter (NIS). NIS uses the sodium gradient generated by the Na^+/K^+-ATPase and transports two sodium ions and one iodide ion into the cell [12, 13]. Certain anions including perchlorate and thiocyanate are competitive inhibitors of NIS. Perchlorate was used in treatment of hyperthyroidism in the past, but because of the rare risk of aplastic anemia, this is no longer the case. Perchlorate is also actively transported by NIS but in an electroneutral manner [22]. Diagnostically, the perchlorate discharge test can be used to determine the degree of iodide organification [23].

In addition to the thyroid gland, NIS is expressed in other tissues such as the gastric mucosa, the salivary glands, and the lactating (but not the non-lactating) mammary gland where it also facilitates active iodide transport [13, 24]. Iodide that is secreted in breast milk serves as a substrate for thyroid hormone synthesis in the nursing newborn [24].

TSH stimulates iodide uptake into follicular cells through several mechanisms. TSH upregulates NIS expression, prolongs NIS half-life, and promotes increased insertion and retention of NIS in the plasma membrane [12].

Iodide also regulates its own accumulation and organification in the thyroid gland [25]. After exposure to moderate and high doses of iodide, NIS mRNA expression decreases [26]. Iodide may also decrease NIS activity and increase NIS turnover [27]. At high intracellular iodide concentration, iodide transiently inhibits the organification process and blocks synthesis of thyroid hormone; this is termed the *Wolff-Chaikoff effect* [28, 29]. This inhibition is temporary as it requires a high intracellular iodine concentration. Due to decreased NIS expression, the intracellular iodine concentration decreases and the inhibitory effect wanes [30].

Individuals with inactivating homozygous or compound heterozygous mutations in the *NIS* gene have impaired iodide uptake and hypothyroidism [12]. These patients often have a diffuse or nodular goiter and minimal or no uptake of radioiodine.

Apical Iodide Efflux, Pendrin, and Anoctamin

TSH stimulates rapid iodide efflux into the follicular lumen and leaves efflux in the basal membrane unchanged [14]. Iodide transport from the apical membrane into the follicular lumen is facilitated by the electrochemical gradient with a negatively charged lumen (Fig. 1.3). Several studies suggest that the anion channel PDS/SLC26A4 may be responsible for iodide efflux at the apical membrane [31, 32]. TSH does not regulate expression of PDS/SLC26A4; however, it rapidly upregulates membrane insertion, which leads to increased iodide efflux from follicular cells [33].

Biallelic mutations in the *PDS/SLC26A4* gene lead to Pendred syndrome, an autosomal recessive disorder defined by sensorineural deafness, impaired iodide organification, and goiter [14]. Iodide efflux can, however, also occur in the absence of pendrin suggesting that other exchangers or channels are involved [14]. Anoctamin 1 (ANO1/TMEM16A), a calcium-activated anion channel, which is also expressed at the apical membrane of thyrocytes, may also be participating in mediating apical efflux [34, 35].

Thyroglobulin: The Matrix for Thyroid Hormone Synthesis

Thyroglobulin (TG) is the matrix upon which thyroxine (T4) and triiodothyronine (T3) are synthesized [18]. During the organification reaction, selected tyrosyl residues in the follicular colloid are iodinated, resulting in the formation of monoiodotyrosines (MIT) and diiodotyrosines (DIT) [11]. Subsequently, in a coupling reaction, some of these iodotyrosines are fused to form T3 or T4. TG is taken up by the follicular cell predominantly via micropinocytosis and digested by lysosomes. Some intact TG is transported to the basolateral membrane by transcytosis and secreted into the blood stream. T4 (about 80%) and T3 (about 20%) are then released into the circulation.

In individuals with biallelic mutations in the *TG* gene, congenital goiter, and depending on the severity of the defect, hypothyroidism, subclinical hypothyroidism, or normal thyroid hormone levels may be present [36]. Serum TG levels may be low, normal, or elevated with elevated radioiodine uptake. Often, the abnormal TG protein is retained in the endoplasmic reticulum leading to a classical endoplasmic reticulum storage disease.

TG is a very specific and sensitive tumor marker in the follow-up of patients with well-differentiated thyroid cancer (Chap. 8) [37]. Antibodies against TG, however, can interfere with these assays.

Thyroperoxidase: The Enzyme Mediating the Organification and Coupling Reactions

Thyroperoxidase (TPO) is a membrane-bound glycoprotein with a heme group located in the follicular lumen. In the presence of hydrogen peroxide (H_2O_2), it catalyzes the oxidation of iodide, which is essential for the iodination of selected tyrosyl residues within thyroglobulin (organification reaction) [15]. In a subsequent step, the coupling reaction, TPO catalyzes the coupling of two iodinated tyrosyl residues, which results in the generation of T3 or T4 (Fig. 1.3) [15]. TSH increases TPO enzyme activity and its insertion into the apical membrane of the follicular cell.

A defect in TPO is a common cause of thyroid hormone synthesis abnormality [38]. Homozygotes or compound heterozygotes for mutations in the *TPO* gene have a partial or total organification defect.

The H_2O_2-Generating System

Hydrogen peroxide (H_2O_2) is necessary for the oxidation of iodide and the organification reaction (Fig. 1.3) [11]. H_2O_2 is generated via two NAPH oxidase systems, DUOX1 and DUOX2. The DUOX oxidase system is redundant such that loss of DUOX2 can be partially compensated by DUOX1. DUOX proteins co-localize with TPO at the apical membrane of the follicular cells. They require specific maturation factors, DUOXA1 and DUOXA2, to transition the protein from the endoplasmic reticulum to the Golgi apparatus and for translocation to the plasma membrane.

Mono- and biallelic mutations in DUOX2 can lead to mild transient or severe congenital hypothyroidism [39].

Hormone Processing and Secretion

TG, after modification by the organification and coupling reactions, enters thyroid follicular cells through micropinocytosis (Fig. 1.3). TG-containing vesicles fuse with lysosomes leading to degradation of TG and release of iodotyrosines (DIT, MIT) and thyroid hormones (T3, T4). T4 and T3 (but only minute amounts of MIT and DIT) are then secreted into the blood stream at the basolateral membrane of thyroid follicular cells. One of the transporters involved in this process is the monocarboxylate transporter 8 (MCT8) [40], which is encoded by a X-chromosomal gene. Males with mutations in MCT8 have a characteristic phenotype termed Allan-Herndon-Dudley syndrome, which includes developmental delay, severe hypotonia, spastic quadriplegia, and dystonic movements [41, 42]. Biochemically, they have low T4 and free T4, elevated T3, low rT3, and normal or slightly elevated TSH levels. Female heterozygotes do not usually have neurological disturbances.

Dehalogenation of MIT and DIT by Dehalogenase I (DEHAL1/IYD)

A large portion of iodotyrosines MIT and DIT are recycled for hormone synthesis and undergo deiodination by a dehalogenase, DEHAL1/IYD, and only a very small portion is released into the bloodstream.

Individuals with biallelic mutations in the *DEHAL1* gene present with large goiters and hypothyroidism [19]. This phenotype is not often evident at birth and thus can be missed on neonatal screening. Affected individuals lose large amounts of iodotyrosines in the urine and have high serum diiodotyrosine levels [19].

Thyroid Hormone Transport

Circulating thyroid hormones are predominantly bound by three plasma proteins: thyroxine-binding globulin (TBG), transthyretin (TTR), and albumin. Only 0.03% of T4 and 0.3% of T3 circulate as free hormone, unbound by proteins [43].

Variations in binding protein concentrations can alter total thyroid hormone levels [43, 44]. This is especially apparent in pregnancy, during which estrogen induces higher circulating TBG levels and consequently total T4 and T3 concentrations (Chap. 4) [45, 46]. Many other physiological changes and drugs can either increase or decrease binding protein concentrations [47]. More rarely, mutations affecting the affinity for thyroid hormone or resulting in increased or decreased concentrations of the binding proteins result in changes in *total* T4 and/or T3 concentrations [48].

Uptake of Thyroid Hormones into Target Cells and Modification by Deiodinases

For a long time, most investigators postulated that thyroid hormones freely enter cells through diffusion. However, it has been formally demonstrated that several transporters mediate thyroid hormone uptake into target cells. They include, among others, the monocarboxylate transporters (MCT8 and MCT10) and the organic anion transporting polypeptide 1(OATP1C1) [17]. After entering the cell, T4 is converted to the more active form, T3, by intracellular 5'-monodeiodination by the deiodinases I and II (DIO1, DIO2), or to the inactive metabolite, reverse T3 (rT3) by 5-monodeiodination through deiodinase III (DIO3) (Fig. 1.4) [9]. T3 ultimately enters the nucleus where it binds to thyroid hormone receptor. About 80% of T3 is metabolized from monodeiodination of T4, and the affinity of the TRs is about tenfold higher for T3 than for T4. For these reasons, T4 is in general considered a prohormone. Deiodinases are tightly regulated as they affect tissue-specific thyroid hormone action by modulating levels of T4 and T3 [49, 50]. Moreover, they display variable expression levels during development, in various tissues, and in disease including critical illness [9, 51].

Thyroid Hormone Action

At the cellular level, thyroid hormone acts on thyroid hormone receptors, which are ligand-regulated nuclear receptors that modify gene transcription [10]. Many other hormones including estrogens, progesterone, androgens, glucocorticoids, and mineralocorticoids also exert their biological effect through nuclear receptors and transcriptional regulation [46]. Two distinct genes, THRA (on chromosome 17) and THRB (on chromosome 3), encode thyroid hormone receptor α (TRα) and β (TRβ), which are present in various isoforms [10]. The TRα1, TRβ1, and TRβ2 isoforms all have high affinity for thyroid hormones, but they display differential expression during development and among various tissues [52].

Thyroid hormone receptors form heterodimers with accessory proteins (e.g., the nuclear receptor retinoic X receptor, RXR) and bind corepressors and coactivators in promoters of target genes (Fig. 1.5a, b) [10, 53]. Depending on the gene, T3 either stimulates or inhibits gene expression. In positively regulated genes, TRs interact with corepressors to deacetylate histones and repress transcription in the absence of T3 (Fig. 1.5a, b). In the presence of T3, the corepressor dissociates, allowing coactivators to bind, resulting in histone acetylation, recruitment of transcription factors, and RNA polymerase II, thereby leading to transcriptional activation. Mechanisms of negative gene regulation, e.g., of the *TSH* and *TRH* genes, are not fully understood [54].

Mutations in TRβ exert a dominant negative effect on the normal allele and result in a condition termed resistance to thyroid hormone β (RTHβ) [55, 56]. This syndrome is characterized by elevated free thyroid hormone levels and an

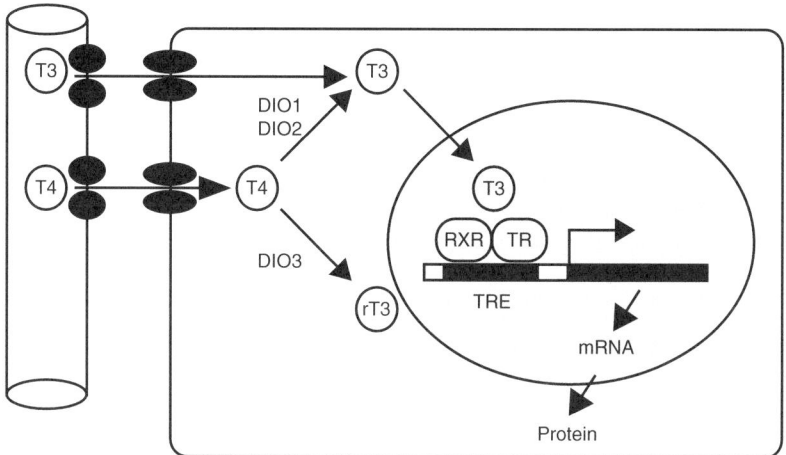

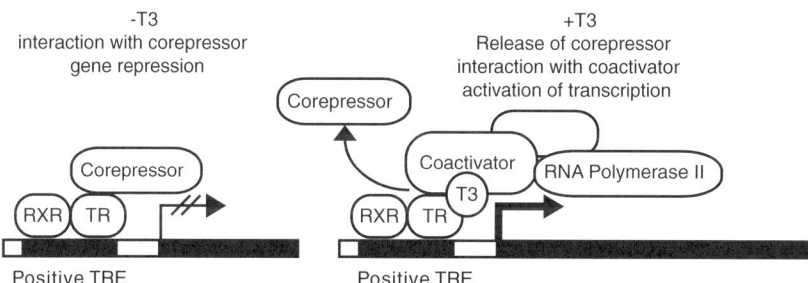

Fig. 1.5 Mechanism of thyroid hormone action on a positively regulated target gene. Upper panel: T4 and T3 enter the target cell by specific amino acid channels such as the monocarboxylate transporters (MCT8 and MCT10) and the organic anion-transporting polypeptide 1(OATP1C1), among others. T4 can be converted by deiodinase 1 and 2 to T3. It then enters the nucleus where it can bind to the cognate nuclear receptor, either TRα or TRβ. The TRs form heterodimers with the nuclear receptor RXR and bind to thyroid hormone response elements in promoters of positively regulated target genes. This interaction leads to changes in transcription and protein expression. Lower panel: In the absence of thyroid hormone, corepressors interact with TR homo- or heterodimers and repress transcription on positively regulate genes. Once T3 binds, the corepressor complex is released, and conformational changes in the receptors lead to interaction of coactivators. They, in turn, recruit factors of the basal transcription apparatus, which results in the activation of gene transcription. RXR, Retinoid X receptor. TR, Thyroid hormone receptor. TRE, thyroid hormone response element. Of note, the mechanisms underlying negative regulation (e.g., of the *TSH beta subunit* gene) are less well understood

inappropriately normal or elevated TSH level. Patients with RTH are less responsive to thyroid hormone in tissues that primarily express TRβ, have elevated T4 and T3 levels due to thyroid hormone resistance, and consequently have increased stimulation in tissues that predominantly express TRα. The clinical presentation varies from isolated abnormalities in thyroid function tests to a constellation of findings including goiter (due to the elevated TSH) and signs of hyper- and hypothyroidism such as tachycardia, learning disabilities, short stature, and delayed bone maturation [57].

The molecular cause of the RTHβ phenotype has been identified through classic linkage studies and the subsequent detection of mutations in TRβ. In contrast, the first mutation in TRα has been identified through whole exome sequencing in a girl with developmental delay, obesity, skeletal dysplasia (evidenced by short stature, delayed closure of fontanels, and epiphyseal dysgenesis), impaired gastrointestinal motility, and mildly abnormal thyroid function [58]. An unbiased next-generation sequencing approach was essential for the discovery of the genetic cause of this phenotype because it was not possible to readily identify a candidate gene that would explain this pattern of abnormalities. Subsequently, several additional TRα mutations have been identified [59, 60]. In this syndrome, now termed RTHα, there is a phenotypic spectrum with patients harboring truncating mutations exhibiting more severe phenotypes and those with missense mutations tending to be less severely affected.

In addition to modifying gene transcription in the cell nucleus, thyroid hormones also have some non-genomic actions affecting the plasma membrane, cytoskeleton, sarcoplasmic reticulum, mitochondrial gene transcription, and contractile elements of the vascular smooth muscle cells [61].

Impact of Thyroid Hormones on the Gonadal Axis

Thyroid hormones affect the gonadal axis resulting in alterations in growth, puberty, and fertility (Chaps. 6, 7, 9, and 10). In addition to impaired longitudinal growth, hypothyroidism in children can impair gonadotropin-releasing hormone (GnRH) release and delay puberty. Primary hypothyroidism can also lead to precocious puberty, possibly due to elevated TSH levels stimulating gonadotropin receptors [46]. In adult women, hypothyroidism can lead to menorrhagia, anovulation, and infertility via changes in sex hormone-binding globulin (SHBG) and sex steroids [62]. Additionally, elevation in thyrotropin-releasing hormone (TRH) due to primary hypothyroidism can induce lactotroph hyperplasia and hyperprolactinemia leading to galactorrhea and menstrual abnormalities. Hyperthyroidism also adversely affects ovulation and may result in irregular menses and infertility [46, 62].

Physiological Changes in the Hypothalamic-Thyroid Axis During Pregnancy

Several physiological changes in thyroid physiology occur during pregnancy, and they impact thyroid function tests, iodide, and thyroid hormone requirements (Chap. 4) [2]. Levels of TBG, total T4, and, to a lesser extent, total T3 are elevated [45, 46]. Accordingly, free T3 and T4 levels are reduced due to increased binding to TBG. See Fig. 1.6. Human chorionic gonadotropin does not only bind to its cognate receptor but also stimulates the TSH receptor. This results in a transient increase in free T4 and a reciprocal lowering of the TSH levels. A robust understanding of these alterations, detailed in Chap. 4, is essential for the interpretation of these frequently ordered tests.

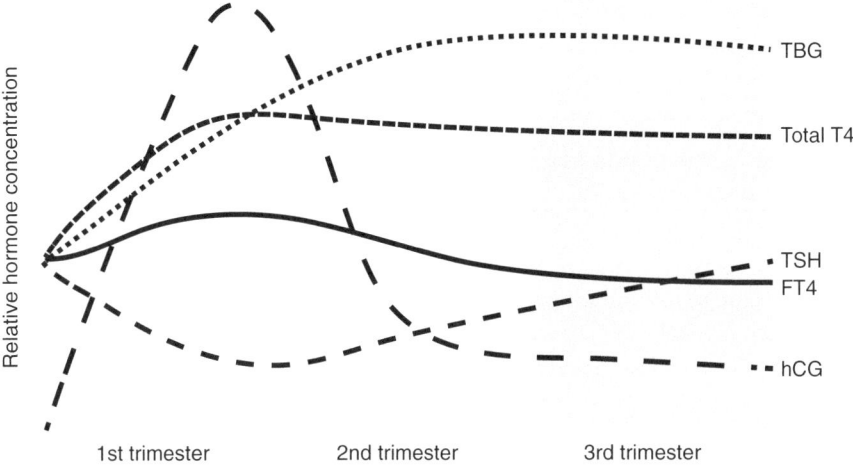

Fig. 1.6 Hormonal changes during pregnancy. Human chorionic gonadotropin (hCG) is structurally similar to thyroid-stimulating hormone (TSH). Therefore, hCG does not only bind to its cognate receptor but also stimulates the TSH receptor. This results in a transient increase in free T4 and a reciprocal lowering of the TSH levels. As hCG levels decline later in pregnancy, maternal TSH levels rise again. Other alterations include an estrogen-mediated increase in thyroxine-binding globulin, which results in increased total T4 concentrations

Clinical Case and Discussion

A 6-year-old girl is referred for evaluation of resting tachycardia and abnormal thyroid function tests. On systematic questioning, she reports frequent bowel movements, and she has difficulties concentrating. On physical examination, her heart rate is 110 bpm, and her thyroid is diffusely enlarged. She has no signs of endocrine ophthalmopathy. Her height is at the 50th percentile, and her weight is at the 20th percentile. Her TSH is mildly elevated at 7.2 mU/l (0.5–4.5), the T4 is 31 mcg/dl (6.0–12.0), and the T3 is 1915 ng/dl (80–178). TSH receptor stimulating antibodies (TSAB) and anti-thyroperoxidase antibodies (TPO-Ab) are negative. What is your differential diagnosis? What type of medical treatment do you recommend?

This patient has elevated peripheral hormones. In this situation, one would typically expect a suppressed TSH due to the negative feedback. However, in this patient, the TSH is inappropriately elevated.

The differential diagnosis includes autonomous secretion of TSH by a pituitary adenoma (TSHoma) or resistance to thyroid hormone β (RTHβ).

In this patient, a MRI of the pituitary showed normal findings. Direct sequencing of the *THRB* gene revealed a de novo point mutation that abolishes binding of T3. Patients with RTHβ are less responsive to thyroid hormone in tissues that primarily express TRβ, have elevated T4 and T3 levels due to thyroid hormone resistance, and consequently have increased stimulation in tissues that predominantly express TRα. The condition can be inherited in an autosomal dominant fashion.

In this patient, beta-blockade was chosen to control her tachycardia. Thyreostatic medication, radioiodine, or thyroidectomy is contraindicated.

The study of rare phenotypes with abnormal thyroid hormone synthesis, thyroid hormone transport, or thyroid hormone action has been instrumental in establishing a thorough mechanistic understanding of these aspects [11, 47, 63].

Acknowledgment Malini Soundarrajan is supported by a Ruth L. Kirschstein National Research Service Award T32 DK007169 from NIH/NIDDK.

References

1. Aoki Y, Belin RM, Clickner R, Jeffries R, Phillips L, Mahaffey KR. Serum TSH and total T4 in the United States population and their association with participant characteristics: National Health and Nutrition Examination Survey (NHANES 1999-2002). Thyroid. 2007;17(12):1211–23.
2. Alexander EK, Pearce EN, Brent GA, Brown RS, Chen H, Dosiou C, et al. 2017 guidelines of the American Thyroid Association for the diagnosis and Management of Thyroid Disease during pregnancy and the postpartum. Thyroid. 2017;27(3):315–89.
3. Maraka S, Singh Ospina NM, O'Keeffe DT, Rodriguez-Gutierrez R, Espinosa De Ycaza AE, Wi CI, et al. Effects of levothyroxine therapy on pregnancy outcomes in women with subclinical hypothyroidism. Thyroid. 2016;26(7):980–6.
4. Cooper DS, Pearce EN. Subclinical hypothyroidism and hypothyroxinemia in pregnancy – still no answers. N Engl J Med. 2017;376(9):876–7.
5. Skudlinski M, Kazlauskaite R, Weintraub B. Thyroid-stimulating hormone and regulation of the thyroid axis. In: DeGroot LJ, Jameson JL, editors. Endocrinology. 2Vols. 5th ed. Philadelphia: Elsevier; 2006, p. 1803–22.
6. Kopp P. The TSH receptor and its role in thyroid disease. Cell Mol Life Sci. 2001;58(9):1301–22.
7. Benvenga S. Thyroid hormone transport proteins and the physiology of hormone binding. In: Braverman L, Utiger R, editors. Werner and Ingbar's the thyroid: a fundamental and clinical text. 9th ed. Philadelphia: Lippincott, Williams & Wilkins; 2005. p. 97–108.
8. Bernal J, Guadano-Ferraz A, Morte B. Thyroid hormone transporters--functions and clinical implications. Nat Rev Endocrinol. 2015;11(7):406–17.
9. Bianco AC, Salvatore D, Gereben B, Berry MJ, Larsen PR. Biochemistry, cellular and molecular biology, and physiological roles of the iodothyronine selenodeiodinases. Endocr Rev. 2002;23(1):38–89.
10. Ortiga-Carvalho TM, Sidhaye AR, Wondisford FE. Thyroid hormone receptors and resistance to thyroid hormone disorders. Nat Rev Endocrinol. 2014;10(10):582–91.

11. Kopp P. Thyroid hormone synthesis: thyroid iodine metabolism. In: Braverman L, Utiger R, editors. Werner and Ingbar's the thyroid: a fundamental and clinical text. 10th ed. Philadelphia: Lippincott, Williams & Wilkins; 2013. p. 48–74.
12. Dohan O, De la Vieja A, Paroder V, Riedel C, Artani M, Reed M, et al. The sodium/iodide symporter (NIS): characterization, regulation, and medical significance. Endocr Rev. 2003;24(1):48–77.
13. Ravera S, Reyna-Neyra A, Ferrandino G, Amzel LM, Carrasco N. The sodium/iodide symporter (NIS): molecular physiology and preclinical and clinical applications. Annu Rev Physiol. 2017;79:261–89.
14. Wemeau JL, Kopp P. Pendred syndrome. Best Pract Res Clin Endocrinol Metab. 2017;31(2):213–24.
15. Taurog A. Hormone synthesis: thyroid iodine metabolism. In: Braverman L, Utiger R, editors. Werner and Ingbar's the thyroid: a fundamental and clinical text. 8th ed. Philadelphia: Lippincott, Williams & Wilkins; 2000. p. 61–85.
16. Moreno JC, Visser TJ. New phenotypes in thyroid dyshormonogenesis: hypothyroidism due to DUOX2 mutations. Endocr Dev. 2007;10:99–117.
17. Visser WE, Friesema EC, Visser TJ. Minireview: thyroid hormone transporters: the knowns and the unknowns. Mol Endocrinol (Baltimore, Md). 2011;25(1):1–14.
18. Di Jeso B, Arvan P. Thyroglobulin from molecular and cellular biology to clinical endocrinology. Endocr Rev. 2016;37(1):2–36.
19. Moreno JC, Klootwijk W, van Toor H, Pinto G, D'Allessandro M, Leger A, et al. Mutations in the iodotyrosine deiodinase gene and hypothyroidism. N Engl J Med. 2008;358(17):1811–8.
20. Martin T, Findlay D, Sexton P. Calcitonin. In: DeGroot LJ, Jameson JL, editors. Endocrinology. 2 vols. 5th ed. Philadelphia: Elsevier; 2006, p. 1419–33.
21. Brandi ML, Gagel RF, Angeli A, Bilezikian JP, Beck-Peccoz P, Bordi C, et al. Guidelines for diagnosis and therapy of MEN type 1 and type 2. J Clin Endocrinol Metab. 2001;86(12):5658–71.
22. Dohan O, Portulano C, Basquin C, Reyna-Neyra A, Amzel LM, Carrasco N. The Na+/I symporter (NIS) mediates electroneutral active transport of the environmental pollutant perchlorate. Proc Natl Acad Sci U S A. 2007;104(51):20250–5.
23. Hilditch TE, Horton PW, McCruden DC, Young RE, Alexander WD. Defects in intrathyroid binding of iodine and the perchlorate discharge test. Acta Endocrinol. 1982;100(2):237–44.
24. Tazebay UH, Wapnir IL, Levy O, Dohan O, Zuckier LS, Zhao QH, et al. The mammary gland iodide transporter is expressed during lactation and in breast cancer. Nat Med. 2000;6(8):871–8.
25. Grollman EF, Smolar A, Ommaya A, Tombaccini D, Santisteban P. Iodine suppression of iodide uptake in FRTL-5 thyroid cells. Endocrinology. 1986;118(6):2477–82.
26. Kogai T, Curcio F, Hyman S, Cornford EM, Brent GA, Hershman JM. Induction of follicle formation in long-term cultured normal human thyroid cells treated with thyrotropin stimulates iodide uptake but not sodium/iodide symporter messenger RNA and protein expression. J Endocrinol. 2000;167(1):125–35.
27. Eng PH, Cardona GR, Previti MC, Chin WW, Braverman LE. Regulation of the sodium iodide symporter by iodide in FRTL-5 cells. Eur J Endocrinol. 2001;144(2):139–44.
28. Wolff J, Chaikoff I. Plasma inorganic iodide as homeostatic regulator of thyroid function. J Biol Chem. 1948;174:555–64.
29. Wolff J, Chaikoff I, Goldberg R, Meier J. The temporary nature of the inhibitory action of excess iodide on organic iodide synthesis in the normal thyroid. Endocrinology. 1949;45:504–13.
30. Braverman LE, Ingbar SH. Changes in thyroidal function during adaptation to large doses of iodide. J Clin Invest. 1963;42:1216–31.
31. Gillam MP, Sidhaye A, Lee EJ, Rutishauser J, Waeber Stephan C, Kopp P. Functional characterization of pendrin in a polarized cell system: evidence for pendrin-mediated apical iodide efflux. J Biol Chem. 2004;279:13004–10.
32. Everett LA, Glaser B, Beck JC, Idol JR, Buchs A, Heyman M, et al. Pendred syndrome is caused by mutations in a putative sulphate transporter gene (PDS). Nat Genet. 1997;17:411–22.

33. Pesce L, Bizhanova A, Caraballo JC, Westphal W, Butti ML, Comellas A, et al. TSH regulates pendrin membrane abundance and enhances iodide efflux in thyroid cells. Endocrinology. 2012;153(1):512–21.
34. Iosco C, Cosentino C, Sirna L, Romano R, Cursano S, Mongia A, et al. Anoctamin 1 is apically expressed on thyroid follicular cells and contributes to ATP- and calcium-activated iodide efflux. Cell Physiol Biochem. 2014;34(3):966–80.
35. Twyffels L, Strickaert A, Virreira M, Massart C, Van Sande J, Wauquier C, et al. Anoctamin-1/TMEM16A is the major apical iodide channel of the thyrocyte. Am J Physiol Cell Physiol. 2014;307(12):C1102–12.
36. Vono-Toniolo J, Rivolta CM, Targovnik HM, Medeiros-Neto G, Kopp P. Naturally occurring mutations in the thyroglobulin gene. Thyroid. 2005;15(9):1021–33.
37. Haugen B, Alexander E, Bible K, Doherty G, Mandel S, Nikiforov Y, et al. 2015 American Thyroid Association management guidelines for adult patients with thyroid nodules and differentiated thyroid cancer. Thyroid. 2016;26:1–133.
38. Bakker B, Bikker H, Vulsma T, de Randamie JS, Wiedijk BM, De Vijlder JJ. Two decades of screening for congenital hypothyroidism in the Netherlands: TPO gene mutations in total iodide organification defects (an update). J Clin Endocrinol Metab. 2000;85:3708–12.
39. Grasberger H, Refetoff S. Genetic causes of congenital hypothyroidism due to dyshormonogenesis. Curr Opin Pediatr. 2011;23(4):421–8.
40. Di Cosmo C, Liao XH, Dumitrescu AM, Philp NJ, Weiss RE, Refetoff S. Mice deficient in MCT8 reveal a mechanism regulating thyroid hormone secretion. J Clin Invest. 2010;120(9):3377–88.
41. Friesema EC, Grueters A, Biebermann H, Krude H, von Moers A, Reeser M, et al. Association between mutations in a thyroid hormone transporter and severe X-linked psychomotor retardation. Lancet (London, England). 2004;364(9443):1435–7.
42. Dumitrescu AM, Liao XH, Best TB, Brockmann K, Refetoff S. A novel syndrome combining thyroid and neurological abnormalities is associated with mutations in a monocarboxylate transporter gene. Am J Hum Genet. 2004;74(1):168–75.
43. Bartalena L, Robbins J. Variations in thyroid hormone transport proteins and their clinical implications. Thyroid. 1992;2(3):237–45.
44. Kopp P. Genetic basis of thyroid disorders. In: Ganten D, Ruekpaul K, editors. Genomics and proteomics in molecular medicine. 2nd ed. Berlin: Springer; 2006. p. 1862–7.
45. Glinoer D, de Nayer P, Bourdoux P, Lemone M, Robyn C, van Steirteghem A, et al. Regulation of maternal thyroid during pregnancy. J Clin Endocrinol Metab. 1990;71(2):276–87.
46. Cooper DS, Ladenson PW. The thyroid gland. In: Gardner DG, Shoback D, editors. Greenspan's basic & clinical endocrinology, 10e. New York: McGraw-Hill Education; 2017.
47. Refetoff S. Thyroid Hormone Serum Transport Proteins. June 7, 2015. In: De Groot LJ, Chrousos G, Dungan K, Feingold KR, Grossman A, Hershman JM, et al., editors. Endotext. South Dartmouth; 2000.
48. Pappa T, Ferrara AM, Refetoff S. Inherited defects of thyroxine-binding proteins. Best Pract Res Clin Endocrinol Metab. 2015;29(5):735–47.
49. Bianco AC. Minireview: cracking the metabolic code for thyroid hormone signaling. Endocrinology. 2011;152(9):3306–11.
50. Williams GR, Bassett JH. Deiodinases: the balance of thyroid hormone: local control of thyroid hormone action: role of type 2 deiodinase. J Endocrinol. 2011;209(3):261–72.
51. Van den Berghe G. Non-thyroidal illness in the ICU: a syndrome with different faces. Thyroid. 2014;24(10):1456–65.
52. Cheng SY, Leonard JL, Davis PJ. Molecular aspects of thyroid hormone actions. Endocr Rev. 2010;31(2):139–70.
53. Astapova I, Hollenberg AN. The in vivo role of nuclear receptor corepressors in thyroid hormone action. Biochim Biophys Acta. 2013;1830(7):3876–81.

54. Ortiga-Carvalho TM, Shibusawa N, Nikrodhanond A, Oliveira KJ, Machado DS, Liao XH, et al. Negative regulation by thyroid hormone receptor requires an intact coactivator-binding surface. J Clin Invest. 2005;115(9):2517–23.
55. Refetoff S. Inherited thyroxine-binding globulin abnormalities in man. Endocr Rev. 1989;10:275–93.
56. Refetoff S, Bassett JH, Beck-Peccoz P, Bernal J, Brent G, Chatterjee K, et al. Classification and proposed nomenclature for inherited defects of thyroid hormone action, cell transport, and metabolism. Thyroid. 2014;24(3):407–9.
57. Refetoff S, Dumitrescu AM. Syndromes of reduced sensitivity to thyroid hormone: genetic defects in hormone receptors, cell transporters and deiodination. Best Pract Res Clin Endocrinol Metab. 2007;21(2):277–305.
58. Bochukova E, Schoenmakers N, Agostini M, Schoenmakers E, Rajanayagam O, Keogh JM, et al. A mutation in the thyroid hormone receptor alpha gene. N Engl J Med. 2012;366(3):243–9.
59. Moran C, Agostini M, McGowan A, Schoenmakers E, Fairall L, Lyons G, et al. Contrasting phenotypes in resistance to thyroid hormone alpha correlate with divergent properties of thyroid hormone receptor alpha1 mutant proteins. Thyroid. 2017;27(7):973–82.
60. van Gucht AL, Meima ME, Zwaveling-Soonawala N, Visser WE, Fliers E, Wennink JM, et al. Resistance to thyroid hormone alpha in an 18-month-old girl: clinical, therapeutic, and molecular characteristics. Thyroid. 2016;26(3):338–46.
61. Davis PJ, Goglia F, Leonard JL. Nongenomic actions of thyroid hormone. Nat Rev Endocrinol. 2016;12(2):111–21.
62. Krassas GE, Poppe K, Glinoer D. Thyroid function and human reproductive health. Endocr Rev. 2010;31(5):702–55.
63. Refetoff S, Weiss RE, Usala SJ. The syndromes of resistance to thyroid hormone. Endocr Rev. 1993;14(3):348–99.

Chapter 2
Hypothyroidism

Vishnu Vardhan Garla, Licy L. Yanes Cardozo, and Lillian Frances Lien

> **Clinical Case**
> A 50-year-old female patient presents to the clinic complaining of fatigue and weight gain. For the past 6 months, she has experienced progressively increasing fatigue associated with a 40 lb. increase in weight. In addition, she complains of hair loss, constipation, and dry skin. She has a past history significant for vitiligo but otherwise unremarkable. Her heart rate is 58 beats per minute, blood pressure is of 140/100, and temperature is 98.4F. Physical exam shows an obese female patient; thyroid exam is significant for a large, non-tender goiter. Laboratory assessment reveals a TSH of 50 mIU/L (reference range 0.27–4.2mIU/L), free T4 of 0.2 ng/dL (0.9–1.7 ng/dl), and TPO antibody of 300 IU/mL (0–3 IU/mL). What is her diagnosis and what treatment should be initiated?

Introduction

Hypothyroidism is due to the deficient production of thyroid hormone. It is classified into primary hypothyroidism, due to decreased production of thyroid hormone from the thyroid gland, and central hypothyroidism, due to decreased stimulation of the thyroid gland secondary to pituitary or hypothalamic disease. Primary hypothyroidism is by far the most common cause of hypothyroidism, accounting for 99% of cases [1].

Hypothyroidism is a common disorder with a strong female preponderance. A study from the United Kingdom reported an incidence of 3.5 women per 1000 population per year and 0.6 men per 1000 population per year [2]. Twenty-year follow-up of the women in that study revealed that among those with thyroid antibodies, the risk of developing hypothyroidism was 4% per year [2, 3].

The clinical features of hypothyroidism reflect a reduction in the rate of various physiological processes due to reduced action of thyroid hormone on the end-organ tissues. Due to the diverse actions of thyroid hormone, hypothyroidism results in a variety of often highly nonspecific symptoms [4].

Laboratory assessment of thyroid-stimulating hormone (TSH) and thyroxine (T4) is widely available; however, various factors can influence the levels of TSH and T4, and a careful assessment of these factors (non-thyroidal illness, medications, age) is essential before diagnosing and treating hypothyroidism. Levothyroxine, the mainstay of treatment in hypothyroidism, is one of the most prescribed medications in the United States [5–7].

Etiology

Etiologies of hypothyroidism can be classified into primary and secondary causes (Box 2.1). Primary hypothyroidism is due to defects in thyroid hormone synthesis or secretion from the thyroid gland itself; it is characterized by a low T4 and a high TSH. The most common cause of hypothyroidism in iodine-sufficient regions is chronic autoimmune hypothyroidism [1].

> **Box 2.1 Causes of Hypothyroidism**
> Primary Hypothyroidism
>
> - Chronic autoimmune hypothyroidism (Hashimoto's hypothyroidism)
> - Iodine deficiency
> - Post-procedure hypothyroidism (postsurgical; post-radioiodine ablation)
> - Congenital hypothyroidism
> - Infiltrative disorders (sarcoidosis, hemochromatosis, Riedel's thyroiditis)
>
> Secondary Hypothyroidism
>
> - Congenital hypopituitarism
> - Post-transsphenoidal surgery or radiation to the pituitary/hypothalamus
> - Infiltrating disorders of the pituitary/hypothalamus (sarcoidosis, lymphoma, metastasis)
>
> Peripheral Causes
>
> - Thyroid hormone resistance
> - Consumptive hypothyroidism

Secondary hypothyroidism is due to pathology in the pituitary gland or, rarely, the hypothalamus. As such, it is characterized by a low T4 and low or normal TSH [8]. The low or "inappropriately" normal TSH reflects the central cause of the disorder, as the pituitary and/or hypothalamus is unable to mount sufficient TSH.

Chronic Autoimmune Hypothyroidism

Autoimmune hypothyroidism can be further divided into two diagnoses based on the presence or absence of a goiter: chronic thyroiditis (Hashimoto's thyroiditis) and chronic atrophic thyroiditis, respectively [9]. The annual incidence of autoimmune hypothyroidism is 4 per 1000 women and 1 per 1000 men [10]. HLA-DR3, HLA-DR4, and HLA-DR5 along with CTLA-4 are associated with autoimmune hypothyroidism [11–13]. These genetic associations also explain the co-occurrence of other autoimmune disorders such as type 1 diabetes, Addison's disease, vitiligo, and pernicious anemia with autoimmune hypothyroidism [14]. It is also speculated that haploinsufficiency of genes on the X chromosome may be responsible for the high incidence of autoimmune hypothyroidism found in patients with Turner's syndrome [15].

Lymphocyte infiltration, atrophy of thyroid follicles, and fibrosis are classically described in autoimmune hypothyroidism. Lymphocyte infiltration is the predominant feature in Hashimoto's hypothyroidism, while marked fibrosis is the hallmark of atrophic thyroiditis. CD8 cells in the lymphocytic infiltrate are primarily responsible for destruction of thyroid follicles [16].

Thyroid peroxidase (TPO) antibodies and anti-thyroglobulin antibodies (TG) are indicators of thyroid autoimmunity. Rarely, antibodies to thyroid hormone receptor (TRab) may exhibit a blocking rather than stimulatory effect and cause hypothyroidism. However, TRab are usually known more for their stimulatory effect in the pathogenesis of Graves' hyperthyroidism [17, 18].

Central Hypothyroidism

Central, also often called "secondary," hypothyroidism occurs when there is decreased thyroid hormone secretion due to decreased stimulation of the thyroid gland. It is characterized by a low T4 and low or inappropriately normal TSH. The low TSH reflects the central cause of the disorder, as it indicates the pituitary and/or hypothalamus is unable to mount sufficient TSH production. It can be isolated, or, more importantly, it can also coexist with other pituitary hormonal abnormalities [1]. Of note, other causes of a non-elevated TSH (non-thyroidal illness, medications) and low T4 level need to be ruled out before making the diagnosis of central hypothyroidism.

Postsurgical or Postablative Hypothyroidism

Hypothyroidism can also occur as a result of a thyroidectomy or a radioiodine ablation procedure. These procedures are often performed necessarily in the treatment of patients with hyperthyroidism or thyroid cancer. In general, these patients have usually been educated in advance of the procedure that they may go on to develop post-procedure hypothyroidism, so they are generally prepared to hear that they may subsequently need lifelong levothyroxine replacement [1].

Pathophysiology and Clinical Features

Thyroid hormone affects the functioning of every organ system in the body, thereby leading to widespread clinical manifestations (Fig. 2.1). However, none of the signs or symptoms alone can be taken as pathognomonic of hypothyroidism, so the probability of the diagnosis increases with the number of signs and symptoms present.

Integumentary System

Thyroid hormone receptors (TR) are found in keratinocytes, fibroblasts, endothelial cells, and erector pili muscle cells. In addition, the skin also expresses deiodinase 2 and 3. Depletion of triiodothyronine (T3) has been shown to increase the transglutaminase levels and decrease the plasminogen activator levels in the keratinocytes which results in increased formation and decreased shedding of cornified envelope manifesting as dry skin [19–22]. Thyroid hormone is also involved in the degradation of hyaluronic acid [23]. Therefore, deficiency of thyroid hormone results in accumulation of hyaluronic acid in the dermis. This, along with increased transcapillary pressure, results in firm and non-pitting dermal edema, classically described as "myxedema." Periorbital edema, facial puffiness, and tongue enlargement are also due to the accumulation of mucopolysaccharides in the dermis. In addition, the accumulation of carotene gives a yellowish hue to the skin best seen on the palms, soles, and nasolabial folds. The skin may also appear pale and cool secondary to hypoperfusion, and rarely ecchymosis may be seen due to the deficiency of clotting factors [24, 25].

Thyroid hormone also affects the initiation and duration of hair growth. Coarse, dry, brittle hair is seen in hypothyroidism. Madarosis (the loss of outer one-third of eyebrows) and slow-growing, brittle nails are observed in hypothyroidism [26, 27].

Besides direct involvement in the skin and hair growth, autoimmune hypothyroidism can be associated with various autoimmune dermatological disorders such as alopecia, vitiligo, pemphigus, and lichen sclerosus [28].

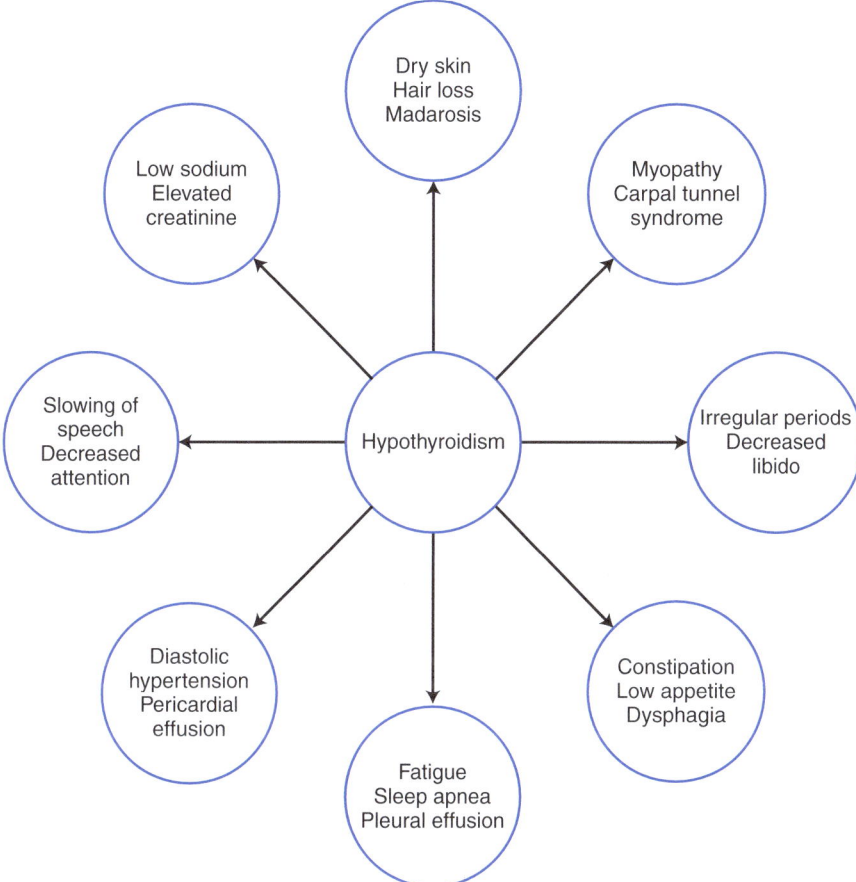

Fig. 2.1 Clinical manifestations of hypothyroidism

Pulmonary System

Hypothyroidism affects the pulmonary system in subtle ways, and the symptoms may be difficult to discern from those caused by obesity. It can decrease respiratory muscular strength, and central respiratory drive resulting in a decrease of vital capacity (VC), oxygen concentration (PaO2), and diffusing capacity of the lung (DLCO) [29]. The decrease in muscular strength could be secondary to decreased activity of the enzyme acid maltase which catalyzes the degradation of glycogen to glucose in the muscle [30]. A change in the balance of slow and fast muscle fibers in the diaphragm has also been implicated as the cause of decreased muscle strength. The pathogenesis of decreased respiratory drive in hypothyroidism is not known [31].

Fatigue and decreased exercise capacity are well described in hypothyroidism. However, it is believed that they are due to a decrease in stroke volume and cardiac output and not pulmonary dysfunction [29]. Pleural effusions, although rare, have been associated with hypothyroidism. They are mostly small, and asymptomatic and can be either transudative or exudative in nature. The mechanisms underlying the pathogenesis of pleural effusions have not been well defined; however, a decrease in diameter and increase in permeability of the pulmonary capillaries have been suspected [32].

Obstructive sleep apnea (OSA) has been known to be associated with hypothyroidism. Increased weight, submucosal accumulation of myxedematous tissue, decreased respiratory drive, and dysfunction of pharyngeal dilator muscles seen in hypothyroidism may predispose to the development of OSA. While it is known that the prevalence of OSA in hypothyroidism is increased, hypothyroidism is seen only in a few cases of OSA. The effect of levothyroxine supplementation on OSA is controversial with studies showing contradictory results [33].

Thyroid hormone has been known to accelerate fetal lung maturation and increase surfactant production. However, using levothyroxine either alone or in combination with glucocorticoids for the prevention of respiratory distress syndrome (RDS) has not been well established [29].

Gastrointestinal System

Decreased motility of the gastrointestinal (GI) tract resulting in constipation is one of the classic features of hypothyroidism. It has been noted that about one in eight hypothyroid patients have three or fewer bowel movements in a week [34]. In elderly patients, this then has to be differentiated from functional constipation secondary to age. Dilation of the entire GI tract can be seen on imaging studies. Pathologically, the colon is leathery and pale with accumulation of myxedematous tissue in the submucosa and muscularis. Several mechanisms have been put forth to explain the intestinal dysmotility in hypothyroidism, including intestinal myopathy, autonomic neuropathy, and altered impulse transmission at the myoneural junction [35]. Intestinal absorption is for the most part intact in hypothyroid patients, but some may develop diarrhea secondary to bacterial overgrowth [36]. It is especially important to note that several medications—including calcium supplements, sucralfate, ferrous sulfate, and bile acid sequestrants—interfere with the absorption of levothyroxine. Providers should be certain to educate their patients that these medications should not be taken at the same time as levothyroxine. Rather, the levothyroxine should be taken at a separate time, several hours apart (i.e., early morning or late at night) from those other potential interfering medications [37]. Dysphagia is a common symptom of hypothyroidism. It could be due to the presence of a goiter compressing the esophagus but can also be related to dysmotility of the esophagus [38, 39].

Hypothyroidism is also associated with mild liver function abnormalities which resolve with thyroid hormone replacement therapy. Decrease in bilirubin excretion and hypotonia of the gall bladder predispose to cholelithiasis. Rarely, central congestive fibrosis of the liver has been reported with hypothyroidism [40–42].

Autoimmune thyroid disease has been associated with pernicious anemia, primary biliary cirrhosis, Addison's disease, and type 1 diabetes mellitus. The triad of Addison's disease, Hashimoto's hypothyroidism, and type 1 diabetes mellitus constitutes autoimmune polyglandular syndrome 2 (APS 2) [35].

Renal System

The thyroid hormone axis and renal physiology are intricately linked. Thyroid hormone not only affects the development of many transport systems in the renal tubule, but it also affects prerenal dynamics by the changes it causes in the cardiovascular system [43].

Hypothyroidism causes a decrease in systolic function secondary to changes in gene transcription which impact myocyte contractility and a delay in diastolic relaxation due to decrease in synthesis of endothelial vasodilators [44]. This, combined with a decrease in sensitivity of the beta-adrenergic receptor and renin release, results in impaired renal autoregulation leading to a decrease in glomerular filtration rate (GFR) [45]. Increased delivery of chloride to the distal tubule due to defective proximal tubule reabsorption affects the activity of the ClC-2 receptors resulting in activation of the tubule glomerular feedback and decreased GFR [46]. A decrease in secretion of erythropoietin leads to a decrease in blood volume [46, 47].

High TSH has been associated with a higher incidence of chronic kidney disease (CKD) in epidemiological studies independent of age, sex, body mass index (BMI), and other comorbidities [48]. Elevated serum creatinine is seen in hypothyroidism which resolves after treatment with levothyroxine. GFR has been known to increase rapidly once thyroid hormone replacement therapy has been started [49]. Shin and colleagues showed that thyroid hormone replacement therapy in patients with subclinical hypothyroidism can slow the progression of CKD, potentially delaying the onset of end-stage renal disease (ESRD) [50].

Hyponatremia is an infrequent finding in hypothyroidism, mostly seen with severe hypothyroidism. This has been attributed to water retention due to decreased renal blood flow and decrease in GFR [51, 52]. The development of hyponatremia develops on the balance between water intake and output, and since these changes are more pronounced in severe hypothyroidism, hyponatremia is more likely in the same.

Autoimmune hypothyroidism has also been associated with immune complex glomerulonephritis, which leads to proteinuria and impaired glomerular filtration [53].

Cardiovascular System

Hypothyroidism can affect the cardiovascular system in a multitude of ways; however, the effects are not as dramatic as seen in hyperthyroidism. Increased vascular resistance and decreased cardiac output are the predominant features.

Increased vascular resistance is due to the lack of the direct vasodilator action of triiodothyronine on the vasculature as well as impaired secretion and action of nitric oxide. This may manifest as increase in diastolic and decrease in systolic blood pressure (narrowed pulse pressure). About 20–40% of hypothyroid patients have high blood pressure. Upon treatment of hypothyroidism, these changes resolve [54].

Thyroid hormone has a direct chronotropic action on the sinoatrial node (SAN), by regulating the pacemaker-related genes and also by stimulating the beta-adrenergic receptors, the lack of which leads to bradycardia as seen in hypothyroidism [57]. Ventricular relaxation and impaired diastolic filling lead to a decrease in stroke volume. Triiodothyronine acts on cardiac myocytes and modulates the expression of genes; these along with changes in myocyte-specific regulatory proteins are responsible for the impaired cardiac contractility seen in hypothyroidism [56].

Pericardial effusions may be seen in association with severe hypothyroidism. They are transudative in nature with a high protein content. On auscultation, heart sounds may be distant, and low-voltage waves may be noted on the electrocardiogram. These effusions may give the appearance of cardiomegaly on chest radiography and resolve with treatment of hypothyroidism [57].

Thyroid hormone plays an important role in cholesterol metabolism. Hypercholesterolemia is commonly observed in hypothyroid patients with increases noted in lipoprotein a (Lpa), low-density lipoprotein (LDL), apoprotein B (Apo B), and total cholesterol [58].

Hematologic System

Thyroid hormone does have some subtle and often overlooked effects on the hematological system. Anemia is a common manifestation among patients with hypothyroidism and may be due to a decrease in erythropoiesis secondary to a decrease in erythropoietin. Bone marrow evaluation is hypocellular in such patients [47, 59]. Iron-deficiency anemia may also occur as a result of menorrhagia and/or achlorhydria. About 10% of patients with autoimmune hypothyroidism have associated pernicious anemia which can give rise to megaloblastic anemia. These patients need thyroid hormone supplementation along with iron or vitamin B12 [60].

In hypothyroidism, the half-lives of factors II, VII, and X are prolonged. This may make patients more resistant to the anticoagulant effect of warfarin, necessitating higher doses. Also, transitioning from heparin to warfarin may take longer. Ristocetin-induced platelet aggregation, which is dependent on factor VIII, may improve with levothyroxine replacement therapy [61].

Neurological System

The effect of thyroid on the neurological system is manifold, especially in infants and neonates in whom hypothyroidism can cause irreversible damage. Neuronal growth, migration, myelination, and synaptogenesis are all affected by thyroid hormone. T3 levels in the brain are tightly regulated, and its receptors are present in the hippocampus, cerebellum, and cortex [62].

Neuropathies are commonly reported in association with hypothyroid patients with the most common mononeuropathy being carpal tunnel syndrome. Carpal tunnel syndrome is due to compression of the median nerve as it passes beneath the flexor retinaculum in the wrist due to myxedema of the perineuronal and synovial tissue. It is characterized by tingling and numbness in the median nerve distribution, the lateral 3.5 fingers [63]. Other reported mononeuropathies include tarsal tunnel syndrome (compression of the posterior tibial nerve) and meralgia paresthetica (compression of the lateral femoral cutaneous nerve). Peripheral neuropathy is far less commonly reported [64, 65].

Cognitive disturbances in hypothyroidism have been noted since the late nineteenth century and were described as "myxedematous madness" [66]. Slowing of speech and decreased attention and concentration are the common symptoms noted in hypothyroidism. However, psychosis, paranoia, and fearfulness can also occur. Among the cognitive functions, memory is most commonly affected. Thyroid hormone replacement therapy can improve but not completely resolve the deficits [67–70].

Hashimoto's encephalopathy is used to describe an encephalopathy characterized by high titers of antithyroid antibodies and responsiveness to glucocorticoid therapy. It can manifest as psychosis or seizures or with stroke-like symptoms. This condition is still poorly described in the current literature, so it must be considered only after ruling out all other identifiable causes of encephalopathy. Cerebrospinal fluid (CSF) analysis shows increased protein but no pleocytosis. Imaging studies are typically normal. Electroencephalogram (EEG) shows a nonspecific excess of slow-wave activity. The treatment usually consists of steroids and thyroid hormone replacement therapy. In case of a lack of response to steroids, immunomodulators like azathioprine can be tried [71].

Reproductive System

Hypothyroidism in males is associated with decreases in sex hormone-binding globulin (SHBG) and total testosterone. Various other androgens—like dehydroepiandrosterone (DHEA), DHEA-S, and androstenedione—are also decreased. This hypogonadism appears to be centrally mediated with normal levels of follicle-stimulating hormone (FSH) and luteinizing hormone (LH); it is suspected that the gonadotropes' response to GnRH (gonadotropin-releasing hormone) is blunted [72].

In hypothyroid women, menstrual irregularities are common (23.4%), with oligomenorrhea being the most common abnormality. A decrease in the clearance and increase in the aromatization of estrone and androstenedione are observed; however, a decrease in SHBG results in more free testosterone and estradiol. Hypothyroidism can be associated with diminished libido and ovulation failure. Gestational hypertension and first trimester abortions also occur more frequently in women with hypothyroidism [73].

Musculoskeletal System

Muscular symptoms are extremely common in patients with hypothyroidism with different series putting their prevalence at 79–100% [74]. Most common symptoms are muscular weakness, cramps, stiffness, and fatigue. Examination may reveal decreased muscle strength and delayed relaxation of deep tendon reflexes; however, in most cases, they are completely normal. Rarely, these myopathic symptoms may be the presenting symptom in hypothyroidism; therefore TSH needs to be checked in patients with unknown myopathy. "Hoffman syndrome" consists of pseudohypertrophy of muscles most commonly the gastrocnemius, deltoid, and trapezius muscles which is characterized by stiffness, cramps, and weakness. Electromyography may show abnormalities with the most common one being low amplitude, short duration, polyphasic motor unit action potentials, fibrillation, and complex repetitive discharges. However, these findings are neither sensitive nor specific. The MM fraction of creatine kinase (CK) may be elevated. Thyroid hormone replacement therapy alleviates the muscular symptoms, pseudohypertrophy, and delayed relaxation of the deep tendon reflexes [75].

Thyroid hormone influences skeletal growth and maturation directly and in conjunction with growth hormone. Hypothyroidism decreases recruitment, differentiation, and activity of bone cells leading to a low bone turnover state. Decreased levels of bone formation markers (osteocalcin, alkaline phosphatase) and resorption markers (urinary hydroxyproline) are observed. Bone mineral density is preserved; however, there may be an increased risk of fracture due to decreased bone repair. This risk is compounded by muscular weakness, leading to an increased risk of falls [76].

Maturation of the skeleton, characterized by the appearance of secondary ossification centers, is dependent on thyroid hormone levels. Deficiency of thyroid hormone leads to a mottled and irregular ossification classically described as stippled epiphysis on radiographs. Hip dislocation, short stature, immature vertebra, scoliosis, and delayed tooth eruption can also be seen [77].

Diagnosis

Diagnosis of Primary Hypothyroidism

Primary hypothyroidism is characterized by an elevated TSH and low T4. The most sensitive assay for the diagnosis of primary hypothyroidism is the third-generation TSH. TSH is a glycoprotein dimeric hormone composed of two subunits (α-GSU and β-TSH). TSH plasma levels exhibit a circadian pattern, with lowest levels in the late afternoon and highest plasma levels during the first hours of sleep [78]. While TSH shows great variability in population studies, individual variation is minimum secondary to a fixed genetic set point. TSH has also been known to increase with age, varies with race, and is affected by numerous medications (Table 2.1) [79]. The

Table 2.1 Medications interfering with thyroid function

Mechanism	Medications
Decreasing TSH secretion	Corticosteroids, bexarotene, ipilimumab, nivolumab, dopamine, octreotide
Blocking the synthesis and release of thyroxine	Methimazole, propylthiouracil, iodine, lithium, perchlorate
Inhibiting conversion of T4 to T3	Corticosteroids, propranolol, propylthiouracil, amiodarone, ipodate/iopanoic acid
Inhibiting absorption of thyroid hormone	Calcium carbonate, iron, sucralfate, colestipol, Metamucil
Increasing metabolism of thyroid hormone	Phenytoin, phenobarbital, rifampin, carbamazepine
Increasing thyroxine-binding globulin	Estrogens, methadone, 5-fluorouracil, heroin, raloxifene
Decreasing thyroxine-binding globulin	Androgens, L-asparaginase, corticosteroids, niacin
Displacement from binding proteins	Aspirin, phenytoin, furosemide, heparin, carbamazepine, salsalate
Thyroiditis	Sunitinib, sorafenib, amiodarone, lithium, IL-2

accuracy of the TSH assay may be affected by other antibodies in the serum like human antimouse antibodies (HAMA) and rheumatoid factor (RF) [80].

T4 is extensively bound (99.97%) to proteins in the serum, mainly to thyroxine-binding globulin and, to a lesser extent, to transthyretin, thyroxine-binding prealbumin, and albumin. This extensive binding makes the measurement of total T4 liable to any factors which affect the binding proteins [81]. Also, it has been reported that after a dose of oral L-thyroxine, there is a transient increase of about 20% in plasmatic thyroid hormone levels for 9 h. Therefore, it may be reasonable to collect blood samples before dosing L-thyroxine [82].

Thyroid function tests need to be interpreted in the context of the patient and not just as stand-alone numbers. In case of a discordance between the clinical picture and biochemical data, one must consider various factors which can confound the interpretation of thyroid function tests (Box 2.2) [83].

Box 2.2 Factors that Can Influence the Interpretation of Thyroid Function Tests
Age
Race
Non-thyroidal illness
Assay interference (HAMA, Rh factor, macro TSH)
Pregnancy
Noncompliance
Malabsorption syndromes
Recent ingestion of levothyroxine
Medications

Diagnosis of Secondary Hypothyroidism

Central, also often called "secondary," hypothyroidism occurs when there is decreased thyroid hormone secretion to decreased stimulation of the thyroid gland. It is characterized by a low T4 and low or inappropriately normal TSH. The low TSH reflects the central cause of the disorder, as it indicates the pituitary and/or hypothalamus is unable to mount sufficient TSH production. It can be isolated, or, importantly, it can also coexist with other pituitary hormonal abnormalities. Therefore, a thorough pituitary evaluation of pituitary function should be performed for these patients [1]. Of note, other causes of a non-elevated TSH and low T4 level (non-thyroidal illness, medications) need to be ruled out before making the diagnosis of central hypothyroidism.

An important caveat to the diagnosis of central hypothyroidism: it is important to check both the TSH and free T4 level to make a proper diagnosis. Diagnostic error can occur when providers check only an isolated TSH level, and it is found to be low. Providers may believe the low TSH is indicative of a diagnosis of hyperthyroidism, which can only be proven if there is a concurrent elevated free T4 level. The correct diagnosis of central hypothyroidism can only be identified when both the low/"inappropriately normal" TSH and low free T4 levels are found concurrently. This is very important since hyperthyroidism is treated with specific medications with potentially dangerous side effects, whereas central hypothyroidism is simply treated with thyroid hormone replacement [1].

Screening

There is no consensus among major organizations regarding screening for thyroid disease in adults. The American Thyroid Association recommends screening at age 35 and every 5 years thereafter. Closer attention should be paid to patients who are at high risk, such as the following: pregnant women, women aged 60 years or older, and subjects with type 1 diabetes mellitus or other autoimmune diseases and a history of neck irradiation or subclinical hypothyroidism [84]. In contrast, the US Preventive Services Task Force does not recommend routine screening for thyroid disease in adults [85].

Management

Although the treatment of both central and primary hypothyroidisms is often thought to be simple, it has been reported that many patients are either over- or under-replaced [86, 87]. In both primary and central hypothyroidisms, treatment should generally aim to restore normal levels of thyroid hormones.

Replacement with T4: Dosing, Adjustment, and Timing

Oral daily administration of levothyroxine (as monotherapy) is the treatment of choice in routine hypothyroidism [81]. In general, young patients and those without cardiac comorbidities can be started on levothyroxine at anticipated full replacement dose [81]:

- In general, 1.6 mcg/kg per day is an appropriate starting dose.
- In patients who have no thyroid tissue left (status-post total thyroidectomy), higher doses may sometimes be needed.
- In patients with subclinical hypothyroidism (discussed separately in more depth below), the elderly, or those with known cardiac disease, lower starting doses may sometimes be more appropriate.

While some degree of clinical improvement is usually noticeable in 3–5 days, in most cases, providers will choose to recheck thyroid function studies and make appropriate dose adjustment at approximately 4–8 weeks after the therapy has been started [81]. Nonetheless, in primary hypothyroidism, achievement of a true normal TSH within the reference range may sometimes take several months.

Levothyroxine is the treatment of choice for thyroid hormone replacement in central hypothyroidism. Importantly, in patients with multiple pituitary deficiencies, other therapies may also be needed. Specifically, a patient with both central hypothyroidism and central adrenal insufficiency would need to have glucocorticoid replacement given before, or at least at the same time as the levothyroxine replacement, in order to prevent an acute adrenal crisis. Providers must also be cautioned: in central hypothyroidism, the TSH level itself cannot be used for monitoring the response to treatment (as is often done in primary hypothyroidism), as it can remain persistently low due to primary/hypothalamic disease. Therefore, monitoring of therapy in central hypothyroidism should be performed with the free T4 level. Ideally, the free T4 needs to be checked before ingesting the daily dose of levothyroxine and should be maintained in the upper half of the normal range [1, 81].

Overtreatment with levothyroxine must be avoided in patients with central hypothyroidism, since these patients may already have a high risk of premature osteoporosis due to associated gonadotroph and growth hormone deficiencies [88].

In all patients on levothyroxine replacement, proper timing of medication administration can be a significant challenge. Studies have shown that levothyroxine absorption is affected by many factors, including other medications (i.e., vitamins and supplements) and food [81]. At a minimum, levothyroxine should be given at least 30–60 min apart from any feeding (whether oral nutrition or enteral nutrition), and expert opinion has suggested taking levothyroxine several hours apart from other medications and supplements. A practical suggestion for the patient is to take other medications in the morning but take the levothyroxine by itself at night.

Replacement in Special Populations

The Patient Who Is Elderly or Has CAD

Elderly patients and any patient with known coronary artery disease should be started on lower than the weight-based doses of levothyroxine (i.e., only 25–50 mcg daily), and doses should be titrated in small increments after 4–6 weeks of therapy [81].

The Patient with Thyroid Cancer

The dosing of levothyroxine in patients with thyroid cancer is complex and beyond the scope of this chapter. However, interested readers will find detailed discussions of dosing in the newest American Thyroid Association guidelines on the management of differentiated thyroid cancer [89].

The Pregnant Patient

Details on management of thyroid disease in the pregnant patient may be found in subsequent chapters. However, safety is paramount, and the following points must always be addressed in the hypothyroid patient who becomes pregnant:

- Patients with known hypothyroidism should already be on a dose of daily levothyroxine replacement. However, as soon as the patient is aware of pregnancy, the dose of levothyroxine should be increased immediately.
- Dose adjustment should be made, ideally with pregnancy trimester-specific goals in mind: If trimester-specific reference ranges for TSH are not available, the following upper normal reference ranges are recommended—first trimester, 2.5 mIU/L; second trimester, 3.0 mIU/L; and third trimester, 3.5 mIU/L [81]. However, it is worth noting that this is an area still undergoing scrutiny, and newer guidelines continue to emerge.

Controversies: Role of T3 Replacement

Although the administration of levothyroxine is the treatment of choice in hypothyroidism, studies have attempted to examine the role of L-triiodothyronine (T3) alone or in combination with levothyroxine (T4).

Effect of monotherapy with oral administration of L-triiodothyronine has been evaluated in small clinical trials. A small short-term study reported that oral administration of L-triiodothyronine three times a day resulted in mild weight loss, decreases in total cholesterol, LDL, and apolipoprotein without differences in cardiovascular function as compared to administration of levothyroxine. Also, a community-based study showed that patients only on thyroxine replacement and biochemically euthyroid displayed a significant impairment in psychological well-being compared to controls of similar age and sex [90].

The possible benefits of substituting 10% of the levothyroxine dosage by L- triiodothyronine were evaluated in a cross-clinical trial. Combination treatment of L-triiodothyronine and levothyroxine for 5 weeks had additional beneficial effects on muscle function and working memory but was also associated with supraphysiological free triiodothyronine (Ft3) concentrations [91]. However, other studies failed to show any additional beneficial effect of combining L-triiodothyronine and levothyroxine [92–94].

The long-term consequences of L-triiodothyronine replacement, alone or in combination with levothyroxine, in routine hypothyroidism remain unclear and unproven. Therefore, it should be emphasized that L-triiodothyronine replacement is not recommended at present. In sum, the management of patients with routine hypothyroidism (as opposed to myxedema crisis, discussed below) should be treatment with levothyroxine monotherapy [81].

Controversies: Armour Thyroid

In addition to the synthetic thyroid hormone replacements [L-triiodothyronine (T3) and levothyroxine (T4)], there is another form of replacement available: desiccated thyroid. Desiccated thyroid most commonly comes from porcine origin and is known as Armour Thyroid. It has a significant bioavailability to both T3 and T4. It must therefore be considered similar to a combination of synthetic L-triiodothyronine and levothyroxine together. At present, there are not sufficient high-quality evidence studies supporting the use of combination therapy with L-triiodothyronine and levothyroxine [81]. The management of patients with routine hypothyroidism should be treatment with levothyroxine monotherapy.

Myxedema Coma

Introduction

Myxedema coma is a life-threatening form of hypothyroidism which can present with significant physiological decompensation [95]. It was first described in 1879 by Ord [96]. It is seen more often in elderly women, although it should be noted that hypothyroidism is approximately eightfold more common in women and is also more common in the latter decades. Most of the patients who develop myxedema coma have a history of long-standing underlying hypothyroidism [95].

Clinical Features

Myxedema coma is particularly alarming in its presentation due to the classic presence of hypothermia and neuropsychiatric manifestations. There is usually a history of some type of precipitating event.

Hypothermia is present in almost all patients, and temperatures have been seen to even go as low as 80°F. In fact, the presenting temperature has prognostic significance with presenting core body temperature less than 90°F portending a worse prognosis [95].

Myxedema coma can be associated with a variety of neuropsychiatric manifestations including depression, psychosis, and memory disturbances. Seizures have also been reported in 25% cases and could be secondary to hypoglycemia or hypoxemia [97].

Myxedema coma can be precipitated by a number of factors including infection, congestive heart failure, cerebrovascular accidents, and certain medications (sedatives, narcotics, amiodarone) which can cause decompensation in a patient with long-standing hypothyroidism.

Respiratory depression is secondary to decreased respiratory center responsiveness to carbon dioxide [98]. The presence of obesity, underlying respiratory infections, and pleural or pericardial effusions can all potentially lead to the development of hypercapnia and respiratory depression. Most patients require mechanical ventilation [99]. Cardiac enlargement could be secondary to dilated ventricles. Hyponatremia is often seen in myxedema coma which can additionally contribute to the altered mental status of the patient [95, 100].

Diagnosis and Treatment of Myxedema Coma

Diagnosis

Early diagnosis is crucial as there is significant mortality (50–60%) associated with this condition. An elderly comatose patient with hypothermia and a long-standing history of hypothyroidism should immediately prompt the examining provider to consider the possible diagnosis of myxedema coma. Physical exam may reveal signs of severe, advanced hypothyroidism such as bradycardia, the presence of a goiter, macroglossia, and delayed reflexes in addition to bradycardia, hypothermia, and hypoventilation [95].

Laboratory evaluation may reveal hyponatremia, anemia, and hyperlipidemia in addition to a high TSH, low T4, and low T3. As a cautionary note, however, approximately 5% of patients with myxedema coma have underlying central hypothyroidism, in which case the TSH levels may be low or inappropriately normal [95, 101].

Treatment

Management of myxedemic coma requires a multipronged approach consisting of correction of electrolyte abnormalities, correction of hypothermia, identification of the precipitating event, and thyroid hormone replacement therapy.

Hypothermia

Hypothermia is the hallmark feature of myxedemic coma. It is of prime importance that temperature be restored to normal as soon as possible. However, it must also be done with caution as rapid temperature restoration may cause vasodilation, potentially lowering blood pressure in an already hypotensive patient. Hypothermia may also mask an underlying infection which may become more evident once the patient's temperature has normalized [95].

Respiratory Depression

Hypoxia and hypercapnia due to respiratory depression are often seen in myxedemic coma. Correction of these abnormalities is essential and may entail the use of mechanical ventilation [102]. Since macroglossia and myxedema of the larynx may be present, it is recommended that intubation be done by an experienced provider.

Hyponatremia

Hyponatremia can potentially contribute to the neuropsychiatric manifestations of myxedemic coma. A conundrum in the treatment of hyponatremia in this context is whether to give fluids for hypotension or restrict fluids for the treatment of hyponatremia. It is recommended that for sodium levels less than 120 mEq/L, 50–100 ml of 3% hypertonic saline may be considered along with furosemide to facilitate water diuresis. Management of hyponatremia must always be done cautiously on a case-by-case basis.

Glucocorticoids

About 5% of patients with myxedema coma have underlying central hypothyroidism, and therefore the provider must remember these are patients who may have coexisting adrenal insufficiency. In addition, even some patients with primary hypothyroidism may have coexisting adrenal insufficiency as part of autoimmune polyglandular syndrome 2 (APS-2). It is therefore recommended that the treatment of myxedema coma must include giving stress-dose hydrocortisone (50–100 mg every 6–8 h) to the patient. This therapeutic plan will prevent against the sudden development of adrenal crisis once thyroid hormone replacement therapy has been instituted [95].

Thyroid Replacement Therapy

Thyroid hormone replacement therapy is the cornerstone therapy in the treatment of myxedema coma. The amounts and proportions of T3 versus T4 therapy, however, have never been truly definitive in the literature. It is usually left to expert opinion rather than evidence, due to the paucity of clinical trial cases and the fact that no well-controlled randomized trials exist. One of the controversies is whether to treat with T4 or T3, each alone, or to use a combination of both.

The purported advantages of using T3 include the ability to bypass the conversion of T4 to T3. In theory, T3 has a quicker onset of action and crosses the blood-brain barrier more easily than T4. However, these potential advantages must be balanced against the very real risk of tachyarrhythmia in the use of T3 and even myocardial infarction [102].

On the other hand, treatment with T4 alone produces less fluctuation in the bioavailable amount of thyroid hormone and thus has a lesser risk of tachyarrhythmia. However, it may not always be sufficient in this potentially life-threatening emergency.

For these reasons, a combination of T4 and T3 has been recommended as treatment for myxedema coma [102]. Both T3 and T4 may need to be given intravenously in the critically ill patient. T4 is dosed daily whereas T3 is given in more frequent intervals each day. Precise dose recommendations are beyond the scope of this chapter given the paucity of high-quality evidence to support specific dosing. The management of myxedema coma cannot be taken as a "one-size-fits-all" regimen, as the patient's cardiovascular status, comorbidities, and concurrent medications must be taken into account [95, 103]. Management requires a critical care setting, and endocrinology consultation, when available, is mandatory.

Subclinical Hypothyroidism

Subclinical hypothyroidism is defined as an elevation in serum TSH levels with a normal (instead of low) T4 level [104].

Subclinical hypothyroidism has an incidence of 3–15% in the general population with a higher incidence in women and the elderly [105, 106]. More importantly, the risk of progression to overt hypothyroidism is 2–6% per year, again with a higher risk in women, the elderly, patients with thyroid peroxidase antibodies (TPO), and those who present with higher TSH and a lower (though still within normal) T4 levels [106].

Since subclinical hypothyroidism is a biochemical diagnosis, many patients are asymptomatic, but some may report fatigue, weight gain, cold intolerance, hair loss, and muscle weakness. Subclinical hypothyroidism is defined as mild if the TSH is 4.5–9 mU/L or severe if the TSH is ≥10 mU/L [107]. Infertility, preeclampsia, and spontaneous abortion occur more frequently in women with subclinical hypothyroidism (Chaps. 6, 9, and 10). Increased demand for thyroid hormone in pregnancy can exacerbate preexisting mild thyroid dysfunction [108].

Observational studies have shown a significant benefit of treating severe subclinical hypothyroidism with a lower risk of heart failure, ischemic heart disease, and all-cause mortality seen in treated as compared to untreated patients. Subgroup analysis has shown the benefit is primarily in those aged less than 70 years. However, data from randomized controlled trials are lacking. A Cochrane meta-analysis has found that treatment with levothyroxine can decrease serum cholesterol levels and carotid intima thickness, but whether this translates into a beneficial effect on cardiovascular events is unknown [109].

Before diagnosing a patient with subclinical hypothyroidism, a transient elevation in TSH due to non-thyroidal illness or drug interactions must be ruled out. It is also recommended that TSH, T4, and thyroid antibodies be repeated in 2–3 months again before making the definitive diagnosis of subclinical hypothyroidism [106]. A significant proportion of patients with TSH <7, were found to have the TSH normalize within 2 years [110].

The decision to treat subclinical hypothyroidism with thyroid hormone replacement therapy is dependent on several factors including the degree of elevation of TSH, age, presence of thyroid peroxidase antibodies (TPO), symptoms suggestive of hypothyroidism, or evidence of heart failure (HF) or atherosclerotic heart disease (AHD). In severe subclinical hypothyroidism (TSH ≥ 10), treatment with levothyroxine should be considered, whereas in mild subclinical hypothyroidism (TSH <10 but greater than the normal limit), treatment is more controversial and may be influenced by symptoms, the presence of TPO antibodies, and the evidence of HF or AHD and plans for pregnancy, particularly in the setting of infertility or recurrent pregnancy loss [81].

Depending on the TSH elevation, a low dose of levothyroxine can be used; often only 25–75 micrograms of levothyroxine is needed as the starting dose. Liothyronine (synthetic T3) has not been evaluated and is not recommended in the treatment of subclinical hypothyroidism [106].

Clinical Case and Discussion
A 50-year-old female patient presents to the clinic complaining of fatigue and weight gain. For the past 6 months, she has experienced progressively increasing fatigue associated with a 40 lb. increase in weight. In addition, she complains of hair loss, constipation, and dry skin. She has a past history significant for vitiligo but otherwise unremarkable. Her heart rate is 58 beats per minute, blood pressure is 140/100, and temperature is 98.4F. Physical exam shows an

obese female patient; thyroid exam is significant for a large, non-tender goiter. Laboratory assessment reveals a TSH of 50 mIU/L (reference range 0.27–4.2 mIU/L), free T4 of 0.2 ng/dL (0.9–1.7 ng/dL), and TPO antibody of 300 IU/mL (0–3 IU/mL). What is her diagnosis, and what treatment should be initiated?

The patient was diagnosed with Hashimoto's thyroiditis as the underlying cause of her hypothyroidism. She was therefore started on levothyroxine monotherapy. She experienced clinically significant improvements in her energy levels, and also her constipation and dry skin resolved. She also lost 10 lb. in 2 months. Reassuringly, her repeat TSH and T4 levels had reached the normal range by the 3-month recheck time point.

References

1. Brent G, Davies T. Hypothyroidism and thyroiditis. In: Melmed S, Polonsky K, Larsen P, Kronenberg H, editors. Williams textbook of endocrinology. 12th ed. Philadelphia: Elsevier; 2011.
2. Vanderpump MP, Tunbridge WM, French JM, Appleton D, Bates D, Clark F, et al. The incidence of thyroid disorders in the community: a twenty-year follow-up of the Whickham survey. Clin Endocrinol. 1995;43:55–68.
3. Vanderpump MP, Tunbridge WM. Epidemiology and prevention of clinical and subclinical hypothyroidism. Thyroid. 2002;12:839–47.
4. Oddie T, Boyd C, Fisher D, Hales I. Incidence of signs and symptoms in thyroid disease. Med J Aust. 1972;2(18):981–6.
5. Zulewski H, Müller B, Exer P, Miserez AR, Staub JJ. Estimation of tissue hypothyroidism by a new clinical score: evaluation of patients with various grades of hypothyroidism and controls. J Clin Endocrinol Metab. 1997 Mar;82(3):771–6.
6. Baskin H, Cobin RH, Duick DS, Gharib H, Guttler RB, Kaplan MM, et al. American association of clinical endocrinologists medical guidelines for clinical practice for the evaluation and treatment of hyperthyroidism and hypothyroidism. Endocr Pract. 2002;8(6):457–69.
7. The 10 most popular prescription drugs in the US. Business Insider [Internet]. 2016 Oct 26 [cited 2017 Nov 27]; Available from: http://www.businessinsider.com/popular-prescription-drugs-us-2016-10.
8. Braverman L, Utiger R. Introduction to hypothyroidism. In: Braverman L, Utiger R, editors. Werner and Ingbar's the thyroid. 9th ed. Philadelphia: Lippincott, William and Wilkins; 2005.
9. Mizukami Y, Michigishi T, Kawato M, Sato T, Nonomura A, Hashimoto T, Matsubara F. Chronic thyroiditis: thyroid function and histologic correlations in 601cases. Hum Pathol. 1992;23(9):980–8.
10. Vanderpump MP, Tunbridge WM, French JM, Appleton D, Bates D, Clark F, Grimley Evans J, Hasan DM, Rodgers H, Tunbridge F, et al. The incidence of thyroid disorders in the community: a twenty-year follow-up of the Whickham survey. Clin Endocrinol. 1995;43(1):55–68.
11. Weissel M, Hofer R, Zasmeta H, Mayr W. HLA-DR and Hashimoto's thyroiditis. Tissue Antigens. 1980;16:256–7.
12. Moens H, Farid N. Hashimoto's thyroiditis is associated with HLA-DRw3. N Engl J Med. 1978;299:133–4.
13. Saverino D, Brizzolara R, Simone R, Chiappori A, Milintenda-Floriani F, Pesce G, Bagnasco M. Soluble CTLA-4 in autoimmune thyroid diseases: relationship with clinical status and possible role in the immune response dysregulation. Clin Immunol. 2007;123(2):190–8.

14. Wiebolt J, Achterbergh R, den Boer A, van der Leij S, Marsch E, Suelmann B, et al. Clustering of additional autoimmunity behaves differently in Hashimoto's patients compared with Graves' patients. Eur J Endocrinol. 2011;164(5):789–94.
15. Jørgensen KT, Rostgaard K, Bache I, Biggar RJ, Nielsen NM, Tommerup N, et al. Autoimmune diseases in women with Turner's syndrome. Arthritis Rheum. 2010;62(3):658–66.
16. Weetman A. Chronic autoimmune thyroiditis. In: Braverman L, Utiger R, editors. Werner and Ingbar's the thyroid. 9th ed. Philadelphia: Lippincott, William and Wilkins; 2005.
17. Bogner U, Kotulla P, Peters H, Schleusener H. Thyroid peroxidase/microsomal antibodies are not identical with thyroid cytotoxic antibodies in autoimmune thyroiditis. Acta Endocrinol. 1990;123(4):431–7.
18. Tahara K, Ishikawa N, Yamamoto K, Hirai A, Ito K, Tamura Y, Yoshida S, Saito Y, Kohn LD. Epitopes for thyroid stimulating and blocking autoantibodies on the extracellular domain of the human thyrotropin receptor. Thyroid. 1997;7(6):867–77.
19. Ahsan MK, Urano Y, Kato S, Oura H, Arase S. Immunohistochemical localization of thyroid hormone nuclear receptors in human hair follicles and in vitro effect of L-triiodothyronine on cultured cells of hair follicles and skin. J Med Investig. 1998;44(3–4):179–84.
20. Törmä H, Rollman O, Vahlquist A. Detection of mRNA transcripts for retinoic acid, vitamin D3, and thyroid hormone (c-erb-A) nuclear receptors in human skin using reverse transcription and polymerase chain reaction. Acta Derm Venereol. 1993;73(2):102–7.
21. Kaplan MM, Gordon PR, Pan CY, Lee JK, Gilchrest BA. Keratinocytes convert thyroxine to triiodothyronine. Ann N Y Acad Sci. 1988;548:56–65.
22. Isseroff RR, Chun KT, Rosenberg RM. Triiodothyronine alters the cornification of cultured human keratinocytes. Br J Dermatol. 1989;120(4):503–10.
23. Yazdanparast P, Carlsson B, Oikarinen A, Risteli J, Faergemann J. A thyroid hormone analogue, triiodothyroacetic acid, corrects corticosteroid-downregulated collagen synthesis. Thyroid. 2004;14(5):345–53.
24. Parving HH, Hansen JM, Nielsen SL, Rossing N, Munck O, Lassen NA. Mechanisms of edema formation in myxedema--increased protein extravasation and relatively slow lymphatic drainage. N Engl J Med. 1979;301(9):460–5.
25. Smith TJ, Bahn RS, Gorman CA. Connective tissue, glycosaminoglycans, and diseases of the thyroid. Endocr Rev. 1989;10(3):366–91.
26. Schell H, Kiesewetter F, Seidel C, von Hintzenstern J. Cell cycle kinetics of human anagen scalp hair bulbs in thyroid disorders determined by DNA flow cytometry. Dermatologica. 1991;182(1):23–6.
27. Mullin GE, Eastern JS. Cutaneous signs of thyroid disease. Am Fam Physician. 1986;34(4):93–8.
28. Burman KD, McKinley-Grant L. Dermatologic aspects of thyroid disease. Clin Dermatol. 2006;24(4):247–55.
29. Ingbar D. The pulmonary system in hypothyroidism. In: Braverman LE, Utiger RD, Werner SC, Ingbar SH, editors. The thyroid: a fundamental and clinical text. 9th ed. Philadelphia: Lippincott Williams and Wilkins; 2005. p. 781.
30. McDaniel HG, Pittman CS, Oh SJ, DiMauro S. Carbohydrate metabolism in hypothyroid myopathy. Metabolism. 1977;26(8):867–73.
31. Kopecká K, Zacharova G, Smerdu V, Soukup T. Slow to fast muscle transformation following heterochronous isotransplantation is influenced by host thyroid hormone status. Histochem Cell Biol. 2014;142(6):677–84.
32. Gottehrer A, Roa J, Stanford GG, Chernow B, Sahn SA. Hypothyroidism and pleural effusions. Chest. 1990;98(5):1130–2.
33. Jha A, Sharma SK, Tandon N, Lakshmy R, Kadhiravan T, Handa KK, Gupta R, Pandey RM, Chaturvedi PK. Thyroxine replacement therapy reverses sleep-disordered breathing in patients with primary hypothyroidism. Sleep Med. 2006;7(1):55–61.
34. Baker JT, Harvey RF. Bowel habit in thyrotoxicosis and hypothyroidism. Br Med J. 1971;1(5744):322–3.
35. Wasan S, Sellin J, Vassilopoulou-Sellin R. The gastrointestinal tract and liver in hypothyroidism. In: Braverman LE, Utiger RD, Werner SC, Ingbar SH, editors. The thyroid: a

fundamental and clinical text. 9th ed. Philadelphia: Lippincott Williams and Wilkins; 2005. p. 796–9.
36. Goldin E, Wengrower D. Diarrhea in hypothyroidism: bacterial overgrowth as a possible etiology. J Clin Gastroenterol. 1990;12(1):98–9.
37. Liwanpo L, Hershman JM. Conditions and drugs interfering with thyroxine absorption. Best Pract Res Clin Endocrinol Metab. 2009;23(6):781–92.
38. İlhan M, Arabaci E, Turgut S, Karaman O, Danalioglu A, Tasan E. Esophagus motility in overt hypothyroidism. J Endocrinol Investig. 2014;37(7):639–44.
39. Eng O, Potdevin L, Davidov T, Lu S, Chen C, Trooskin S. Does nodule size predict compressive symptoms in patients with thyroid nodules? Gland Surg. 2014;3(4):232–6.
40. Van Steenbergen W, Fevery J, De Vos R, Leyten R, Heirwegh KP, De Groote J. Thyroid hormones and the hepatic handling of bilirubin. I. Effects of hypothyroidism and hyperthyroidism on the hepatic transport of bilirubin mono- and diconjugates in the Wistar rat. Hepatology. 1989;9(2):314–21.
41. de Castro F, Bonacini M, Walden JM, Schubert TT. Myxedema ascites. Report of two cases and review of the literature. J Clin Gastroenterol. 1991;13(4):411–4.
42. Wang Y, Yu X, Zhao QZ, Zheng S, Qing WJ, Miao CD, Sanjay J. Thyroid dysfunction, either hyper or hypothyroidism, promotes gallstone formation by different mechanisms. J Zhejiang Univ Sci B. 2016;17(7):515–25.
43. Kaptein E. The kidney and electrolyte metabolism in hypothyroidism. In: Braverman LE, Utiger RD, Werner SC, Ingbar SH, editors. The thyroid: a fundamental and clinical text. 9th ed. Philadelphia: Lippincott Williams and Wilkins; 2005. p. 789.
44. Diekman MJ, Harms MP, Endert E, Wieling W, Wiersinga WM. Endocrine factors related to changes in total peripheral vascular resistance after treatment of thyrotoxic and hypothyroid patients. Eur J Endocrinol. 2001;144(4):339–46.
45. Sabio JM, Rodriguez-Maresca M, Luna JD, del RC G, Vargas F. Vascular reactivity to vasoconstrictors in aorta and renal vasculature of hyperthyroid and hypothyroid rats. Pharmacology. 1994;49:257–64.
46. van Hoek I, Daminet S. Interactions between thyroid and kidney function in pathological conditions of these organ systems: a review. Gen Comp Endocrinol. 2009;160(3):205–15.
47. Das KC, Mukherjee M, Sarkar TK, Dash RJ, Rastogi GK. Erythropoiesis and erythropoietin in hypo- and hyperthyroidism. J Clin Endocrinol Metab. 1975;40:211–20.
48. Sun MT, Hsiao FC, Su SC, Pei D, Hung YJ. Thyrotropin as an independent factor of renal function and chronic kidney disease in normoglycemic euthyroid adults. Endocr Res. 2012;37(3):110–6.
49. Hataya Y, Igarashi S, Yamashita T, Komatsu Y. Thyroid hormone replacement therapy for primary hypothyroidism leads to significant improvement of renal function in chronic kidney disease patients. Clin Exp Nephrol. 2013;4:525–31.
50. Shin DH, Lee MJ, Lee HS, Oh HJ, Ko KI, Kim CH, et al. Thyroid hormone replacement therapy attenuates the decline of renal function in chronic kidney disease patients with subclinical hypothyroidism. Thyroid. 2013;6:654–61.
51. Macaron C, Famuyiwa O. Hyponatremia of hypothyroidism. Appropriate suppression of antidiuretic hormone levels. Arch Intern Med. 1978;138(5):820–2.
52. Skowsky WR, Kikuchi TA. The role of vasopressin in the impaired water excretion of myxedema. Am J Med. 1978;64(4):613–21.
53. Santoro D, Vadalà C, Siligato R, Buemi M, Benvenga S. Autoimmune thyroiditis and glomerulopathies. Front Endocrinol (Lausanne). 2017;2(8):119.
54. Klein I, Danzi S. Thyroid disease and the heart. Circulation. 2007;116(15):1725–35.
55. Sun Z, Ojamaa K, Coetzee WA, Artman M, Klein I. Effects of thyroid hormone on action potential and repolarization currents in rat ventricular myocytes. Am J Physiol Endocrinol Metab. 2000;278:E302–7.
56. Klein I, Ojamaa K. Thyroid hormone and the cardiovascular system. N Engl J Med. 2001;344:501.

57. Kabadi UM, Kumar SP. Pericardial effusion in primary hypothyroidism. Am Heart J. 1990;120(6 Pt 1):1393–5.
58. Biondi B, Klein I. Hypothyroidism as a risk factor for cardiovascular disease. Endocrine. 2004;24(1):1–13.
59. Axelrod AR, Berman L. The bone marrow in hyperthyroidism and hypothyroidism. Blood. 1951;6:436–53.
60. Szczepanek-Parulska E, Hernik A, Ruchała M. Anemia in thyroid diseases. Pol Arch Intern Med. 2017;127(5):352–60.
61. Marqusee E, Mandel S. The blood in hypothyroidism. In: Braverman LE, Utiger RD, Werner SC, Ingbar SH, editors. The thyroid: a fundamental and clinical text. 9th ed. Philadelphia: Lippincott Williams and Wilkins; 2005. p. 803–5.
62. Bernal J. Thyroid hormones in brain development and function. In: De Groot LJ, Chrousos G, Dungan K, Feingold KR, Grossman A, Hershman JM, Koch C, Korbonits M, McLachlan R, New M, Purnell J, Rebar R, Singer F, Vinik A, editors. Endotext [Internet]. South Dartmouth (MA): MDText.com, Inc.; 2000. 2 Sep 2015.
63. Palumbo CF, Szabo RM, Olmsted SL. The effects of hypothyroidism and thyroid replacement on the development of carpal tunnel syndrome. J Hand Surg Am. 2000;5(4):734–9.
64. Schwartz MS, Mackworth-Young CG, McKeran R. The tarsal tunnel syndrome in hypothyroidism. J Neurol Neurosurg Psychiatry. 1983;46:440.
65. Suarez G, Sabin TD. Meralgia parasthetica and hypothyroidism. Ann Intern Med. 1990;112:149.
66. Asher R. Myxedematous madness. BMJ. 1949;2:555.
67. Whybrow P, Bauer M. Behavioral and psychiatric aspects of hypothyroidism. In: Braverman LE, Utiger RD, Werner SC, Ingbar SH, editors. The thyroid: a fundamental and clinical text. 9th ed. Philadelphia: Lippincott Williams and Wilkins; 2005. p. 842.
68. Burmeister LA, Ganguli M, Dodge HH, Toczek T, DeKosky ST, Nebes RD. Hypothyroidism and cognition: preliminary evidence for a specific defect in memory. Thyroid. 2001;11(12):1177–85.
69. Samuels MH. Psychiatric and cognitive manifestations of hypothyroidism. Curr Opin Endocrinol Diabetes Obes. 2014;21(5):377–83.
70. Ueno S, Tsuboi S, Fujimaki M, Eguchi H, Machida Y, Hattori N, Miwa H. Acute psychosis as an initial manifestation of hypothyroidism: a case report. J Med Case Rep. 2015; 17(9):264.
71. Montagna G, Imperiali M, Agazzi P, D'Aurizio F, Tozzoli R, Feldt-Rasmussen U, Giovanella L. Hashimoto's encephalopathy: a rare proteiform disorder. Autoimmun Rev. 2016;15(5):466–76.
72. Krassas GE, Pontikides N. Male reproductive function in relation with thyroid alterations. Best Pract Res Clin Endocrinol Metab. 2004;18(2):183–95.
73. Krassas GE. Thyroid disease and female reproduction. Fertil Steril. 2000;74(6):1063–70.
74. Gardner D. The neuromuscular system and brain in hypothyroidism. In: Braverman LE, Utiger RD, Werner SC, Ingbar SH, editors. The thyroid: a fundamental and clinical text. 9th ed. Philadelphia: Lippincott Williams and Wilkins; 2005. p. 836.
75. Sindoni A, Rodolico C, Pappalardo MA, Portaro S, Benvenga S. Hypothyroid myopathy: a peculiar clinical presentation of thyroid failure. Review of the literature. Rev Endocr Metab Disord. 2016;17(4):499–519.
76. Gittoes N, Sheppard M. The skeletal system and brain in hypothyroidism. In: Braverman LE, Utiger RD, Werner SC, Ingbar SH, editors. The thyroid: a fundamental and clinical text. 9th ed. Philadelphia: Lippincott Williams and Wilkins; 2005. p. 830.
77. Williams GR, Bassett JHD. Thyroid diseases and bone health. J Endocrinol Investig. 2018;41(1):99–109.
78. Brabant G, Ocran K, Ranft U, von Zur Mühlen A, Hesch RD. Physiological regulation of thyrotropin. Biochimie. 1989;71(2):293–301.
79. Surks MI, Boucai L. Age- and race-based serum thyrotropin reference limits. J Clin Endocrinol Metab. 2010;95(2):496–502.

80. Després N, Grant AM. Antibody interference in thyroid assays: a potential for clinical misinformation. Clin Chem. 1998;44(3):440–54.
81. Garber JR, Cobin RH, Gharib H, Hennessey JV, Klein I, Mechanick JI, Pessah-Pollack R, Singer PA, Woeber KA. American Association of Clinical Endocrinologists and American Thyroid Association Taskforce on hypothyroidism in adults. Clinical practice guidelines for hypothyroidism in adults: cosponsored by the American Association of Clinical Endocrinologists and the American Thyroid Association. Endocr Pract. 2012;18(6):988–1028.
82. Ain KB, Pucino F, Shiver TM, Banks SM. Thyroid hormone levels affected by time of blood sampling in thyroxine-treated patients. Thyroid. 1993;3:81–5.
83. Koulouri O, Moran C, Halsall D, Chatterjee K, Gurnell M. Pitfalls in the measurement and interpretation of thyroid function tests. Best Pract Res Clin Endocrinol Metab. 2013;27(6):745–62.
84. Ladenson PW, Singer PA, Ain KB, Bagchi N, Bigos ST, Levy EG, Smith SA, Daniels GH, Cohen HD. American Thyroid Association guidelines for detection of thyroid dysfunction. Arch Intern Med. 2000 June 12;160(11):1573–5.
85. Helfand M, U.S. Preventive Services Task Force. Screening for subclinical thyroid dysfunction in nonpregnant adults: a summary of the evidence for the U.S. Preventive Services Task Force. Ann Intern Med. 2004;140(2):128–41.
86. Parle JV, Franklyn JA, Cross KW, Jones SR, Sheppard MC. Thyroxine prescription in the community: serum thyroid stimulating hormone level assays as an indicator of undertreatment or overtreatment. Br J Gen Pract. 1993;43(368):107–9.
87. De Whalley P. Do abnormal thyroid stimulating hormone level values result in treatment changes? A study of patients on thyroxine in one general practice. Br J Gen Pract. 1995;45(391):93–5.
88. Mosekilde L, Eriksen EF, Charles P. Effects of thyroid hormones on bone and mineral metabolism. Endocrinol Metab Clin N Am. 1990;19(1):35–63.
89. Haugen BR, Alexander EK, Bible KC, Doherty GM, Mandel SJ, Nikiforov YE, Pacini F, Randolph GW, Sawka AM, Schlumberger M, Schuff KG, Sherman SI, Sosa JA, Steward DL, Tuttle RM, Wartofsky L. 2015 American Thyroid Association management guidelines for adult patients with thyroid nodules and differentiated thyroid Cancer: the American Thyroid Association guidelines task force on thyroid nodules and differentiated thyroid Cancer. Thyroid. 2016;26(1):1–133.
90. Saravanan P, Chau WF, Roberts N, Vedhara K, Greenwood R, Dayan CM. Psychological well-being in patients on 'adequate' doses of l-thyroxine: results of a large, controlled community-based questionnaire study. Clin Endocrinol. 2002;57(5):577–85.
91. Slawik M, Klawitter B, Meiser E, Schories M, Zwermann O, Borm K, Peper M, Lubrich B, Hug MJ, Nauck M, Olschewski M, Beuschlein F, Reincke M. Thyroid hormone replacement for central hypothyroidism: a randomized controlled trial comparing two doses of thyroxine (T4) with a combination of T4 and triiodothyronine. J Clin Endocrinol Metab. 2007;92(11):4115–22.
92. Escobar-Morreale HF, Botella-Carretero JI, Gómez-Bueno M, Galán JM, Barrios V, Sancho J. Thyroid hormone replacement therapy in primary hypothyroidism: a randomized trial comparing L-thyroxine plus liothyronine with L-thyroxine alone. Ann Intern Med. 2005;142(6):412–24.
93. Siegmund W, Spieker K, Weike AI, Giessmann T, Modess C, Dabers T, Kirsch G, Sänger E, Engel G, Hamm AO, Nauck M, Meng W. Replacement therapy with levothyroxine plus triiodothyronine (bioavailable molar ratio 14: 1) is not superior to thyroxine alone to improve Well-being and cognitive performance in hypothyroidism. Clin Endocrinol. 2004;60(6):750–7.
94. Ma C, Xie J, Huang X, Wang G, Wang Y, Wang X, Zuo S. Thyroxine alone or thyroxine plus triiodothyronine replacement therapy for hypothyroidism. Nucl Med Commun. 2009;30(8):586–93.
95. Wartofsky L. Myxedema coma. Endocrinol Metab Clin N Am. 2006;35(4):687–98. vii-viii
96. Ord WM. Report of a committee of the Clinical Society of London to investigate the subject of myxoedema. Trans Clin Soc (Lond). 1888; (Suppl):21.

97. Sanders V. Neurologic manifestations of myxedema. N Engl J Med. 1962;266:547–51.
98. Zwillich CW, Pierson DJ, Hofeldt FD, Lufkin EG, Weil JV. Ventilatory control in myxedema and hypothyroidism. N Engl J Med. 1975;292:662–5.
99. Yamamoto T. Delayed respiratory failure during the treatment of myxedema coma. Endocrinol Jpn. 1984;31:769–75.
100. DeRubertis FR Jr, Michelis MF, Bloom MG, Mintz DH, Field JB, Davis BB. Impaired water excretion in myxedema. Am J Med. 1971;51:41–53.
101. Wartofsky L, Burman KD. Alterations in thyroid function in patients with systemic illness: the euthyroid sick syndrome. Endocr Rev. 1982;3:164–217.
102. Wartofsky L. Myxedema Coma. In: Braverman LE, Utiger RD, Werner SC, Ingbar SH, editors. The thyroid: a fundamental and clinical text. 9th ed. Philadelphia: Lippincott Williams and Wilkins; 2005. p. 850.
103. Brent G, Davies T. Hypothyroidism and thyroiditis. In: Melmed S, Polonsky K, Larsen P, Kronenberg H, editors. Williams textbook of endocrinology. 12th ed. Philadelphia: Elsevier; 2011. p. 431–3.
104. Canaris GJ, Manowitz NR, Mayor G, Ridgway EC. The Colorado thyroid disease prevalence study. Arch Intern Med. 2000;160:526–34.
105. Vanderpump MP, Tunbridge WM, French JM, Appleton D, Bates D, Clark F, et al. The incidence of thyroid disorders in the community: a twenty year follow-up of the Whickham survey. Clin Endocrinol. 1995;43:55–68.
106. Peeters RP. Subclinical hypothyroidism. N Engl J Med. 2017;377(14):1404.
107. Cooper DS, Biondi B. Subclinical thyroid disease. Lancet. 2012;379:1142–54.
108. Chan S, Boelaert K. Optimal management of hypothyroidism, hypothyroxinaemia and euthyroid TPO antibody positivity preconception and in pregnancy. Clin Endocrinol. 2015;82(3):313–26.
109. Villar HC, Saconato H, Valente O, Atallah AN. Thyroid hormone replacement for subclinical hypothyroidism. Cochrane Database Syst Rev. 2007;3:CD003419.
110. Somwaru LL, Rariy CM, Arnold AM, Cappola AR. The natural history of subclinical hypothyroidism in the elderly: the cardiovascular health study. J Clin Endocrinol Metab. 2012;97(6):1962–9.

Chapter 3
Thyrotoxicosis

Adva Eisenberg, Rebecca Herbst, and Tracy L. Setji

Abbreviations

AIT	Amiodarone-induced thyrotoxicosis
ATA	American Thyroid Association
ATD	Antithyroid drugs
FT3	Free triiodothyronine
FT4	Free thyroxine
GO	Graves' orbitopathy
LFTs	Liver function tests
MMI	Methimazole
MNG	Multinodular goiter
PTU	Propylthiouracil
RAI	Radioactive iodine
SSKI	Saturated solution of potassium iodide
TA	Toxic adenoma
TBG	Thyroxine-binding globulin
TFTs	Thyroid function tests
TMNG	Toxic multinodular goiter
TRAb	Thyrotropin receptor antibody
TSH	Thyroid-stimulating hormone
WBC	White blood cell

A. Eisenberg (✉) · R. Herbst · T. L. Setji
Duke University Medical Center, Division of Endocrinology, Metabolism, and Nutrition, Department of Medicine, Durham, NC, USA
e-mail: adva.eisenberg@duke.edu

> **Clinical Case**
>
> A 33-year-old African American female is referred by her primary care provider for a new diagnosis of hyperthyroidism after presenting with a 10 pound weight loss, palpitations, loose stools, and nervousness. Her thyroid-stimulating hormone (TSH) was <0.01 mIU/L (reference range 0.34–5.66 mIU/L), and her free thyroxine (FT4) was 1.95 ng/dL (reference range 0.52–1.21 ng/dL). Her provider started treatment with atenolol 25 milligrams daily; no further work-up has been done. She has a history of asthma as a child, currently experiences 1–2 flares annually requiring use of a rescue albuterol inhaler. Her mother has hypothyroidism treated with levothyroxine.
>
> Vital signs include temperature 37.0 °C, heart rate 90 beats per minute, blood pressure 135/70 mm/Hg, and respirations 14 breaths/min. Physical exam is notable for mild bilateral proptosis (~2 mm), lid lag, a diffusely enlarged and smooth goiter with a detectable thyroid bruit, regular heart rhythm, mild fine tremor of the outstretched hands, warm moist skin, and brisk reflexes. You suspect Graves' disease and confirm this diagnosis with an elevated serum thyrotropin receptor antibody (TRAb) of 3.85 IU/L (reference range 0.00–1.75). You also check a free triiodothyronine (FT3) level which is elevated at 5.88 pg/mL (reference range 2.20–3.80).
>
> The patient is recently married and desires conception in the next 2 years. How do you counsel her about her various treatment options both in the immediate future and long term?

Epidemiology of Hyperthyroidism

Globally, dietary iodine intake has a profound impact on the regional prevalence of thyroid disease. Both low and high iodine intake can affect thyroid function and may lead to anatomic adaptations of the thyroid gland, such as "goiter." In areas of iodine insufficiency, the gland can compensate for low substrate availability with chronic thyroid hyperactivity [1]. This can result in excess growth of the gland which increases the risk for mutations that can cause autonomous thyroid hormone production. Nearly one-third of the world's population lives in areas that are at high risk for iodine insufficiency. These places tend to be remote, often in mountainous areas with low amounts of iodine in the soil [2]. Thyroid goiters can become endemic when dietary iodine intake is less than 25 micrograms per day, and the prevalence of goiter is up to 80% in severely iodine-deficient areas [2]. For these reasons, the World Health Organization recommends that all food-grade salt is fortified with iodine [3].

In the United States and other iodine-sufficient areas, autoimmune disease and toxic multinodular goiter are the most common causes of thyrotoxicosis. In iodine-replete areas, the prevalence of thyrotoxicosis of any cause is 1–2% in women and

0.1–0.2% in men [4]. There are some data to suggest that the incidence of thyrotoxicosis is increasing in women but is not changing in men [2].

There are several risk factors that can influence the incidence and severity of thyroid disease. Excessive iodine intake or iodine exposure, such as with amiodarone or contrast dye, can precipitate Graves' disease and autonomous nodular disease. Graves' disease has also been associated with the immune reconstitution phase of highly active antiretroviral therapy [5]. Smoking increases the risk for autoimmune hyperthyroidism and is particularly important in the setting of Graves' orbitopathy (or ophthalmopathy, GO). Smokers with Graves' disease have at least a twofold increased risk for developing GO as compared to nonsmokers with Graves' disease [6]. Pregnancy profoundly affects thyroid hormone homeostasis and pathology and is discussed in detail in Chap. 7. Further, postpartum thyroiditis is defined by de novo thyroiditis that occurs within 1 year of pregnancy and affects 5.4% of the general population [7].

Etiologies of Thyrotoxicosis

Diffuse autoimmune hyperthyroidism, or Graves' disease, accounts for approximately 60–80% of thyrotoxicosis. It is caused by activating thyrotropin receptor antibodies (TRAb) that cause overproduction of thyroid hormone. The hallmark features of Graves' disease include hyperthyroidism, thyroid goiter, orbitopathy, and, less commonly, dermopathy. Risk factors include a family history of Graves' disease, a personal history of other autoimmune disease, and tobacco use. The typical age of onset is 20–50 years, but it also occurs in the elderly [8]. Graves' disease is about ten times more common in women than in men [8].

The second most common cause for thyrotoxicosis is hyperthyroidism (defined as increased thyroid hormone synthesis) from a toxic multinodular goiter (MNG). These are often polyclonal nodules that are thought to be caused by a hyperplastic response to local factors. The nodules can also be monoclonal, caused by mutations that confer a selective growth advantage [8]. The exact cause for the development of autonomous hormone production in MNGs remains to be elucidated. Typically, hyperthyroidism from a toxic MNG is less severe and progresses less rapidly than hyperthyroidism from Graves' disease. As in Graves' disease, acute exposure to iodine (such as contrast dye) or chronic exposure to high amounts of iodine (such as in amiodarone) can precipitate clinically evident hyperthyroidism.

A toxic adenoma, or a solitary autonomous nodule, is caused by mutations that stimulate TSH receptor signaling and induce constitutive activation of the cyclic AMP (adenosine monophosphate) pathway [9]. The degree of hyperthyroidism from toxic adenoma is relatively mild and often is suspected by the presence of a large, palpable nodule. A single autonomous nodule is less common than toxic MNG.

Thyroiditis is a generic term for thyrotoxicosis caused by inflammatory destruction of the thyroid gland with subsequent release of preformed thyroid hormone. This process is differentiated from hyperthyroidism in that there is usually not an associated increase in thyroid hormone synthesis. However, there can be "mixed" cases in which both hyperthyroid and destructive processes coexist; an example of this is mixed type 1 and type 2 amiodarone-induced thyrotoxicosis. There are many different causes for thyroiditis, including postpartum thyroiditis, subacute thyroiditis (also called "silent" or "painless" thyroiditis), de Quervain's thyroiditis (painful thyroiditis related to viral infection), suppurative thyroiditis (infectious process, presumed bacterial or fungal), radiation thyroiditis, and palpation thyroiditis. Additionally, several medications can cause thyroiditis, including amiodarone and iodinated contrast. The Jod-Basedow phenomenon refers to rapid production and release of thyroid hormone following the rapid uptake of excess iodine.

Amiodarone has become an increasingly common cause of thyroid disease due to its frequent use as an effective antiarrhythmic medication. People taking amiodarone are at risk for both hyperthyroidism and hypothyroidism which can occur at any time during, or even after, treatment. A 200 mg dose of amiodarone contains approximately 20–40 times more iodine than the typical American diet provides. Also, the drug is stored in adipose tissue which allows its effect on the thyroid to persist for months, even greater than a year, after the medication has been discontinued. Amiodarone-induced thyrotoxicosis (AIT) is unique in that it is more common in men than in women; this may simply be due to the higher use of this medication in the male population. The prevalence of AIT and the type of AIT are influenced by the iodine status in the area. Iodine-insufficient areas are thought to be at an increased risk for type 1 AIT which refers to hyperthyroidism caused by the sudden, high iodine load. However, type 2 AIT is independent of iodine status as it is caused by direct toxic effects of the drug which leads to destructive thyroiditis, without continued thyroid hormone production [10].

Ectopic sources of thyroid hormone production, such as struma ovarii or functional metastatic thyroid cancer, are rare causes of thyrotoxicosis. Struma ovarii refers to a mature ovarian teratoma that is primarily composed of thyroid tissue. Rarely, these are malignant [11]. Also rare are processes that lead to beta human chorionic gonadotropin stimulation of the TSH receptor, including choriocarcinoma, hydatidiform mole, or hyperemesis gravidarum [12]. TSH-producing pituitary adenomas are rare causes for hyperthyroidism that present with a normal or even elevated serum TSH. "TSHomas" account for only 1–2% of all pituitary tumors [13]. Finally, exogenous thyroid hormone intake, either factitious or iatrogenic, must be considered in the differential of thyrotoxicosis [8]. Table 3.1 outlines the etiologies of thyrotoxicosis.

Clinical Presentation

Systemic Symptoms

Active thyroid hormone affects nearly every organ; thus, high thyroid hormone levels can cause a myriad of symptoms (Table 3.2). The clinical signs and symptoms are similar among all causes of thyrotoxicosis, and they are largely based on the

3 Thyrotoxicosis

Table 3.1 Etiologies of thyrotoxicosis

Hyperthyroidism (increased thyroid hormone synthesis)	*Thyroiditis* (destructive release of preformed thyroid hormone)	*Extra-thyroidal thyrotoxicosis*
Graves' disease	Subacute de Quervain's thyroiditis (viral)	Exogenous thyroid hormone intake
Toxic multinodular goiter	Radiation-induced thyroiditis	Functional thyroid metastases
Solitary toxic adenoma	Acute, suppurative thyroiditis (bacterial)	Struma ovarii
TSH-producing pituitary adenoma	Palpation-induced thyroiditis	–
TSH receptor stimulation by hCG (trophoblastic disease, transient hyperthyroidism in pregnancy)	Painless thyroiditis (also called subacute lymphocytic thyroiditis)	–
Amiodarone-induced thyrotoxicosis, type 1	Medication-induced thyroiditis (amiodarone, interferon)	–
–	Postpartum thyroiditis	–

Table 3.2 Clinical manifestations of thyrotoxicosis

Cardiovascular	Metabolism	Sympathetic nervous system	Nervous system	Musculoskeletal	Gastrointestinal
Decreased resting peripheral vascular resistance	Heat intolerance +/− elevated body temperature	Increased sympathetic tone	Fine tremor (hands, tongue, eyelids)	Weakness	Increased appetite
Tachycardia (increased sympathetic activity, decreased parasympathetic activity)	Muscle wasting, muscle weakness, hypoalbuminemia (net protein loss)	Increased sensitivity to catecholamines	Nervousness, restlessness, hyperkinesia	Fatigability	Diarrhea
Supraventricular tachyarrhythmia	Increased insulin turnover	–	Emotional lability, rarely mania, paranoia, schizoid reactions	Graves' disease is associated with myasthenia gravis	Hepatic dysfunction (in severe thyrotoxicosis)
Increased cardiac output, increased stroke volume, increased inotropy, increased ventricular mass	Increased lipolysis, increased free fatty acids; decreased cholesterol levels	–	–	Periodic paralysis of hypokalemia	–
Increased pulse pressure	Increased bone turnover	–	–	–	–

degree of thyrotoxicosis. However, it should be noted that the severity of the clinical presentation does not necessarily correlate with the degree of lab abnormalities. Further, because increased thyroid hormone production and/or release may occur over months, the condition may go unnoticed for a prolonged period of time.

The active form of thyroid hormone, triiodothyronine or T3, mediates its cellular actions, including activation of nuclear receptors that regulate gene expression as well as nongenomic and pleiotropic effects. In general, T3 increases basal metabolic rate and increases tissue thermogenesis [12]. T3 also has profound effects on the cardiovascular system as it decreases systemic vascular resistance, increases sympathetic tone while decreasing parasympathetic tone, increases pulse pressure, and increases both chronotropy and inotropy. It is estimated that about 15% of cases of atrial fibrillation are caused by thyrotoxicosis [14] and 10–25% of patients with thyrotoxicosis have atrial fibrillation [15]. Other supraventricular arrhythmias can also occur with hyperthyroidism. Thyroid hormone has effects similar to, but separate from, catecholamines, so they can be additive. Additionally, thyrotoxicosis leads to an increased sensitivity of the body (particularly cardiomyocytes and adipocytes) to sympathetic stimulation [4].

Classically, people with thyrotoxicosis present with one or more of the following: palpitations, tremor, diaphoresis, restlessness, insomnia, anxiety, heat intolerance, weight loss, and hyperdefecation. People often describe an increase in appetite and increase in food intake; however, this may not be enough to compensate for the increased metabolic rate so still often results in loss of weight. Hyperthyroidism may also present with myopathy, usually proximal muscle weakness, due to a loss of muscle mass. This is caused by the hypermetabolic state that leads to degradation of protein. Other metabolic changes that can occur include a net increased rate of lipolysis which can manifest as decreased cholesterol, decreased triglycerides, and increased levels of free fatty acids. Thyrotoxicosis may worsen diabetes control due to the increased metabolism of insulin. Also, people may develop evidence of volume overload, including lower extremity edema, even without other findings of overt heart failure. Older individuals, however, may experience "apathetic" or "masked" symptoms of thyrotoxicosis. These cases can be less clinically evident as they tend to have fewer adrenergic signs and may have minimal symptoms altogether. Thyroid disease should be considered in any elderly patient with unexplained depression, apathy, or cognitive change [16].

Thyroid storm refers to clinically severe and life-threatening thyrotoxicosis. This is considered an endocrine emergency as its rapid identification and treatment are critical. Mortality rates from thyroid storm range from 8% to 25% [12]. There are scoring systems, such as the Burch-Wartofsky diagnostic criteria, which are used to systematically evaluate the severity and breadth of thyrotoxicosis [17] (Table 3.3). These are helpful with diagnosis as well as to guide treatment strategies and prognostication. Also, it is critical to recognize "impending thyroid storm" which again speaks to the nature of the hyperthyroid spectrum and the fluidity of the diagnosis. Important clinical parameters to consider in cases of severe hyperthyroidism include body temperature, changes in mental status, cardiovascular status, potential gastrointestinal symptoms or lab abnormalities, and identification of a potential precipitating event (such as discontinuing thionamide medication) [18].

Table 3.3 The Burch-Wartofsky Point Scale for the diagnosis of thyroid storm

Criteria		Points
Thermoregulatory dysfunction (temperature, degrees Celsius)	37.2–37.7	5
	37.8–38.3	10
	38.4–38.8	15
	38.9–39.3	20
	39.4–39.9	25
	>40.0	30
Cardiovascular tachycardia (beats per minute)	90–109	5
	110–119	10
	120–129	15
	130–139	20
	>140	25
	Atrial fibrillation	Absent, 0; present, 10
Congestive heart failure (if absent, 0 points)	Mild (pedal edema)	5
	Moderate (bibasilar rales)	10
	Severe (pulmonary edema)	15
Gastrointestinal-hepatic dysfunction (if absent, 0 points)	Moderate (diarrhea, abdominal pain, nausea, vomiting)	10
	Severe (jaundice)	20
Central nervous system Disturbance (if absent, 0 points)	Mild (agitation)	10
	Moderate (delirium, psychosis, extreme lethargy)	20
	Severe (seizure, come)	30
Precipitation event	–	No: 0; yes: 10

Adapted with permission from Burch and Wartofsky [17]
Total score, ≥ 45 likely thyroid storm; 25–44 impending storm; < 25 storm unlikely

Thyroid Examination

The thyroid examination can vary greatly among patients with thyrotoxicosis and provide valuable insight into the etiology of thyrotoxicosis. Patients with Graves' disease often have enlarged smooth glands with a bruit. Nodules can be palpated in patients with Graves' disease, MNG, or a solitary nodule. In thyroiditis, the gland can range from an acutely firm and tender gland suggesting de Quervain's (granulomatous thyroiditis) to a painless gland consistent with painless or subacute thyroiditis. Less commonly, suppurative or infectious thyroiditis can present with fever, pain, edema, dysphagia, and/or dysphonia. Finally, Riedel's thyroiditis, a rare cause of thyroiditis in which there is fibrosis of the thyroid gland as part of a systemic process related to IgG4 disease, presents with a hard, fixed thyroid gland and either hypothyroidism or thyrotoxicosis. In addition to causing abnormal thyroid levels, structural disease from a large goiter or MNG may cause compressive symptoms such as dysphagia, voice hoarseness, and compression of the trachea, particularly when in the supine position. These compressive symptoms are indications for surgical referral.

Eye Examination

Graves' orbitopathy (GO) is a potentially sight-threatening eye disease that is present to some degree in 25–70% of people with Graves' hyperthyroidism [19–21]. Although much remains unknown about GO, current research supports that it is an autoimmune process similar to that seen in the thyroid gland itself. All patients with GO have detectable TRAb, and the levels of antibodies correlate with the severity and prognosis of the eye disease. Recent data have demonstrated that orbital fibroblasts are the target cells or autoantigens in GO. Symptoms can vary drastically between patients and may include a dry/gritty sensation, diplopia, ptosis, conjunctivitis, increased lacrimation, and a sensation of retro-orbital pressure. More severe disease can manifest with inflammation, severe pain, and corneal ulceration. Pathologically, this results from enlargement of the muscles and adipose tissue of the orbit. GO most commonly occurs during periods of hyperthyroidism, but it can be seen in euthyroid or hypothyroid states and can present many years before or after thyroid disease. It should be noted that GO should be differentiated from lid lag and "stare" which can be seen in thyrotoxicosis of any etiology because these findings result from increased sympathetic tone as opposed to structural deposition disease [21].

Laboratory Evaluation to Distinguish Etiology

Thyroid Function Studies

In patients with clinical signs and/or symptoms that raise concern for thyroid disease, the biochemical diagnostic process begins with basic thyroid labs. TSH is the most sensitive and most specific of these tests. Large changes in TSH are caused by much smaller changes in thyroid hormone levels [22]. If TSH is abnormal, thyroid hormone levels should be obtained. Most thyroid guidelines recommend free thyroxine (FT4) and total triiodothyronine (TT3) as the most accurate assessment of each hormone status. The vast majority of serum thyroid hormone is in the inactive, protein-bound state. In fact, 99.98% of T4 and 99.7% of T3 is protein-bound [8]. Therefore, the total thyroid hormone levels are greatly affected by the amount of available thyroxine-binding globulin (TBG), transthyretin, and albumin. In patients with protein abnormalities, such as hypoalbuminemia, liver failure, or androgen use, free hormone levels are more clinically useful. Also, TBG can be increased in some settings, such as pregnancy, estrogen, methadone, or heroin use and hepatitis.

A suppressed TSH with elevated thyroid hormone(s) indicates primary thyrotoxicosis or disease of the thyroid gland itself as opposed to the hypothalamus or pituitary. If a patient is clinically thyrotoxic with a normal or elevated TSH and elevated thyroid hormone levels, a hypothalamic and/or pituitary process, thyroid hormone resistance, or ectopic TSH production (very rare) should be considered. In addition, TSH is often downregulated during periods of systemic illness, presumably as part of a physiologic protective mechanism. This condition is referred to as "non-thyroidal illness" or "sick euthyroid syndrome." Associated lab findings in non-thyroidal illness include low or normal free and total thyroid hormones and elevated reverse T3.

Thyroid Uptake and Scan

After establishing the diagnosis of primary thyrotoxicosis with suppressed TSH and elevated thyroid hormones, the next step is to determine the etiology. An important initial distinction is to assess whether the abnormality is caused by increased hormone synthesis ("hyperthyroidism") or by release of preformed thyroid hormone ("thyrotoxicosis without hyperthyroidism"). A thyroid uptake and scan, a radiologic procedure in which the subject is given radiolabeled iodine and then imaged to determine the degree and distribution of uptake by thyroid tissue, is useful in this setting. A high radioactive iodine uptake indicates that increased hormone synthesis is the underlying etiology. Alternatively, low uptake supports a state of thyroid gland destruction and release of preformed hormone. However, it is important to remember that, in patients with recent iodine exposure (such as contrast dye) or amiodarone use within the past 12–18 months, the uptake may be inaccurate (falsely low) due to pre-procedure supra-saturation with iodine.

High Uptake Etiologies

Etiologies of thyrotoxicosis from hyperthyroidism (high uptake) include Graves' disease and autonomous hormone production from nodular disease. Elevated iodine uptake in a diffuse, homogeneous pattern indicates Graves' disease, whereas focal or asymmetric uptake suggests nodular disease. Alternatively, thyrotropin receptor antibodies (TRAb) could be checked as this is a highly sensitive, and specific, test for Graves' disease [23]. A thyroid ultrasound can give pertinent structural information, as to the presence and characteristics of any nodules, which may be diagnostically useful. In some institutions, ultrasound with color flow Doppler images can help to distinguish hyperthyroidism (increased Doppler flow) versus destructive thyroiditis (low Doppler flow).

Low Uptake Etiologies

If thyroid uptake of iodine is very low or if the patient has negative TRAb with low Doppler flow on ultrasound, a diagnosis of thyroiditis is most likely. Other, less common, considerations for low iodine uptake include ectopic or exogenous hyperthyroidism. Both ectopic and exogenous T3 and T4 intake react with the thyroid hormone assay and suppress endogenous TSH. Serum thyroglobulin levels can be helpful to identify exogenous thyroid hormone intake, either iatrogenic or factitious. Because thyroglobulin is an endogenous precursor to thyroid hormones, the only cause for low thyroglobulin in the setting of thyrotoxicosis is exogenous intake.

Determining Etiology in Presence of Amiodarone

When amiodarone-related thyrotoxicosis is suspected, studies should be obtained to help determine if the pathophysiology is from increased hormone synthesis (referred to as type 1 AIT) or from hormone release (type 2 AIT). This distinction is important as the two pathologies are treated differently. Helpful studies include thyroid ultrasound with Doppler and thyroid antibodies. A nodular gland or positive antibodies suggest underlying thyroid disease (previously quiescent or subclinical) which can predispose patients to type 1 AIT. Findings such as low Doppler flow on ultrasound, negative TRAb, and normal gland structure are suggestive of type 2 AIT. As will be discussed later in this chapter, differentiating the two types is not always possible.

Important Considerations for Thyroid Labs

There are several important lab artifacts that should be considered, particularly in the setting of discordant TFTs. A common finding in hospitalized patients is "euthyroid hyperthyroxinemia" which refers to lab findings of normal TSH with elevated FT4. This can be due to an in vitro effect of heparin, caused by the activation of lipoprotein lipase which releases free fatty acids that displace T4 from it binding globulins in the test tube [22]. Furosemide, salicylate, and some antiepileptics can also cause displacement of thyroid hormone from the binding globulin which causes falsely elevated free hormone values. Biotin, a commonly used over-the-counter B vitamin that is marketed for strengthening hair and nails, can cause either falsely high or low free thyroid hormone results; the effect depends on the type of assay that is used [24]. Patients should be instructed to hold biotin for at least 2 days prior to having thyroid labs drawn. Common inpatient medications, such as steroids and dopamine, can suppress TSH. Also, heterophile antibody interference can cause significant false elevations in TSH assays. Sometimes TFTs may be discordant (e.g., low TSH with low FT4) or clinically discordant (labs suggestive of hyperthyroidism, whereas patient clinically appears hypothyroid). In these cases, it is important to consider possible lab interference from medications and/or supplements, iodine exposure, and possible binding globulin abnormalities (such as hypoalbuminemia in critically or chronically ill patients). When discordant labs are present, consideration should be given to the following diagnoses: subclinical thyroid disease, central hypothyroidism or hyperthyroidism, resistance to thyroid hormone, non-thyroidal illness (including acute psychiatric disease), malabsorption or nonadherence with thyroid medication, and recent treatment for functional thyroid disease (note that TSH changes will lag behind thyroid hormone lab changes) [22].

Diagnosing thyroid pathology during pregnancy can be challenging as one must consider the normal, physiologic changes of TFTs during pregnancy. Thus this topic is covered in detail in Chap. 7.

Other lab abnormalities that may raise consideration for thyroid disease or provide supportive data for thyrotoxicosis include hypercalcemia, normocytic anemia, elevated (bone specific) alkaline phosphatase, low cholesterol, and abnormal liver function tests.

Treatment of Hyperthyroidism

Symptomatic Management

Beta-blockers are the standard first-line agents for symptomatic management of hyperthyroidism regardless of the underlying etiology. They are especially important for patients who are elderly, have comorbid cardiovascular disease, or have a resting heart rate over 90 beats per minute [12]. Propranolol (at doses >160 mg/day) has the specific advantage of weakly blocking conversion of T4 to T3 via a mechanism independent of its effect on catecholamine pathways [4, 12].

Active bronchospastic lung disease is a relative contraindication to beta-blocker use since there is insufficient beta 1-receptor specificity at the high doses typically needed to control thyrotoxicosis (e.g., 160–320 mg/day of propranolol). Higher doses may be required because drug clearance is increased in hyperthyroidism [25]. In such patients, an agent with relative beta 1-receptor specificity may be considered with close monitoring for respiratory decompensation [12]. Other relative contraindications to beta-blocker use include decompensated heart failure and Raynaud's phenomenon, in which case the nondihydropyridine calcium channel blockers (i.e., verapamil and diltiazem) can be used for rate control [4, 12, 25]. In patients who are critically ill, intravenous use of propranolol or the cardioselective beta-blocker esmolol is preferred because of the rapid onset and short duration of action [25].

Treatment of Hyperthyroidism Secondary to Graves' Disease

Treatment of Graves' disease almost always starts with administration of an antithyroid drug (ATD), which can be used for exclusive management or as a bridge to definitive treatment with radioactive iodine (RAI) or thyroidectomy. Table 3.4 compares the three potential treatment modalities along with their pregnancy considerations (which are addressed in more detail in Chap. 7). The presence of Graves' orbitopathy (GO) is also a special consideration and thus is further discussed in its own section.

Table 3.4 Treatment options for Graves' disease

Treatment modality	Indications and benefits	Contraindications	Pregnancy considerations
ATD	No associated surgical risks Can be used in the presence of orbitopathy If remission achieved, avoids need for long-term thyroid hormone replacement	Known severe adverse reaction to ATD Baseline significant lab abnormality (relative contraindication; see text)	PTU should be used in first trimester of pregnancy, MMI recommended in the second and third trimesters
RAI	No associated surgical risks Can be used in patients with previously operated or externally irradiated necks Most cost-effective option	Pregnancy Lactation Thyroid cancer	Can be used for definitive management in women planning pregnancy in the future but must wait >6 months post-RAI to conceive Transient increase in TRAb levels post-RAI often followed by long-term persistence; transplacental passage must be considered
Surgery	Can be used in the presence of orbitopathy Can relieve compressive symptoms in large goiters Preferred option if thyroid malignancy confirmed or suspected Coexisting hyperparathyroidism requiring surgery	Significant medical comorbidities or limited life expectancy Previous neck operation or external radiation increasing surgical risk	Can be used for definitive management in women planning pregnancy often with quicker normalization in thyroid function than RAI as well as decrease in TRAb levels over time If surgery required during pregnancy, ideally performed in the second trimester

Data from: Melmed et al. [4]; and Ross et al. [12]
ATD antithyroid drug, *MMI* methimazole, *PTU* propylthiouracil, *RAI* radioactive iodine

Antithyroid Drugs for Graves' Disease

The thionamide drugs methimazole (MMI) and propylthiouracil (PTU) block thyroid hormone synthesis by inhibiting the actions of thyroid peroxidase; PTU additionally inhibits peripheral conversion of T4–T3. MMI should always be used as a first-line therapy due to the higher risk of hepatotoxicity with PTU. However, PTU is used during the first trimester of pregnancy as well as during the treatment of thyroid storm. Further, PTU may be considered in patients with minor adverse effects from MMI who decline or are not candidates for RAI or surgery [12].

Starting doses of MMI are usually between 10–40 mg daily until patients are biochemically euthyroid, at which point the dose can be reduced by 30–50% until a maintenance range of 5–10 mg daily is reached [12, 26]. Higher initial doses (i.e., 60–80 mg daily) do not improve remission rates and are not recommended due to the increased risk of adverse effects. Although the duration of action of MMI is less than 24 h, a single daily dose helps maximize adherence and is typically sufficient to treat milder cases, as well as during maintenance therapy [4]. If rapid control is required for more severe hyperthyroidism, twice-daily dosing may be more efficient [12]. PTU has a shorter duration of action than MMI and is typically divided into two or three daily doses. The biologic activity of PTU on a weight basis is 1:10 to 1:20 that of methimazole [4], with starting doses ranging from 50 to 150 mg three times daily, followed by maintenance dosing of 50 mg two to three times daily [12].

Thyroid function tests including free T4 and free or total T3 (depending on lab availability) should be obtained within 2–6 weeks of initiating therapy followed by every 4–6 weeks until the patient is euthyroid. Serum T3 levels are important to assess because some patients will normalize their free T4 but have ongoing elevations in free T3 ("T3 thyrotoxicosis"). Serum TSH can remain suppressed for 1–2 months after starting therapy and is not a useful marker to follow initially [12, 25]. Once euthyroidism is achieved with the minimal dose of medication, evaluations can be spaced out to every 2–3 months for the first 6 months. If a patient is receiving long-term MMI (>18 months), this interval can be increased to every 6 months [12].

Adverse Effects of ATD Therapy

Minor adverse effects such as pruritic rash and arthralgias occur in approximately 5% of patients taking methimazole and typically begin within the first few weeks of initiating therapy. A mild rash may self-resolve or be treated with antihistamines with continuation of ATD therapy but occasionally may be severe enough to require drug withdrawal [12, 25]. Such patients can be switched to PTU though 30–50% will experience a similar reaction [25].

The primary three rare but dangerous side effects of ATD are outlined below:

1. *Agranulocytosis.* While extremely uncommon (0.1–0.3% of patients on therapy) [4], agranulocytosis can be life-threatening. The risk is higher in older patients and with higher doses of MMI (rare at doses <10 mg) [4, 25]. PTU at any dose appears to be more likely to cause agranulocytosis compared with low doses of MMI [12]. Notably, most cases of agranulocytosis develop within the first 90 days of therapy. In the case of agranulocytosis with either MMI or PTU, use of the other medication is contraindicated due to the risk of cross-reactivity [4, 12].
2. *Hepatotoxicity.* This side effect is also very rare with an incidence of <0.1% [25]. MMI has classically been described as causing cholestatic injury with PTU causing hepatocellular toxicity, though both patterns have been described with MMI. Liver toxicity from PTU tends to be more severe and has caused hepatic failure requiring liver transplant. In fact, it is the third most common cause of drug-related liver failure, accounting for 10% of all drug-related liver transplants, with children appearing to be more susceptible than adults [4, 12]. Similar to agranulocytosis, the majority of cases develop within the first 120 days of

therapy. Except in cases of severe PTU-induced hepatotoxicity, MMI can be used without ill effects [12, 27, 28].
3. *Vasculitis*. PTU and less commonly MMI have been associated with perinuclear antineutrophil cytoplasmic antibody (p-ANCA)-positive small-vessel vasculitis as well as drug-induced lupus. ANCA-positive vasculitis is more common in patients of Asian ethnicity [4, 12]. Unlike the aforementioned effects which tend to occur near the start of treatment, the risk of vasculitis is associated with the length of therapy. It tends to improve with cessation of the offending drug, though immunosuppressive therapy has been required [12].

Monitoring of ATD Therapy

Baseline liver function tests (LFTs) including transaminases, bilirubin, and alkaline phosphatase and a white blood cell (WBC) count with differential should be measured prior to starting ATD treatment for comparison with future labs if needed, though it is important to mention that both mild leukopenia and LFT abnormalities are fairly common in patients with Graves' disease, with up to 30% of patients having a mild elevation in LFTs [25, 29]. Mild baseline liver disease or LFT abnormalities are not necessarily a contraindication to ATD therapy but should be monitored over time for normalization; a rising alkaline phosphatase with improvement in all other parameters typically represents an origin from bone as opposed to the liver [30], while rising transaminases or bilirubin should be concerning for drug toxicity.

Although there is no evidence that baseline neutropenia or liver disease increases the risk of complications from ATDs, the recommendation by the task force from the most recent American Thyroid Association (ATA) guidelines is that a baseline absolute neutrophil count less than <1000/mm3 or liver transaminase enzyme levels >fivefold above the upper limit of normal should prompt consideration of alternative treatments [12].

A WBC with differential should always be checked if a patient taking an ATD presents with a fever or pharyngitis. However, there is insufficient evidence to recommend for or against routine monitoring of WBC counts in patients taking ATD because the incidence of agranulocytosis is extremely low and develops over the course of days. There is also insufficient evidence to recommend for or against routine monitoring of LFTs in patients taking ATD since this practice has not been found to prevent severe hepatotoxicity [12]. However, patients should be instructed on the potential adverse effects of ATD, preferably with information also provided in writing, and they should be advised to stop therapy immediately and notify their provider if any concerning symptoms develop including pruritic rash, jaundice, acholic stools, dark urine, arthralgias, abdominal pain, nausea, fatigue, fever, or pharyngitis [12]. ATD therapy should be stopped if transaminase levels (found incidentally or measured as clinically indicated) reach >3 times the upper limit of normal or if levels elevated at the onset of therapy increase further. After stopping the drug, LFTs should be monitored weekly until there is evidence of resolution.

Cessation of Therapy

Before considering stopping the therapy, measurement of thyroid receptor antibody (TRAb) levels is recommended to prognosticate which patients may be successfully tapered off medication: in patients with elevated TRAb, relapse rates are between 80% and 100%, while in patients with lower levels, relapse rates are around 20–30% [12, 31, 32]. Additional factors that predict a lower chance of remission include male gender, smoking (especially in men), and large goiter size (>80 g) [12].

MMI should be continued for a minimum of 12–18 months and can be discontinued after that time frame if TSH and TRAb levels are normal [12]. Therapeutic durations longer than 18 months have not been shown to increase remission rates [4]. A patient is considered to be in remission if TSH, free T4, and total T3 levels remain normal for 1 year after stopping ATD therapy [12]. Thyroid function tests should be measured every few months in the first year after discontinuation to monitor for early relapse, since approximately 75% of relapses occur in the first 3 months after withdrawal of therapy [4]. They should be measured at least annually after that because relapses can occur many years later [12, 31] and some patients may eventually become hypothyroid.

Radioactive Iodine for Graves' Disease

Radioactive iodine ablation is a form of radiation in which radioactive iodine is administered to destroy the thyroid gland. The destruction of thyroid tissue from RAI occasionally results in transient worsening of thyrotoxicosis for the first few weeks following therapy [25], while rare, thyroid storm has been reported following RAI [33]. For this reason, pretreatment with MMI should be considered for high-risk patients (i.e., elderly, cardiovascular disease). Patients will need to hold the medication a minimum of 2–3 days before the procedure. In high-risk patients, the use of beta-blockers as well as resumption of MMI 3–7 days following the procedure should also be considered [12]. A pregnancy test should be obtained within 48 h before treatment with RAI in any woman of childbearing potential [12]. In addition, any suspicious appearing nodules on ultrasound should be biopsied as indicated per guidelines prior to RAI, with reconsideration for surgery for any high-suspicion nodules or confirmed thyroid malignancy [12].

Thyroid function tests including free T4, free or total T3, and TSH should be monitored every 4–6 weeks for the first several months following RAI therapy until the patient becomes hypothyroid. If hyperthyroidism is still present after 6 months and the patient is symptomatic, treatment can be repeated, usually with about 1.5 times the initial dose of iodine [4]. Initiation and early titration of thyroid hormone replacement should be based on free hormone levels because the rise in TSH may lag following a long period of suppression. Complete weight-based replacement of 1.6 mcg/kg/day is not always required if there is residual endogenous thyroid function [12]. Close monitoring should continue until a stable dose is established. Most patients become hypothyroid by 16 weeks [34]. There is a well-described post-RAI surge in TRAb levels that tends to peak at around 3 months but can persist for many years, thought to be due to RAI-associated leakage of thyroid antigens [35]. This may be a particular consideration for those with thyroid eye disease as well as those considering pregnancy due to the transplacental passage of these antibodies [25].

Thyroidectomy for Graves' Disease

Surgical therapy is often recommended for patients with large goiters or obstructive manifestations. Computerized tomography or magnetic resonance imaging can be useful to characterize the extent of the goiter and any tracheal narrowing [4]. Prior to undergoing thyroidectomy, patients should be pretreated with ATD with the goal of achieving euthyroidism, which helps minimize operative risk as well as the risk of precipitating thyroid storm from the stress of surgery, anesthesia, or palpation thyroiditis during surgery [12]. Adjunctive use of beta-blockers is also recommended. Pretreatment with saturated solution of potassium iodide (SSKI) at a dose of 50–100 mg (1–2 drops or 0.05–0.1 mL) three times daily should start 10 days before surgery, which inhibits thyroid hormone synthesis and secretion and can also reduce thyroid size and vascularity [12].

Hypocalcemia related to hypoparathyroidism is one of the most common postoperative complications, with transient gland "stunning" from ischemia occurring in up to 25% of cases and more serious injury or gland removal leading to permanent damage occurring in approximately 4% of cases [25]. Other complications include recurrent or superior laryngeal nerve injury (leading to hoarseness or complete vocal cord paralysis with more serious injury), bleeding, and complications from general anesthesia. Studies have shown that higher surgical volume is tied to better patient outcomes [12].

Serum calcium and 25-hydroxy vitamin D levels should be measured prior to surgery and repleted as necessary to minimize the risk of postoperative hypocalcemia from hypoparathyroidism and/or hungry bone syndrome. Preoperative use of calcitriol should be considered for those at higher risk for hypoparathyroidism [12]. Standardized postoperative protocols for oral calcium and calcitriol replacement have been shown to decrease the incidence of hypocalcemic symptoms and need for intravenous calcium replacement [12]. Supplementation can be tapered off postoperatively based on serial monitoring of levels.

Thyroid hormone replacement should be started immediately postoperatively at standard weight-based dosing, with the exception of elderly patients who may require less. Serum TSH should be assessed 6–8 weeks postoperatively to allow time for steady-state concentrations to be achieved.

Treatment of Graves' Disease with Orbitopathy

RAI therapy is a known risk factor for precipitating or worsening GO, likely at least in part related to the increased surge in autoimmunity against the thyrotropin receptor [35]. This risk is highest in smokers, untreated hyperthyroidism, high pretreatment TRAb levels (>8.8 IU/L, normal <1.75 IU/L,), and delayed treatment of hypothyroidism after therapy [12, 36]. Smoking is the most significant of these risk factors, and both firsthand and secondhand smoking exposure can play a role.

Prophylactic use of glucocorticoids can help minimize the risk of GO. The decision whether to use glucocorticoids depends on each patient's individual risk profile which should be measured against the risk for adverse effects from steroid therapy (e.g., uncontrolled diabetes, immunocompromised state, osteoporosis, psychiatric illness, etc.) [12]. The dose of corticosteroids validated in a randomized clinical trial for GO prophylaxis is the equivalent of prednisone 0.4–0.5 mg/kg per day, started 1–3 days after RAI administration, continued for 1 month, and then tapered over 2 months [37]. However, one retrospective cohort study suggested that lower doses and shorter duration of oral prednisone (approximately 0.2 mg/kg per day for 6 weeks) may be comparable for preventing worsening of GO in patients with baseline mild or absent eye disease [38].

Guidelines differ and clinical judgment should always be instituted, but in general, corticosteroid prophylaxis is recommended in patients with mild Graves' orbitopathy and risk factors for worsening disease and in patients with moderate Graves' orbitopathy regardless of risk factors. RAI should be avoided in those with active and moderate to severe Graves' orbitopathy [12, 25].

Treatment of Toxic Multinodular Goiter or Toxic Adenoma

The three treatment modalities available for toxic multinodular goiter (TMNG) and toxic adenoma (TA) are the same as those described for Graves' disease, and thus treatment considerations are fairly similar (Table 3.4). However, since nodular disease is generally a progressive condition that does not revert spontaneously, RAI or thyroidectomy is preferred for long-term management since ATD alone cannot induce remission. The risk of treatment failure is overall much higher for RAI therapy (20% for TMNG and 6–18% for TA) compared with surgery (<1%). A toxic adenoma can often be treated with lobectomy or hemithyroidectomy which can potentially prevent development of hypothyroidism and can often be performed on an outpatient basis or even under local anesthesia [4]. Following thyroid lobectomy for TA, thyroid hormone replacement is required in approximately 15–20% of patients [12, 39]. In selected situations, long-term treatment with methimazole may be reasonable, such as in poor surgical candidates who reside in a nursing home or long-term care facility where radiation safety guidelines cannot be observed [12]. Fortunately, the dose of MMI required to achieve euthyroidism in TMNG or TA patients is typically low (5–10 mg/d).

If RAI is chosen, pretreatment with MMI followed by resumption of medication 3–7 days following RAI should be considered for high-risk patients, similar to Graves' disease [12]. For those choosing to undergo surgery, preoperative SSKI is typically not recommended. The theoretical risk of exacerbating the hyperthyroidism from the iodine load outweighs the benefits, since the thyrotoxicosis with TA and TMNG is typically milder than Graves' disease and thus pretreatment with ATD and beta-blockers is sufficient [12]. Posttreatment monitoring after RAI or surgery is similar to that discussed for Graves' disease.

Treatment of Thyroid Storm

The diagnosis of thyroid storm is ultimately a clinical one though scoring systems exist as discussed earlier in this chapter. If clinical suspicion is high, the benefits generally outweigh the risks to treat the patient aggressively as true thyroid storm. The need for close vital sign monitoring typically necessitates admission to an intensive care unit. Management consists of a combination of supportive therapy, treatment of underlying precipitants, and direct treatment of the thyrotoxicosis. Sequential therapy is thus typically needed including ATD, inorganic iodide, beta-blockers, and corticosteroids; see Table 3.5 [12].

Thyroid storm is one of the only instances in which the use of PTU is recommended over MMI due to its ability to decrease conversion of T4 to the more active T3 hormone. This effect is more apparent at dosages greater than 600 mg/day [4]. If a patient is unable to tolerate oral intake, a gastric tube may be used; rectal administration has also been described. Additional measures aimed at blocking peripheral T4–T3 conversion include corticosteroids and beta-blockers (namely, propranolol) at higher doses [4, 12]. Particularly if the use of first-line agents is contraindicated, adjunctive use of cholestyramine has been described which binds thyroid hormones in the intestine and thereby increases their fecal excretion [40]. In critically ill patients who fail to improve or have contraindications to first-line therapies, plasmapheresis or surgery can be used as salvage therapies [12, 41].

Table 3.5 Treatment of thyroid storm

Medication	Dose	Mechanism of action
Thionamides: PTU (preferred) or MMI	*PTU*: 200–250 mg PO q 4 h (1200–1500 mg daily); can load with 600–1000 mg dose *MMI*: 20 mg PO q 4 h or 30 mg q 6 h	Both block new thyroid hormone synthesis PTU also inhibits T4–T3 conversion
Beta-blockers: Propranolol or Esmolol	*Propranolol*: IV (1 mg/min) if needed, then PO 60–80 mg q 4 h *Esmolol*: IV bolus 250–500 ug/kg followed by gtt 50–100 ug/kg/min	Both help block beta-adrenergic stimulation Propranolol at high doses inhibits T4–T3 conversion
Glucocorticoids: Dexamethasone or Hydrocortisone	*Dexamethasone*: 2 mg q6h PO or IV *Hydrocortisone*: 100 mg IV q 8 h	Block conversion of T4–T3 Treat relative adrenal insufficiency if present
Iodine[a]: Lugol's solution or SSKI	*Lugol's solution*: 8–10 drops q 6–8 h *SSKI*: 5 drops every 6 h	Block new hormone synthesis Block release of thyroid hormone

Data from: Melmed et al. [4]; and Ross et al. [12]
MMI methimazole, *PTU* propylthiouracil, *SSKI* saturated solution of potassium iodide
[a]Iodine should be given a *minimum* of 1 h after thionamide initiation to prevent the synthesis of additional thyroid hormone from the administered iodine

Treatment of Subclinical Hyperthyroidism

Prior to committing a patient to therapy, the first step is to rule out a transient lab abnormality with repeat thyroid function tests at 3–6 months, since many patients will have normal TSH on follow-up without intervention. A shorter interval of 2–6 weeks may be considered for patients at high risk of complications [12].

Evidence for treating subclinical hyperthyroidism is overall inconclusive, and there are few randomized trials demonstrating clear improvement in outcomes. The majority of evidence comes from small uncontrolled studies that showed improvement in surrogate markers such as bone mineral density, cardiac structure and function, and frequency of ectopic heart beats, but there are less data for clinically meaningful endpoints such as rate of cardiovascular events, atrial fibrillation, and fractures [12]. In general, patients with TSH persistently <0.1 mU/L should be treated as the risk of developing overt hyperthyroidism is higher when the TSH is fully suppressed as compared to a TSH that is low but detectable. The exception to this is in young, asymptomatic healthy patients, in whom a monitoring strategy is reasonable. For patients with TSH 0.1–0.4 mU/L, age, comorbidities, presence of symptoms, and personal preferences should all be considered. In older patients, postmenopausal osteoporosis and cardiac disease are the main indications for which treatment should be considered, while infertility or menstrual disorders are important in younger women [4]. In borderline cases, a trial of beta-blocker can assess whether symptomatic therapy alone is adequate [12]. If treatment is chosen, management is the same as for overt hyperthyroidism from the same cause.

Treatment of Amiodarone-Induced Thyrotoxicosis

The decision whether to discontinue amiodarone should be based on the severity of the underlying arrhythmia measured against the severity of thyroid dysfunction as well as the viability of alternate antiarrhythmics, and thus consultation with the patient's cardiologist is recommended. In the case of refractory or life-threatening arrhythmias, most experts agree that the patient's cardiac status should take precedence. In these cases, amiodarone should be continued with simultaneous treatment of the thyroid abnormality. Even in such cases, discontinuation of amiodarone is controversial since it may have T3-antagonistic properties and inhibit T4–T3 conversion at the cardiac level so that withdrawal could in theory lead to cardiac decompensation. Furthermore, due to its fat-soluble properties, the medication has an extremely long half-life of 50–60 days [4], and therefore its effects can last for months even following discontinuation [12].

MMI should be used for clear-cut cases of type 1 amiodarone-induced thyrotoxicosis (AIT) due to underlying Graves' or nodular disease, while corticosteroids should be used to treat clear-cut cases of type 2 AIT due to destructive thyroiditis. However, this distinction is not always easy to make, and many patients present with overlap features. Combination therapy with MMI and steroids is often employed in patients with severe thyrotoxicosis, those at high risk for complications or in those who fail to improve after a trial of monotherapy. After resolution of the initial hyperthyroidism, patients should be monitored for progression to hypothyroidism, particularly after a course of suspected destructive thyroiditis (i.e., type 2 AIT) [12].

The recommended starting dose of MMI is 40 mg once daily until euthyroidism is achieved, which can take on the order of 3–6 months. The recommended starting dose of corticosteroids is the equivalent of 40 mg prednisone daily for 2–4 weeks, followed by a slow taper over 2–3 months. Patients with inadequate response to dual therapy or whose cardiac condition is likely to require lifelong amiodarone therapy should be considered for thyroidectomy [4]. Although thyroidectomy in this setting has a very high morbidity and mortality rate (9%), there is an even higher mortality rate if surgery is postponed or deferred [12, 42].

Treatment of Thyroiditis

There are several forms of thyroiditis which all have in common a low uptake on nuclear medicine uptake and scan. There is no role for ATD therapy in such cases as production of new thyroid hormone is already suppressed [12]. Patients with mild symptoms due to subacute thyroiditis should be managed conservatively with beta-blockers and nonsteroidal anti-inflammatory agents; corticosteroids should be given if patients fail to respond to anti-inflammatories or present with moderate to severe pain and/or thyrotoxic symptoms [12]. Recommended dosing is prednisone 40 mg daily for 1–2 weeks followed by a taper over 2–4 weeks or longer, depending upon clinical response [12]. Patients with symptoms from painless thyroiditis should be treated with beta-blockers alone. Thyroid hormone replacement should be started during the hypothyroid phase if TSH reaches >10 mIU/L, but it should be tapered off after 3–6 months of therapy to monitor for recovery of thyroid function [12].

Clinical Case and Discussion

A 33-year-old African American female is referred by her primary care provider for a new diagnosis of hyperthyroidism after presenting with a 10 pound weight loss, palpitations, loose stools, and nervousness. Her thyroid-stimulating hormone (TSH) was <0.01 mIU/L (reference range 0.34–5.66 mIU/L), and her free thyroxine (FT4) was 1.95 ng/dL (reference range 0.52–1.21 ng/dL). Her provider started treatment with atenolol 25 milligrams daily; no further work-up has been done. She has a history of asthma as a child, currently experiences 1–2 flares annually requiring use of a rescue albuterol inhaler. Her mother has hypothyroidism treated with levothyroxine.

Vital signs include temperature 37.0 °C, heart rate 90 beats per minute, blood pressure 135/70 mm/Hg, and respirations 14 breaths/min. Physical exam is notable for mild bilateral proptosis (~2 mm), lid lag, a diffusely enlarged and smooth goiter with a detectable thyroid bruit, regular heart rhythm, mild fine tremor of the outstretched hands, warm moist skin, and brisk reflexes. You suspect Graves' disease and confirm this diagnosis with an elevated serum thyrotropin receptor antibody (TRAb) of 3.85 IU/L (reference range 0.00–1.75). You also check a free triiodothyronine (FT3) level which is elevated at 5.88 pg/mL (reference range 2.20–3.80).

The patient is recently married and desires conception in the next 2 years. How do you counsel her about her various treatment options both in the immediate future and long term?

In order to provide immediate therapeutic and symptomatic benefit, the patient should be started on therapy with a thionamide, such as methimazole 20 milligrams daily. She should be counseled on the potential adverse effects of methimazole including agranulocytosis, vasculitis, arthralgias, liver injury, and rash. She should be instructed to stop the medication and notify her provider if she develops a fever, sore throat, rash, nausea, vomiting, yellowing of the skin, or abdominal pain. These instructions should be provided both verbally and in writing and reviewed at each follow-up visit. She should be counseled to use a reliable form of contraception until her hyperthyroidism is treated, both due to the potential adverse effects on pregnancy from uncontrolled hyperthyroidism and due to the potential teratogenicity of methimazole.

For long-term management, her options include 12–18 months of methimazole therapy with monitoring to see if she goes into spontaneous remission. This would be a reasonable option since initial antibody level is only mildly elevated. This option may delay her plans for conception; however, it may allow her to conceive without the risk of thionamide use and with close monitoring only throughout pregnancy. An alternative option would be to restore her to euthyroidism with methimazole and then switch to PTU as soon as she becomes pregnant and throughout the first trimester. Definitive treatment options include thyroidectomy, which would provide the most rapid control though comes with the associated risks of general anesthesia and surgery, and RAI ablation. However, pregnancy should be avoided for 6 months following RAI, and levothyroxine dosing should be stabilized prior to pursuing pregnancy. Further, RAI ablation does not reduce serum levels of TRAb. Whatever the patient's choice, she will need close follow-up with both obstetrical and endocrinological management throughout her pregnancy.

References

1. Laurberg P, Cerqueira C, Ovesen L, Rasmussen LB, Perrild H, Andersen S, et al. Iodine intake as a determinant of thyroid disorders in populations. Best Pract Res Clin Endocrinol Metab. 2010;24(1):13–27.
2. Vanderpump MPJ. The epidemiology of thyroid disease. Br Med Bull. 2011;99(1):39–51.
3. WHO. Guideline: fortification of food-grade salt with iodine for the prevention and control of iodine deficiency disorders. Geneva: World Health Organization; 2014. [cited 2017 10/4/2017]. Available from: https://www.ncbi.nlm.nih.gov/books/NBK254243/.
4. Melmed S, Polonsky KS, Reed Larsen P, Kronenberg HM. Williams textbook of endocrinology. 13th ed. Philadelphia: Elsevier Health Sciences; 2016.
5. Weetman A. Immune reconstitution syndrome and the thyroid. Best Pract Res Clin Endocrinol Metab. 2009;23(6):693–702.
6. Thornton J, Kelly S, Harrison R, Edwards R. Cigarette smoking and thyroid eye disease: a systematic review. Eye. 2007;21(9):1135.
7. Stagnaro-Green A, Abalovich M, Alexander E, Azizi F, Mestman J, Negro R, et al. Guidelines of the American Thyroid Association for the diagnosis and management of thyroid disease during pregnancy and postpartum. Thyroid. 2011;21(10):1081–125.
8. Longo D, Fauci A, Kasper D. Harrison's principles of internal medicine. 18th ed. New York: The McGraw-Hill Company; 2011. Available at: /accessmedicine com/content aspx.
9. Tonacchera M, Chiovato L, Pinchera A, Agretti P, Fiore E, Cetani F, et al. Hyperfunctioning thyroid nodules in toxic multinodular goiter share activating thyrotropin receptor mutations with solitary toxic adenoma. J Clin Endocrinol Metabol. 1998;83(2):492–8.
10. Basaria S, Cooper DS. Amiodarone and the thyroid. Am J Med. 2005;118(7):706–14.
11. Wei S, Baloch ZW, LiVolsi VA. Pathology of struma ovarii: a report of 96 cases. Endocr Pathol. 2015;26(4):342–8.
12. Ross DS, Burch HB, Cooper DS, Greenlee MC, Laurberg P, Maia AL, et al. 2016 American thyroid association guidelines for diagnosis and management of hyperthyroidism and other causes of thyrotoxicosis. Thyroid. 2016;26(10):1343–421.
13. Rotermund R, Riedel N, Burkhardt T, Matschke J, Schmidt NO, Aberle J, et al. Surgical treatment and outcome of TSH-producing pituitary adenomas. Acta Neurochirurgica. 2017;159(7):1219–26.
14. Kahaly GJ, Dillmann WH. Thyroid hormone action in the heart. Endocr Rev. 2005;26(5):704–28.
15. Devidi M, Buddam A, Dacha S, Rao DS. Atrial fibrillation and its association with endocrine disorders. J Atr Fibrillation. 2014;6(5):959.
16. Mooradian AD. Asymptomatic hyperthyroidism in older adults. Drugs Aging. 2008;25(5):371–80.
17. Burch HB, Wartofsky L. Life-threatening thyrotoxicosis. Thyroid storm. Endocrinol Metab Clin N Am. 1993;22(2):263–77.
18. Nayak B, Burman K. Thyrotoxicosis and thyroid storm. Endocrinol Metab Clin. 2006;35(4):663–86.
19. Hiromatsu Y, Eguchi H, Tani J, Kasaoka M, Teshima Y. Graves' ophthalmopathy: epidemiology and natural history. Intern Med. 2014;53(5):353–60.
20. Menconi F, Marcocci C, Marinò M. Diagnosis and classification of Graves' disease. Autoimmun Rev. 2014;13(4):398–402.
21. Bahn RS. Graves' ophthalmopathy. N Engl J Med. 2010;362(8):726–38.
22. Koulouri O, Moran C, Halsall D, Chatterjee K, Gurnell M. Pitfalls in the measurement and interpretation of thyroid function tests. Best Pract Res Clin Endocrinol Metab. 2013;27(6):745–62.
23. Barbesino G, Tomer Y. Clinical utility of TSH receptor antibodies. J Clin Endocrinol Metabol. 2013;98(6):2247–55.

24. Samarasinghe S, Meah F, Singh V, Basit A, Emanuele N, Emanuele MA, et al. Biotin interference with routine clinical immunoassays: understand the causes and mitigate the risks. Endocr Pract. 2017;23(8):989–98.
25. Burch HB, Cooper DS. Management of Graves disease: a review. JAMA. 2015;314(23):2544.
26. Cooper DS. Antithyroid drugs. N Engl J Med. 2005;352(9):905–17.
27. Weiss M, Hassin D, Bank H. Propylthiouracil-induced hepatic damage. Arch Intern Med. 1980;140(9):1184–5.
28. Waseem M, Seshadri KG, Kabadi UM. Successful outcome with methimazole and lithium combination therapy for propylthiouracil-induced hepatotoxicity. Endocr Pract. 1998;4(4):197–200.
29. Huang MJ, Liaw Y. Clinical associations between thyroid and liver diseases. J Gastroenterol Hepatol. 1995;10(3):344–50.
30. Cooper DS, Kaplan MM, Ridgway EC, Maloof F, Daniels GH. Alkaline phosphatase isoenzyme patterns in hyperthyroidism. Ann Intern Med. 1979;90(2):164–8.
31. Carella C, Mazziotti G, Sorvillo F, Piscopo M, Cioffi M, Pilla P, et al. Serum thyrotropin receptor antibodies concentrations in patients with Graves' disease before, at the end of methimazole treatment, and after drug withdrawal: evidence that the activity of thyrotropin receptor antibody and/or thyroid response modify during the observation period. Thyroid. 2006;16(3):295–302.
32. Laurberg P, Wallin G, Tallstedt L, Abraham-Nordling M, Lundell G, Tørring O. TSH-receptor autoimmunity in Graves' disease after therapy with anti-thyroid drugs, surgery, or radioiodine: a 5-year prospective randomized study. Eur J Endocrinol. 2008;158(1):69–75.
33. McDermott MT, Kidd GS, Dodson LE, Hofeldt FD. Radioiodine-induced thyroid storm: case report and literature review. Am J Med. 1983;75(2):353–9.
34. Stan MN, Durski JM, Brito JP, Bhagra S, Thapa P, Bahn RS. Cohort study on radioactive iodine–induced hypothyroidism: implications for Graves' ophthalmopathy and optimal timing for thyroid hormone assessment. Thyroid. 2013;23(5):620–5.
35. Ponto KA, Zang S, Kahaly GJ. The tale of radioiodine and Graves' orbitopathy. Thyroid. 2010;20(7):785–93.
36. Eckstein AK, Plicht M, Lax H, Neuhäuser M, Mann K, Lederbogen S, et al. Thyrotropin receptor autoantibodies are independent risk factors for Graves' ophthalmopathy and help to predict severity and outcome of the disease. J Clin Endocrinol Metabol. 2006;91(9):3464–70.
37. Stan MN, Garrity JA, Bahn RS. The evaluation and treatment of graves ophthalmopathy. Med Clin N Am. 2012;96(2):311–28.
38. Lai A, Sassi L, Compri E, Marino F, Sivelli P, Piantanida E, et al. Lower dose prednisone prevents radioiodine-associated exacerbation of initially mild or absent Graves' orbitopathy: a retrospective cohort study. J Clin Endocrinol Metabol. 2010;95(3):1333–7.
39. Stoll SJ, Pitt SC, Liu J, Schaefer S, Sippel RS, Chen H. Thyroid hormone replacement after thyroid lobectomy. Surgery. 2009;146(4):554–60.
40. Kaykhaei MA, Shams M, Sadegholvad A, Dabbaghmanesh MH, Omrani GR. Low doses of cholestyramine in the treatment of hyperthyroidism. Endocrine. 2008;34(1–3):52–5.
41. Muller C, Perrin P, Faller B, Richter S, Chantrel F. Role of plasma exchange in the thyroid storm. Ther Apher Dial. 2011;15(6):522–31.
42. Houghton SG, Farley DR, Brennan MD, van Heerden JA, Thompson GB, Grant CS. Surgical management of amiodarone-associated thyrotoxicosis: Mayo Clinic experience. World J Surg. 2004;28(11):1083–7.

Chapter 4
Thyroid Function and Pregnancy

Nathan King and Lia A. Bernardi

> **Clinical Case**
> A 27-year-old female, gravida 1 and para 0, at 10 weeks' gestational age presents with persistent nausea and vomiting for 2 days. She has been experiencing intermittent nausea and vomiting for several weeks but recently has been unable to keep solid food or water down. On exam, she appears dehydrated with dry lips and skin and has ongoing emesis. Otherwise, her exam is unremarkable, with normal vital signs, no palpable goiter, and no ophthalmopathy. Her labs are notable for slight hypokalemia of 3.4 mEq as well as a urinalysis with greater than 80 ketones and a specific gravity of 1.032. She is admitted for intravenous hydration and parenteral antiemetic therapy. Further testing reveals a TSH of 0.04 mIU/L, FT4 index of 13.0 mcg/dL, and a serum HCG of 450,000 mIU/mL. What is the most likely diagnosis? Is antithyroid therapy indicated in this case?

N. King
Northwestern University, Feinberg School of Medicine, Department of Obstetrics and Gynecology, Chicago, IL, USA

L. A. Bernardi (✉)
Northwestern University, Feinberg School of Medicine, Division of Reproductive Endocrinology and Infertility, Department of Obstetrics and Gynecology, Chicago, IL, USA
e-mail: lia.bernardi@northwestern.edu

© Springer Nature Switzerland AG 2019
J. L. Eaton (ed.), *Thyroid Disease and Reproduction*,
https://doi.org/10.1007/978-3-319-99079-8_4

Physiologic Changes of the Thyroid Gland During Pregnancy

Iodine Requirement During Pregnancy

During pregnancy, increased vascularity occurs within the thyroid gland, and a subsequent increase in thyroid size ensues [1]. On average, compared to prepregnancy, the thyroid gland volume increases by 30% [2]. This increase in volume is accompanied by a nearly 50% increase in the production of the active thyroid hormones, thyroxine (T4), and triiodothyronine (T3), resulting in a 50% increase in the iodine requirement [3]. Concurrently, iodine clearance increases along with the increased glomerular filtration rate of pregnancy. Additionally, as discussed in Chap. 5, iodide and iodothyronines are shunted to the fetal-placental unit. These physiologic changes result in increased susceptibility to iodine deficiency and its consequences [4]. For this reason, the World Health Organization (WHO) recommends 250ug per day of iodine intake in the preconception and pregnant state [5]. In comparison, the WHO recommends 150ug per day for nonpregnant adults and adolescents [6]. In the United States, women can typically achieve the recommended intake with 150ug of supplemental iodine [3, 7]. In countries where iodine repletion is not standard, pregnant women must be monitored closely for thyroid dysfunction as they are at a greatly elevated risk of goiter development as a consequence of iodine deficiency [4].

hCG and Its Impact on the Hypothalamic-Pituitary-Thyroid (HPT) Axis

There are several physiologic explanations for the changes in thyroid gland function that occur during pregnancy. Human chorionic gonadotropin (hCG) rises exponentially throughout the first trimester and then remains present throughout pregnancy at varying levels. Molecular homology between hCG and thyroid-stimulating hormone (TSH) allows for significant cross-reactivity at the level of their respective receptors [8, 9]. hCG has approximately 1/4000th the thyrotropic activity of TSH itself [8, 9]. Thus, in the presence of high hCG levels, which peak around 10 weeks' gestation, thyroid gland activity is significantly increased.

In circumstances where hCG levels greatly exceed those found during a normal gestation, such as in trophoblastic disease, multiple gestations, or the presence of hCG-secreting tumors, hCG alone may be enough to cause clinical hyperthyroidism [10]. This phenomenon is termed as gestational transient thyrotoxicosis (GTT), and as expected, its peak incidence occurs around 10–12 weeks' gestation, at the time of the hCG peak described earlier [11]. In contrast to other etiologies of clinical hyperthyroidism, most notably Graves' disease, GTT does not present with the characteristic symptoms of thyrotoxicosis such as goiter, ophthalmopathy, tachycardia, and tremor [11]. It does, however, commonly cause hyperemesis gravidarum, with persistent nausea and vomiting that is atypical of alternative etiologies of hyperthyroidism [12]. Additionally, it is accompanied by modest elevations in free T4 concentration, and T3 levels may be normal, while those with Graves' disease typically have more pronounced elevations in both free T4 and T3. Ultimately, given the progressive drop in hCG levels, GTT usually resolves by 14–16 weeks' gestation and typically requires no treatment [11, 12]. When symptoms do not resolve, alternative diagnoses must be considered.

Another less well-known thyroid-stimulating hormone specific to pregnancy is human chorionic thyrotropin (HCT). Also produced by the placenta, this hormone has direct stimulating effects on the TSH receptors of the maternal thyroid. It is also believed to cause an increase in thyroid gland function, though its physiologic role is less defined than hCG [8, 9].

Despite the relationship between hCG and thyroid function, healthy women generally remain euthyroid throughout gestation due to compensatory mechanisms. The most important of these is the downregulation of the hypothalamic-pituitary-thyroid (HPT) axis. Given the cross-reactivity of the described thyrotropic molecules produced by the placenta, TSH production is simultaneously downregulated at the level of the pituitary. This creates an inverse relationship between hCG and TSH throughout pregnancy. As hCG plateaus in the second and third trimesters, TSH trends back toward, but does not quite reach, nonpregnant values (Fig. 4.1) [13, 14].

This becomes important as the ranges of normal TSH during pregnancy differ not only from those in the non-gravid state, but also by trimester [11, 12]. The 2017 guidelines of the American Thyroid Association highlight this complex relationship [3]. Variations in TSH levels during pregnancy are evident when comparisons are made between different ethnic and racial groups, those with multiple gestations, and women of various body mass indexes (BMI) [3]. Thus, it is recommended that when possible, reference ranges for each trimester should be made by assessment of local population-based data from individuals with adequate iodine intake who do not have a history of thyroid disease or measurable anti-TPO antibodies. When this assessment is unfeasible or data are unavailable, the ATA provides approximate expected changes in TSH. In the late first trimester, between 7 and 12 weeks' gestation, the lower reference range value of TSH can decrease by as much as 0.4 mU/L,

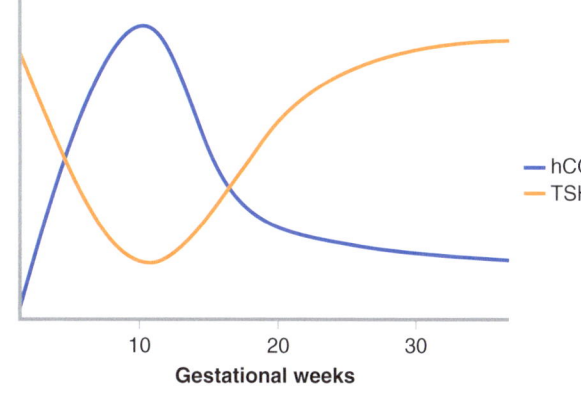

Fig. 4.1 Changes in hCG and TSH levels during pregnancy [13, 14]. (Adapted with permission of Wolters Kluwer from Speroff and Fritz [30])

which includes some normal pregnancies with undetectable TSH [3]. The upper reference range is expected to decrease by approximately 0.5 mU/L during this same period, yielding an upper limit of approximately 4.0 mU/L [3]. There are no specific suggestions for the 2nd or 3rd trimester other than that a gradual trend toward the normal, nonpregnant reference ranges that should be expected.

Regulation of Thyroid Hormone Levels by Thyroxine-Binding Globulin (TBG)

An increase in serum levels of thyroxine-binding globulin (TBG) is another important mechanism that is responsible for the changes in the function of the thyroid gland during pregnancy. TBG is the major transporter, along with transthyretin and serum albumin, of T4 and T3 in the bloodstream. It regulates the amount of active, or free, T4 and T3, given that any thyroid hormone bound to TBG is unable to bind to its receptor. Consequently, a greater amount of TBG present in serum equates to a greater binding capacity for T3 and T4 and thus a decrease in circulating free T3 and T4 (Fig. 4.2) [13, 15]. The rise in TBG, however, is unrelated to hCG levels or thyroid function itself. Instead, the increase in TBG results from the increasing estrogen levels during pregnancy. Estrogen stimulates the synthetic function of the liver, thereby causing increased production of TBG. Estrogen also stimulates increased glycosylation of TBG, leading to

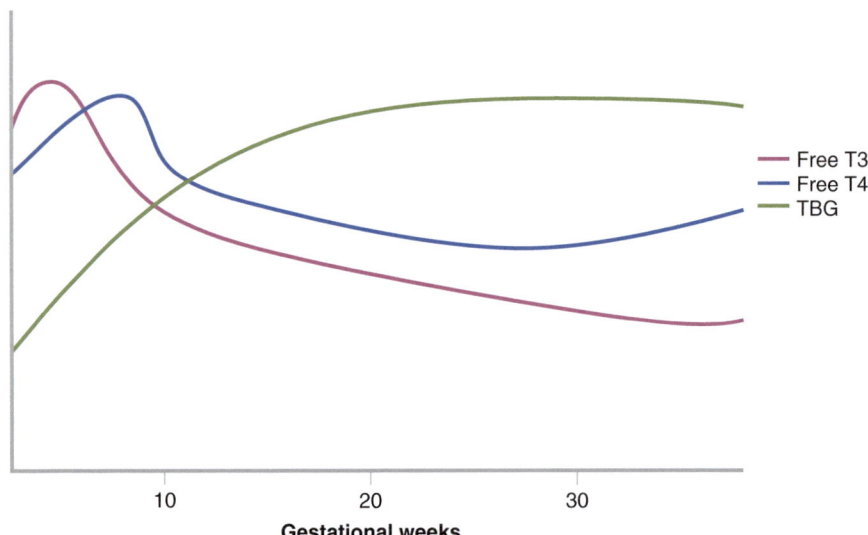

Fig. 4.2 Changes in free T4, free T3, and TBG throughout pregnancy [13, 15]. (Adapted with permission of Wolters Kluwer from Speroff and Fritz [30])

decreased clearance of TBG from the circulation. Levels of TBG plateau at the end of the first trimester remain consistently elevated throughout the remainder of pregnancy (Fig. 4.2) [13, 15].

Changes in Free T4 Levels Measured by Immunometric Assays

The changes in TBG and other serum proteins during pregnancy have implications for the common laboratory assays used to measure thyroxine levels. The most clinically important thyroxine level is free T4 (FT4). This is because FT4 is the biologically active form of thyroxine, which is responsible for the downstream effects of thyroid hormone and the manifestations of aberrant thyroid function. However, FT4 only accounts for approximately 0.03% of total T4 (TT4) levels [3]. Thus, testing for only FT4 is challenging in the presence of much higher levels of bound T4, and gold-standard testing with ultrafiltration involves numerous time-consuming and expensive tests. As a result, the most commonly used test nationwide is an indirect analog immunoassay, which is quicker and more feasible but relies on equilibrium standards determined in nonpregnant individuals. Consequently, this testing is prone to error in the face of altered equilibriums, which are seen in pregnancy owing to the drastic changes in maternal serum TBG, as well as other protein and fatty acid concentrations. While this problem may be addressed by setting pregnancy and trimester-specific reference ranges for each laboratory's own unique immunoassay test, this approach is impractical [3].

Conversely, the accuracy of measurements of TT4 and the subsequent FT4 index have not been found to be affected by these same physiological changes in maternal serum. Thus, both these measurements have been suggested by the ATA as reliable means for measuring thyroid hormone during pregnancy [3].

TT4 is known to increase throughout pregnancy from 7 to 16 gestational weeks, and changes are highly predictable. At 16 weeks' gestation, the TT4 level is expected to be 50% higher than the nonpregnant level, and this increase is maintained throughout the remainder of pregnancy. Therefore, the reference range for TT4 after 16 weeks' gestation can be appropriately adjusted with the same 50% increase. If measuring TT4 levels between 7 and 16 weeks, however, the ATA recommends adjusting the reference range based on an expected 5% increase in the TT4 level per gestational week completed after week 7 (i.e., 5% higher at week 8, 10% higher at week 9, etc.) [3].

The FT4 index is an indirect measurement of FT4 calculated by the quotient of TT4 and the thyroid-binding index (TBI). The TBI is a separate test of the thyroxine-binding capacity, calculated through a thyroxine-uptake assay, and thus accounts for any changes in the concentrations of TBG and other thyroxine-binding protein, as known to occur in maternal serum. Thus, calculation of the FT4 index accounts for both the changes in maternal proteins and as maternal TT4 levels and is suggested by the ATA to be preferred to the measurement of FT4 by immunologic assay during pregnancy [3].

Summary

In conclusion, the complex balance achieved by the various physiologic changes experienced during pregnancy results in a euthyroid state for mothers with normally functioning thyroid glands. In women with thyroid dysfunction, however, the impact of pregnancy on thyroid function can worsen their underlying disease. Overt hypothyroidism or hyperthyroidism during pregnancy is pathologic and should be evaluated and treated accordingly with special attention to maternal and fetal well-being, as detailed in Chaps. 6 and 7.

Maternal Thyroid Function and Fetal Development

The normal changes in thyroid function in the gravid state are important for many aspects of fetal development, especially in the first trimester [11, 16]. Most notably, the fetal brain, which begins forming at around 4 weeks' gestation, requires thyroid hormone for normal development [17]. Specifically, thyroid hormone has been found to play a role in synaptogenesis, creation of dendrites and axons, myelination, and neuronal migration [18]. The development of the fetal pituitary-thyroid system, however, is not complete until 12–14 weeks' gestation [19, 20]. Until then, fetal development relies on the transfer of maternal T4 for proper development [16, 20]. The maternal-fetal transfer of thyroid hormone is described in detail in Chap. 5.

Screening for Maternal Thyroid Dysfunction

Routine screening for maternal thyroid dysfunction in the preconception period or during pregnancy remains controversial. Overt thyroid dysfunction, which encompasses clinical hyperthyroidism and hypothyroidism, is rare in pregnant women. Clinical hyperthyroidism, defined as a TSH below the normal range and a free T4 above the normal range, affects approximately 0.2% of pregnancies [21]. Clinical hypothyroidism, defined as a TSH that is above the normal range and a free T4 that is below the normal range, is slightly more prevalent, occurring in up to 1% of pregnancies [22]. Both of these clinical entities cause a wide range of symptoms in affected patients, and these symptoms should prompt testing if noted either in the preconception period or during pregnancy. Treatment of overt thyroid dysfunction is highly recommended for women who are pregnant or considering pregnancy. The adverse outcomes associated with both clinical hyperthyroidism and hypothyroidism have been well studied and are described in Chaps. 6 and 7. Identifying affected patients, therefore, is of utmost importance [23].

On the other hand, universal screening of all pregnant women, regardless of symptoms, would yield a substantial increase in the diagnosis of subclinical thyroid dysfunction. In order for a screening test to be recommended, it must not only be able to identify a majority of patients with a specific ailment, but also allow for a clinically beneficial intervention to be enacted. Several studies have shown that subclinical hyperthyroidism is not associated with adverse obstetrical and neonatal complications [22, 24, 25]. Thus, although screening may identify patients with subclinical disease, no treatment is warranted in these individuals. Subclinical hypothyroidism, however, is much more nuanced and controversial, as discussed in Chaps. 6, 9, and 10. Existing literature supports an association between subclinical hypothyroidism and adverse perinatal outcomes, such as preeclampsia, preterm birth, abruption placentae, and gestational diabetes; however, evidence for a treatment benefit are sparse [24, 25].

Given the conflicting data, universal thyroid screening remains a topic of controversy. Table 4.1 summarizes the recommendations for screening of asymptomatic patients during pregnancy and in the preconception period. The American Congress of Obstetricians and Gynecologists (ACOG) and the American Association of Clinical Endocrinologists (AACE) recommend against universal screening for thyroid disease in pregnancy, anchoring on the lack of benefit found from treating subclinical disease [26, 27]. The American Association of Clinical Endocrinologists does recommend "aggressive case finding," though not universal screening, in women who are planning pregnancy [28]. The American Thyroid Association and the Endocrine Society make no clear recommendation for or against universal screening, citing insufficient evidence [3, 29]. The Endocrine Society recommends against universal preconception screening for thyroid disease, given that no clear benefit has been proven from detection or treatment of subclinical hypothyroidism prior to pregnancy [29]. However, it does specify numerous patient characteristics that confer a higher risk of thyroid dysfunction and warrant prepregnancy screening. These characteristics, which encompass a large portion of reproductive-aged women, include the following: age greater than 30, morbid obesity (BMI greater

Table 4.1 Consensus of professional medical organizations on universal screening for thyroid dysfunction during pregnancy and preconception

	ACOG [26]	The Endocrine Society [29]	ATA [3]	AACE [27]
Universal screening in pregnancy	Not recommended	No consensus	No recommendation, insufficient evidence	Not recommended
Universal preconception screening	Not addressed	Not recommended	No recommendation, insufficient evidence	"Aggressive case finding" but not universal screening

Data from References: [3, 26, 27, 29]
ACOG The American College of Obstetricians and Gynecologists, *ATA* American Thyroid Association, *AACE* American Association of Clinical Endocrinologists

than or equal to 40), family history of thyroid dysfunction, presence of a goiter, thyroid antibody positivity, symptoms or clinical signs of thyroid hypofunction, history of type 1 diabetes or other autoimmune disease, infertility, personal history of miscarriage or preterm delivery, and those with history of head or neck irradiation. The American Thyroid Association cites insufficient evidence to make a recommendation for or against universal preconception screening but does advocate for screening in patients utilizing assisted-reproductive therapies or those with a history of positive anti-TPO antibodies [3]. Similar to the Endocrine Society, the ATA also recommends screening for patients at higher risk of having thyroid dysfunction, which includes all of the characteristics previously listed.

Overall, although screening asymptomatic pregnant women is not harmful, it may not be cost-effective, and clear evidence that proves definitive benefit and strongly supports universal screening is lacking. Testing patients defined at higher risk for thyroid disease, however, is more strongly supported by the literature. All of the aforementioned organizational bodies strongly recommend screening women with any symptoms that may be attributable to thyroid dysfunction [3, 26, 27, 29]. Recommendations are likely to continuing adapting as future clinical studies aim to further address these questions.

Clinical Case and Discussion

A 27-year-old female, gravida 1 para 0, at 10 weeks' gestational age presents with persistent nausea and vomiting for 2 days. She has been experiencing intermittent nausea for several weeks but recently has been unable to keep solid food or water down. On exam, she appears dehydrated with dry lips and skin and has ongoing emesis. Otherwise, her exam is unremarkable, with normal vital signs, no palpable goiter, and no ophthalmopathy. Her labs are notable for slight hypokalemia of 3.4 mEq as well as a urinalysis with greater than 80 ketones and a specific gravity of 1.032. She is admitted for intravenous hydration and parenteral antiemetic therapy. Further testing reveals a TSH of 0.04 mIU/L, FT4 index of 13.0 mcg/dL, and a serum HCG of 450,000mIU/mL. What is the most likely diagnosis? Is antithyroid therapy indicated in this case?

The patient's symptoms are indicative of hyperemesis gravidarum, which is associated with gestational transient thyrotoxicosis (GTT). She has no objective or subjective signs associated with hyperthyroidism of other etiologies, such as tachycardia, ophthalmopathy, or goiter. Her TSH is low, but within normal limits for the first trimester, and she does not have anti-TPO antibodies. Her high hCG also lends toward this diagnosis, given its affinity for TSH receptors as described in the chapter. Antithyroid therapy is not indicated in this case. Aside from patients with extreme variants of GTT that result in severe thyrotoxicosis or thyroid storm, patients should not be treated with antithyroid drugs as the condition is self-limited and not associated with adverse maternal and fetal outcomes. The patient should expect her condition to improve at around 14–16-week gestational age, secondary to a decline in hCG.

References

1. Glinoer D. The regulation of thyroid function in pregnancy: pathways of endocrine adaptation from physiology to pathology. Endocr Rev. 1997;18:404–33.
2. Fister P, Gaberscek S, Zaletel K, Krhin B, Gersak K, Hojker S. Thyroid volume changes during pregnancy and after delivery in an iodine-sufficient Republic of Slovenia. Eur J Obstet Gynecol Reprod Biol. 2009;145:45–8.
3. Alexander E, Pearce E, Brent G, Brown R, Chen H, Dosiou C, Grobman W, Laurberg P, Lazarus J, Mandel S, Peeters R, Sullivan S. 2017 guidelines of the American Thyroid Association for the diagnosis and management of thyroid disease during pregnancy and the postpartum. Thyroid. 2017;27:315–93.
4. Smyth PP, Hetherton AMT, Smith DF, Radcliff M, O'Herlihy C. Maternal iodine status and thyroid volume during pregnancy: correlation with neonatal iodine intake. J Clin Endocrinol Metab. 1997;82:2840–3.
5. WHO Secretariat, Andersson M, de Benoist B, Delange F, Zupan J. Prevention and control of iodine deficiency in pregnant and lactating women and in children less than 2-years-old: conclusions and recommendations of the technical consultation. Public Health Nutr. 2007;10(12A):1606–11.
6. World Health Organization. United Nations Children's Fund & International Council for the Control of Iodine Deficiency Disorders. Assessment of iodine deficiency disorders and monitoring their elimination. 3rd ed. Geneva: WHO; 2007.
7. Berghout A, Wiersinga W. Thyroid size and thyroid function during pregnancy: an analysis. Eur J Endocrinol. 1998;138:536–42.
8. Kennedy R, Darne J. The role of hCG in regulation of the thyroid gland in normal and abnormal pregnancy. Obstet Gynecol. 1991;78:298–307.
9. Ballabio M, Poshyachinda M, Ekins RP. Pregnancy-induced changes in thyroid function: role of human chorionic gonadotropin as putative regulator of maternal thyroid. J Clin Endocrinol Metab. 1991;73:824–31.
10. Kimura M, Amino N, Tamaki H, Ito E, Mitsuda N, Miyai K, Tanizawa O. Gestational thyrotoxicosis and hyperemesis gravidarum: possible role of hCG with higher stimulating activity. Clin Endocrinol. 1993;38:345–50.
11. Goldman AM, Mestman JH. Transient non-autoimmune hyperthyroidism of early pregnancy. J Thyroid Res. 2011;2011:1424–13.
12. Goodwin TM, Montoro M, Mestman JH. Transient hyperthyroidism and hyperemesis gravidarum: clinical aspects. Am J Obstet Gynecol. 1992;167:648.
13. Glinoer D, DeNayer P, Bourdoux P, Lemone M, Robyn C, Van Steirteghem A, Kinthaert J, Lejeune B. Regulation of maternal thyroid during pregnancy. J Clin Endocrinol Metab. 1990;71:276–87.
14. Dashe JS, Casey BM, Wells CE, McIntire DD, Byrd EW, Leveno KJ, Cunningham FG. Thyroid-stimulating hormone in singleton and twin pregnancy: importance of gestational age-specific ranges. Obstet Gynecol. 2006;106:753–7.
15. Berghout A, Ended E, Ross A, Hogerzeil HV, Smits NJ, Wiersinga WM. Thyroid function and thyroid size in normal pregnant women living in an iodine replete area. Clin Endocrinol. 1994;41:375–9.
16. Kimura M, Amino N, Tamaki H, Mitsuda N, Miyai K, Tanizawa O. Physiologic thyroid activation in normal early pregnancy is induced by circulating hCG. Obstet Gynecol. 1990;75:775–8.
17. Calvo RM, Jauniaux E, Gulbis B, Asuncion M, Gervy C, Contempre B, Morreale de Escobar G. Fetal tissues are exposed to biologically relevant free thyroxine concentrations during early phases of development. J Clin Endocrinol Metab. 2002;87:1768–77.
18. Bernal J. Thyroid hormone receptors in brain development and function. Nat Clin Pract Endocrinol Metab. 2007;3:249–59.
19. Thorpe-Beeston J, Nicolaides K, McGregor A. Fetal thyroid function. Thyroid. 1992;2:207.
20. Burrow GN, Fisher DA, Larsen PR. Maternal and fetal thyroid function. N Engl J Med. 1994;331:1072–8.

21. Ecker JL, Musci TJ. Thyroid function and disease in pregnancy. Curr Probl Obstet Gynecol Fertil. 2000;23:109–22.
22. Casey BM, Leveno KJ. Thyroid disease in pregnancy. Obstet Gynecol. 2006;108:1283–92.
23. Abalovich M, Gutierrez S, Alcaraz G, Maccallini G, Garcia A, Levalle O. Overt and subclinical hypothyroidism complicating pregnancy. Thyroid. 2002;12:63–8.
24. Tudela CM, Casey BM, McIntire DD, Cunningham FG. Relationship of subclinical thyroid disease to the incidence of gestational diabetes. Obstet Gynecol. 2012;119:983–8.
25. Wilson KL, Casey BM, McIntire DD, Halvorson LM, Cunningham FG. Subclinical thyroid disease and the incidence of hypertension in pregnancy. Obstet Gynecol. 2012;119:315–20.
26. Practice Bulletin of the American College of Obstetricians and Gynecologists. Thyroid disease in pregnancy. Number 148, 2015.
27. Garber J, Cobin R, Gharib H, Hennessey J, Klein I, Mechanick J, Pessah-Pollack R, Singer PA, Woeber KA. Clinical practice guidelines for hypothyroidism in adults: cosponsored by the American Association of Clinical Endocrinologists and the American Thyroid Association. Endocr Pract. 2012;18:988–102.
28. Stagnaro-Green A, Abalovich M, Alexander E, Azizi F, Mestman J, Negro R, Nixon A, Pearce EN, Soldin OP, Sullivan S, Wiersinga W. 2011 guidelines of the American Thyroid Association for the diagnosis and management of thyroid disease during pregnancy and postpartum. Thyroid. 2011;21:1081–125.
29. De Groot L, Abalovich M, Alexander E, Amino N, Barbour L, Cobin R, Eastman CJ, Lazarus JH, Luton D, Mandel SJ, Mestman J, Rovet J, Sullivan S. Management of thyroid dysfunction during pregnancy and postpartum: an Endocrine Society clinical practice guideline. J Clin Endocrinol Metab. 2012;97:2543–65.
30. Speroff L, Fritz MA. Clinical gynecologic endocrinology and infertility. 8th ed. Philadelphia: Lippincott Williams & Wilkins; 2010.

Chapter 5
Fetal and Neonatal Thyroid Physiology

Laura C. Page and Robert W. Benjamin

Clinical Case
A 7-day-old male infant is referred to the pediatric endocrine clinic after his newborn screen returns positive for congenital hypothyroidism. He was born at term by spontaneous vaginal delivery, with a birth weight of 3.4 kg, and has been vigorous with breastfeeding. His newborn screen, drawn at 36 h of life, reveals TSH >100 mIU/L and T4 4.2 mcg/dL.

The infant is alert and interactive with no dysmorphic features. No goiter is appreciated. Serum thyroid studies confirm primary hypothyroidism, with TSH 245 mIU/L, T4 3.6 mcg/dL, and fT4 0.58 ng/dL. Thyroid scintigraphy using iodine-123 (I^{123}) reveals no uptake of I^{123} by thyroid tissue. A thyroid ultrasound shows a thyroid gland in the normal location. What is the most likely explanation for this infant's findings? What is the expected course?

Introduction

Thyroid hormone is vital to fetal and neonatal neurodevelopment. The thyroid gland is the first endocrine organ to develop, but the fetus requires thyroid hormone before the gland is able to produce it. Thus, the fetus relies on maternal thyroid hormone until approximately 16 weeks gestation. Maternal thyroid dysfunction can have profound effects on the fetus and neonate, ranging from lower IQ and impaired psychomotor development to increased mortality [1–4].

L. C. Page (✉) · R. W. Benjamin
Duke University Medical Center, Department of Pediatrics, Durham, NC, USA
e-mail: laura.page@duke.edu

In this chapter, we explore thyroid embryology and fetal thyroid physiology, highlighting contributions of the mother and placenta to the fetus and neonate. We then describe neonatal thyroid physiology and pathophysiology, including a discussion of neonatal thyroid disorders.

Given the critical role of thyroid hormone in neurodevelopment, fetal and neonatal thyroid physiology is an area of active research and continued advancement. Newborn screening has allowed for early detection and treatment of congenital hypothyroidism, thereby preventing morbidity in numerous infants [5]. Additionally, new genetic approaches have enhanced our understanding of many neonatal thyroid disorders [6–8]. Despite these accomplishments, certain topics remain elusive. Controversies, such as using levothyroxine to treat mild, transient perturbations in thyroid levels of premature infants, require further investigation [9].

Embryology

The main anlage of the thyroid gland, formed by the thickening and then outpouching of the foregut endoderm at the base of the future tongue, becomes apparent just after 3 weeks gestation [10, 11] (Table 5.1). Downward growth brings the anlage close to the developing heart, which it then follows caudally toward the anterior neck [12]. As the anlage descends, the thyroglossal duct serves as a remnant connection to the pharyngeal floor. The duct then involutes by 6 weeks gestation, leaving behind the foramen cecum, which is a small dimple in the posterior third of the tongue [10].

The main anlage reaches its final position by approximately 8 weeks gestation [10]. As it grows, the anlage begins to fuse with two lateral ultimobranchial bodies, which allows the gland to assume its bilobate shape [11]. It is generally accepted that the ultimobranchial bodies contain C-cell progenitors, while the main anlage gives rise to the follicular cells [11]. However, evaluation of individuals with aberrant thyroid migration, such as lingual thyroid, suggests these roles may be somewhat fluid [13, 14]. Thyroid follicles appear around 10 weeks gestation and contain colloid by 11–12 weeks [10, 12].

Table 5.1 Thyroid gland morphogenesis

	Approximate gestational age
Main anlage appears	21 days
Main anlage descent into the neck begins	24 days
Thyroglossal duct dissolution	35 days
Main anlage descent complete	50 days
Main anlage fuses with UB bodies	60 days
Folliculogenesis	70 days
Colloid present	80 days

UB ultimobranchial bodies

Although TSH is commonly recognized as a major controller of the thyroid gland and thyroid hormone production, thyroid gland organogenesis occurs independently of TSH [15]. As noted later in this chapter, TSH is not detected until approximately 14 weeks gestation, which is well after the gland has formed and started to synthesize thyroid hormone. Instead, morphogenesis requires the expression of four transcription factors: Nkx2–1, Pax8, Foxe1, and Hhex [11, 10]. While the individual transcription factors drive differentiation of other tissues, the unified action of all four appears to be unique to thyroid gland development [11].

Fetal Thyroid Physiology

Maternal-Fetal Interaction

Maternal TSH and TRH have little effect on fetal thyroid function, as the placenta is essentially impermeable to TSH, and while TRH can cross to the fetus, it is at such low physiologic concentrations that its impact is insignificant [16, 17]. However, maternal T4 crosses the placenta and serves as the fetus' sole source for thyroid hormone early in gestation (Fig. 5.1). The transfer of maternal T4 occurs via placental thyroid hormone transporters, including monocarboxylate transporters (MCTs), L-type amino acid transporters (LATs), and organic anion transporters (OATPs). These transporters have varying levels of expression in the placental cell layers and, in some cases, competitively bind other ligands as well [18]. The purpose of the transporters' ostensible redundancy, apart from protecting fetal thyroid hormone supply, is not well understood.

Despite the high expression of thyroid hormone transporters in the placenta, the amount of maternal thyroid hormone that reaches the fetus is relatively low. Maternal thyroid hormone passage to the fetus is highly regulated by placental iodothyronine deiodinases, which are enzymes that remove an iodine moiety from thyroid hormone. Placental deiodinase type 2 (D2) and deiodinase type 3 (D3) convert T4 to T3 and reverse T3 (rT3), respectively [19]. Notably, the activity of D3 in the placenta is approximately 200 times greater than D2, making it an important barrier to prevent fetal overexposure to maternal thyroid hormone [19]. Meanwhile, placental production of thyroid binding proteins transthyretin (TTR) and albumin partly offsets this effect by shuttling maternal T4 between transporters and protecting it from D3 [20].

Although maternal thyroid hormone contribution to the fetus is generally thought to be negligible by 16 weeks gestation, it continues to serve an important role for fetuses with thyroid agenesis and thyroid hormone synthesis defects. At birth, T4 levels in infants with total organification defects are approximately one third to one half those of normal neonates [21]. These levels decline to undetectable by about 2 weeks of life [21]. Placental D3 activity is normal in severely hypothyroid newborns [19], implying a different mechanism is responsible for the increased maternal contribution.

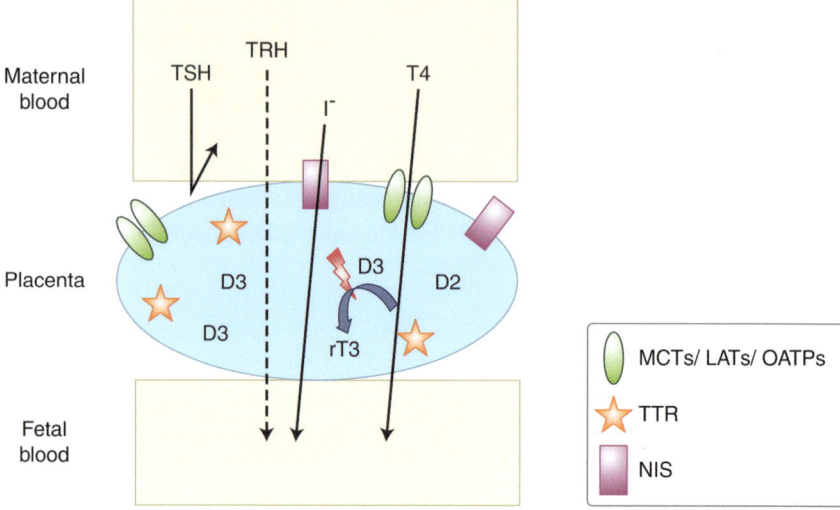

Fig. 5.1 Schematic depicting maternal thyroid hormone transfer early in gestation. The placenta is impermeable to maternal TSH. Maternal TRH can traverse the placenta, but its effect is negligible due to low concentrations. Maternal T4 crosses the placenta through placental thyroid hormone transporters including MCTs, LATs, and OATPs. Once in the placenta, T4 may be converted to rT3 by D3 or may be carried to the fetal blood by placental TTR. The placenta additionally allows passage of maternal iodide through the NIS. D2 deiodinase type 2, D3 deiodinase type 3, I⁻ iodide, NIS sodium iodide symporter, T4 thyroxine, rT3 reverse T3, TTR transthyretin, MCTs monocarboxylate transporters, LATs L-type amino acid transporters, OATPs organic anion transporters

In addition to transporting maternal T4, the placenta promotes transfer of maternal iodide to the fetus through the sodium iodide symporter (NIS) [22]. Placental NIS, along with the iodothyronine deiodinases, provides the iodide needed for the fetal thyroid gland to synthesize thyroid hormone. Thus, maternal iodine status is critical to normal fetal thyroid function, and efforts have targeted maternal iodine repletion as a strategy to reduce congenital hypothyroidism [3, 23].

Development of Fetal Thyroid Function

The fetal thyroid gland is able to concentrate iodide by approximately 11 weeks gestation and begins to synthesize thyroid hormone at approximately 12 weeks gestation [24] (Fig. 5.2). Interestingly, this initial thyroid hormone production is independent of the pituitary input, as fetal TSH does not appear until about 12 weeks gestation [24]. In fact, the first detectable hypothalamic-pituitary-thyroid (HPT) axis hormone is TRH. Production in the fetal hypothalamus occurs around 8 weeks gestation, but secretion by the fetal gut and pancreas as well as the placenta begins even earlier [25–28]. Unlike T4, T3, and TSH, which are relatively low during the

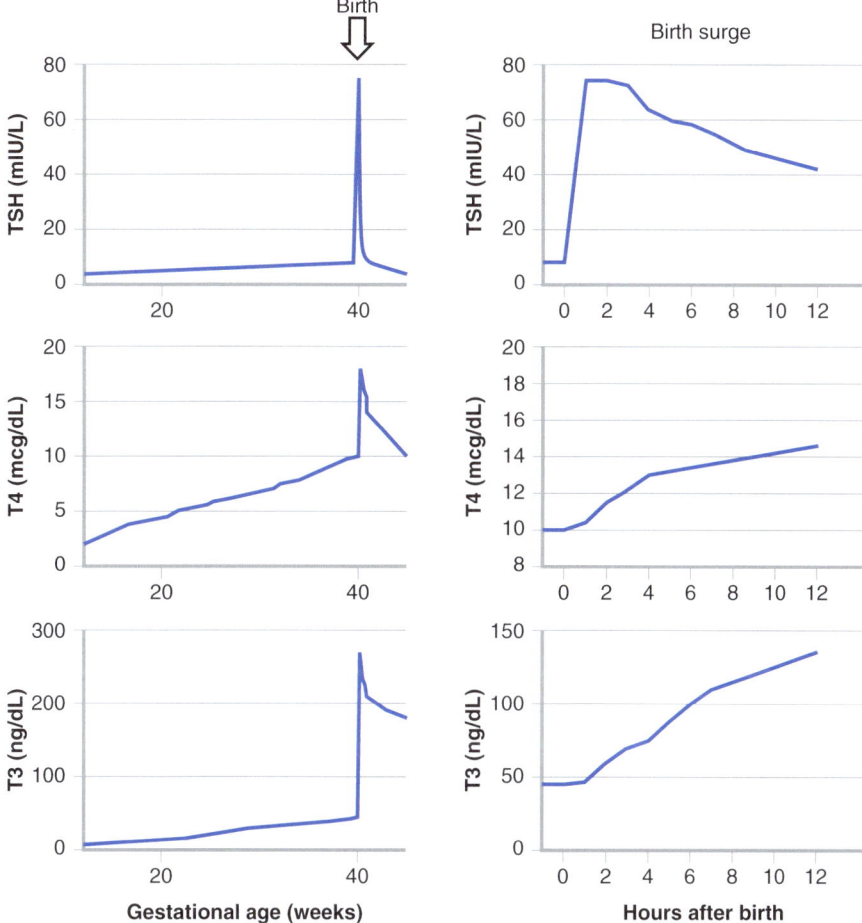

Fig. 5.2 Changes in fetal TSH and thyroid hormone concentrations during gestation and immediately after birth. Fetal TSH, T4, and T3 production begin around 12 weeks gestation. Initially, levels of each of these hormones are low, but TSH and T4 rise over time, surpassing normal adult levels. T3 stays low throughout gestation due to high levels of D3. Exposure to the cold environment after birth stimulates a rapid surge in TSH, which is soon followed by a rise in T4 and T3 levels. TSH levels fall and normalize over the first week of life, while T4 and T3 levels remain elevated until approximately 4 weeks of life. This figure is meant to serve as a stylized depiction of the changes in fetal and neonatal TSH, T4, and T3 levels over time

first half of gestation, fetal TRH is elevated compared to maternal levels. In addition to the extrahypothalamic contributions, the elevated levels reflect decreased TRH degradation in fetal serum [29].

TSH concentrations rise steadily from a mean of approximately 4 mU/L at 12 weeks gestation to 8 mU/L at 40 weeks [30] (Fig. 5.2). Fetal TSH levels are elevated compared to maternal levels from approximately 26 weeks gestation onwards [24]. Fetal T4 levels rise under the influence of TSH as well as increasing levels of thyroxine-binding globulin (TBG), which is made by the liver [24]. Mean total T4 levels are approximately 2 mcg/dL at 12 weeks and 10 mcg/dL at 40 weeks, while free T4 levels increase from 0.1 ng/dL at 12 weeks to 2 ng/dL at 40 weeks [24, 30, 31]. By 36 weeks gestation, fetal T4, fT4, and TBG have reached mean adult levels [24].

Although T3 levels also rise with increasing gestational age, they remain low overall, even late in gestation [24, 30]. Mean T3 increases from 6 ng/dL at 12 weeks to 45 ng/dL at 40 weeks, well below the mean for nonpregnant adults, which is 136 ng/dL [24, 31]. T3 promotes thermogenesis and catabolism processes detrimental to a developing fetus; therefore, its levels are tightly regulated. T3 suppression is accomplished through high levels of D3 along with low expression of deiodinase type 1 (D1) [28, 32]. D1 converts T4 to T3 primarily in the liver, kidney, and thyroid; thus, decreased levels complement the elevated levels of D3. Because D1 additionally inactivates sulfated conjugates of T4, fetal levels of sulfated iodothyronines are elevated [33]. Notably, certain areas, such as the fetal cerebral cortex, have higher T3 concentrations [34]. The reasons behind these differences are discussed later in this chapter.

The HPT axis continues to develop throughout gestation. During the second and third trimesters, TSH stimulates T4 production and thyroid gland growth as expected, but its levels are elevated overall [24]. This higher TSH set point may be consistent with the immature HPT axis. Similarly, TSH and T4 levels rise concurrently until birth [24]. However, the feedback circuits are at least partly intact early in the third trimester. Deviations in TSH levels are detected in hypothyroid and hyperthyroid fetuses by approximately 28 weeks gestation [35, 36]. Furthermore, exogenous TRH administered to pregnant women results in increased fetal TSH in fetuses 24–35 weeks gestation [16, 37]. The HPT axis is thought to fully mature 1–2 months after birth [24, 38].

Role of Thyroid Hormones in Fetal Neurodevelopment

To enter the fetal brain, thyroid hormone must cross the blood-brain barrier (BBB). This process is facilitated by transporter proteins, similar to transport of maternal thyroid hormone across the placenta. Both MCT8 and OATP1C1 are found in fetal brains, with MCT8 likely serving as the predominant transporter [39]. Based on animal and human studies, it is currently believed that MCT8 permits thyroid hormone entry across the BBB into the brain endothelial cells [40]. Thyroid hormone then enters the astrocytes, possibly through OATP1C1 [40].

Unlike most fetal tissues, the cerebral cortex has elevated levels of D2 and low levels of D3, which results in increased T3 concentrations [34]. D2 is detected in the cerebral cortex, specifically the glial cells such as astrocytes, even in the first trimester [41, 42]. The T3 generated in the astrocytes is transported to neurons, although the specific transporter protein is currently unknown [40, 43]. By mid-gestation, T3 levels in the cerebral cortex exceed those of adults [34]. In contrast, D2 activity is low, and D3 activity is elevated in the cerebellum. Accordingly, T3 levels remain low in this area of the fetal brain [34].

Thyroid hormone action relies on nuclear thyroid hormone protein receptors (TRs), which are detected in the brain by 10 weeks gestation [44]. Thyroid hormone, particularly T3, regulates a number of nervous tissue genes and is critical for fetal brain maturation. While the exact mechanisms have not yet been defined, T3 likely plays a major role in neuronal migration and differentiation, myelination, and synaptogenesis [43, 45, 46]. Thus, alterations in fetal T3 levels can have profound impacts on brain development.

Neonatal Thyroid Physiology

Exposure to the cold, extrauterine environment at delivery stimulates TRH release from the neonatal hypothalamus and results in a dramatic TSH surge. TSH peaks at approximately 30 min of life, with levels reaching 60–80 mU/L [28, 31] (Fig. 5.2). The TSH surge stimulates a rise in T4 and T3, which begins in the first hours after birth and peaks in the second day of life [28, 47]. T4 levels reach 10–22 mcg/dL (fT4 2–5 ng/dL), and maximum T3 levels are approximately 250 ng/dL [31].

In addition to TSH stimulation, a shift in the predominating deiodinases after birth facilitates the T3 rise. D3 activity is decreased by the removal of the placenta, while D1 activity rises [28]. D2 activity in brown adipose tissue and the consequent increase in T3 are vital for thermogenesis, which allows the neonate to maintain normal body temperature after birth [48].

Under the feedback inhibition of rising T4 and T3, TSH levels fall, reaching typical infant levels by approximately 1 week of life [31, 47]. Conversely, T4 and T3 levels remain elevated for the first several weeks after birth [31, 47]. Even after this period, T4, fT4, and T3 levels remain elevated compared to older children and adults. Thus, age-appropriate reference ranges are crucial for identifying and managing mild cases of congenital hypothyroidism.

Neonatal Thyroid Disorders

Introduction

Neonatal thyroid disorders are common and are usually treatable. Early detection and appropriate management are critical to prevent morbidity, including neurodevelopmental sequelae. In this section, we will review causes of abnormal thyroid studies in premature infants followed by a discussion of the clinical presentation, etiologies, diagnosis, and management of congenital hypothyroidism as well as neonatal Graves' disease.

Prematurity and the Thyroid

Hypothyroidism is common in premature infants. The physiologic surge of TSH and T4 that follows delivery is blunted in premature infants compared to those born at term. In premature infants born before 31 weeks, T4 concentrations may fall during the first weeks of life, in contrast to the steady rise seen in term infants. This fall may be particularly pronounced in extremely premature and/or critically ill infants, with undetectable T4 levels reported in some neonates who ultimately do not require thyroid hormone replacement.

Typically, the hypothyroidism found in premature infants is transient, unless an underlying defect is present. Immaturity of the HPT axis is the most common cause of hypothyroidism in prematurity and is referred to as transient hypothyroxinemia of prematurity (THOP). THOP affects approximately 50% of infants born before 28 weeks [49] with laboratory findings of low T4 and T3 and inappropriately normal or low TSH levels. Despite the importance of thyroid hormone for neurodevelopment, there is currently little evidence to support levothyroxine treatment for infants with THOP.

Premature infants have additional risks factors for abnormal thyroid labs. These infants are often critically ill, which may result in low T4 and T3 levels with low TSH due to non-thyroidal illness. Confounding the picture further, these infants may be on pressors (such as dopamine) and glucocorticoids, which suppress TSH release and present a clinical picture similar to THOP. Premature infants are more susceptible to hypothyroidism from iodine deficiency given their reduced iodine stores. Because they cannot adequately compensate for an increased iodine load until approximately 36 weeks gestation, they are also at risk for transient hypothyroidism caused by iodine excess [49]. Finally, interpretation of thyroid panels in premature infants can be difficult as total T4 may be relatively lower than free T4 levels, owing to immaturity of the liver and reduced concentrations of thyroid-binding transport proteins.

Interestingly, premature infants with low birth weight (<1500 grams) are at increased risk of congenital hypothyroidism (CH), defined as the deficiency or absence of thyroid hormone at birth. The incidence of CH has been estimated to be as high as 1 in 400 in this population. Because the TSH is often low at birth and rises as the infant approaches term, newborn screening (NBS) only detects CH in approximately one third of these infants. Extremely low birth weight infants (<1000 grams) are at even higher risk for CH with delayed TSH rise [50]. To ensure that such cases are not missed, many NICUs repeat NBS in these infants between 2 and 4 weeks of age.

Congenital Hypothyroidism

Classification and Epidemiology

As described above, CH is the deficiency or absence of thyroid hormone at birth. Thyroid hormone is essential for brain myelination in the fetal, neonatal, and infantile periods; thus, early identification and treatment of CH is critical for neurodevelopmental outcome. CH may be permanent, requiring thyroid replacement for life or may be transient. It may also be classified as primary or central. Primary hypothyroidism reflects deficiency in thyroid synthesis due to a defect within the thyroid gland, while central CH refers to a defect in thyroid synthesis from pituitary (secondary) or hypothalamic (tertiary) dysfunction.

Over the past 20 years, the incidence of CH has risen to 1 in 2000 [51]. This dramatic increase likely reflects improved newborn screening (NBS) methods more than environmental factors. Notably, ethnic differences in CH incidence exist, with Asian, Native American, and Hispanic populations having increased likelihood compared to American White or Black infants [51].

Clinical Presentation

The clinical features of CH are often subtle and may be easily overlooked. Some maternal thyroid hormone crosses the placenta and is used by the fetus [21], and many infants with CH are able to make small amounts of thyroid hormone, making the diagnosis challenging [52]. Infants with CH are usually born at term, though in up to 20%, pregnancy may extend to 42 weeks [53]. While many are asymptomatic, some infants with CH may be lethargic after birth and may sleep through the night earlier than expected. Parents may note decreased energy with feeding, hoarse cry, hypothermia, and constipation. Physical features may include a goiter, cold and mottled skin, umbilical hernia, and prolonged jaundice, which is caused by decreased maturation of hepatic glucuronyl transferase [51]. There may be relevant history of maternal autoimmune thyroid disease, surgery, radioiodine exposure, and/or medications. Additionally unusual maternal diets or supplements may result in elevated or low maternal iodide levels.

Causes of Transient CH

Transient CH may be caused by neonatal and/or maternal factors. Neonatal factors include iodine deficiency or excess, hepatic hemangiomas, and loss of function (LOF) mutations in genes involved in thyroid synthesis (*DUOX2* or *DUOXA2*). Maternal factors causing transient CH include iodine deficiency or excess, transplacental passage of thyrotropin receptor-blocking antibodies, and maternal use of antithyroid medication [51].

Iodine Deficiency

Iodine deficiency is the leading cause of CH worldwide, accounting for the much higher incidence of transient CH in Europe (1:100) compared to the United States (1:50,000) [51]. Iodine deficiency causing maternal hypothyroidism during pregnancy results in insufficient maternally derived thyroid hormone for the fetus early in gestation and leaves the fetus unable to synthesize adequate thyroid hormone in the second and third trimesters. Affected neonates are often profoundly hypothyroid at birth and have severe mental retardation, which is not reversed with early initiation of thyroid hormone replacement. Premature infants are particularly susceptible to iodine deficiency due to decreased iodine stores and to increased demands for iodine in the extrauterine environment [54].

Iodine Excess

Iodine excess can also cause transient CH. Iodine excess may result from maternal dietary intake of iodide, medication use (such as amiodarone and lithium), or exposure to iodinated contrast agents (used for radiologic studies) [55]. Neonatal exposure to iodinated contrast or to topical iodine-containing antiseptics may also lead to iodine excess. Infants, particularly premature infants, are more susceptible to iodine overdose compared to older children due to increased skin absorption and decreased renal clearance of iodine. Iodine excess leads to transient CH through inhibition of TPO-mediated uptake and organification of iodine (termed the Wolff-Chaikoff effect) and inhibition of thyroglobulin (TG) proteolysis [56]. In most infants, the thyroid eventually compensates for the higher iodine content by decreasing expression of the NIS, thereby decreasing the intracellular iodine pool [57]. This compensation results in resumption of normal TPO function and thyroid hormone synthesis.

Maternal Hyperthyroidism

Maternal use of the antithyroid medications methimazole (MMI) and propylthiouracil (PTU) may lead to transient neonatal hypothyroidism. In some cases, this hypothyroidism may result in a goiter with respiratory compromise [58]. Clearance of the drug from the infant's circulation typically occurs within the first week of life, and replacement therapy with levothyroxine is not usually required. However, these infants still require careful monitoring once maternal medications have cleared circulation given the risk of a delayed-onset neonatal Graves' disease.

Additionally, women with Graves' disease may have blocking antibodies that cause transient hypothyroidism in the infant. Maternal thyrotropin receptor antibodies (TRAbs) can cross the placenta freely and bind avidly to the fetal and neonatal thyrotropin receptors. Importantly, TRAbs may be found in women who have been successfully treated for Graves' disease. Maternal TRAbs may have no effect on fetal/neonatal thyroid function (N-TRAbs), may cause primary hyperthyroidism (TSAbs), or may cause transient primary hypothyroidism (TBAbs) [59]. Because TBAbs may persist for several months, treatment with levothyroxine is usually required. TBAbs may also be seen in mothers with the non-goitrous form of chronic lymphocytic thyroiditis (primary myxedema) [58]. These mothers may be unaware of their hypothyroidism, which can lead to permanent neurodevelopmental deficits in the infant if the hypothyroidism is present throughout gestation.

Rarely, infants born to mothers with hyperthyroidism may have transient central hypothyroidism. Elevated thyroid hormone exposure in utero leads to fetal suppression of TRH and TSH, which continues in infancy. TBAb titers are not usually markedly elevated in these infants. The hypothyroidism is may be self-limited and not require treatment, although case reports have described children affected for years [58].

Hepatic Hemangiomas

Hepatic hemangiomas usually manifest in the first 6 months of life and are the most common benign hepatic tumors of infancy [60]. They may be an incidental finding or manifest with abdominal distention, hepatomegaly, intra-abdominal bleeding, cholestasis, and/or heart failure. Infants with these tumors can have transient hypothyroidism due to increased activity of D3, resulting in elevated levels of inactive rT3. This consumptive hypothyroidism can be severe but usually resolves with successful treatment of the hemangioma [60].

Mutations in DUOX2 and DUOXA2

The DUOX proteins (DUOX1 and DUOX2) are involved in the synthesis of hydrogen peroxide (H_2O_2), which is required for the oxidation of iodide to iodine. The *DUOXA2* gene encodes a protein involved in DUOX2 transport and cell-surface expression. Inactivating mutation in the *DUOX2* gene or in *DUOXA2* results in reduced H_2O_2 synthesis and iodine deficiency [61, 62]. *DUOXA2* mutations are a rare cause of transient congenital hypothyroidism, with fewer than ten cases described to date. They are inherited in an autosomal recessive manner. *DUOXA2* mutations have wide phenotypic variability, with some individuals euthyroid and others having severe congenital hypothyroidism. Monoallelic mutations in *DUOX2* are inherited in an autosomal dominant fashion and have been associated with transient CH. The transient nature of the hypothyroidism with *DUOXA2* and *DUOX2* mutations is likely due to the higher demands for thyroid hormone synthesis in neonates and infants compared to older children and may also reflect compensatory increased activity of DUOX1 proteins. Biallelic *DUOX2* mutations have an autosomal recessive inheritance and are associated with more severe, permanent CH. However, genotype-phenotype correlation is variable, and transient CH has been described in individuals with biallelic *DUOX2* mutations [61].

Causes of Permanent Congenital Hypothyroidism

In the United States and other areas of the world with sufficient iodine availability, the most common etiology of permanent congenital hypothyroidism is thyroid dysgenesis (TD), accounting for approximately 85% of CH. Thyroid dyshormonogenesis refers to inborn errors of thyroid synthesis and accounts for approximately 10% of CH cases in the United States. Central hypothyroidism is an underrecognized and underdiagnosed cause of CH, resulting from insufficient TRH, TSH, or both. Patients with central CH may have multiple pituitary hormone deficiencies.

Thyroid Dysgenesis

In TD, hypoplastic thyroid tissue is more common than complete absence of thyroid tissue (agenesis) and is often associated with an ectopic gland owing to arrested migration [58]. Ectopic thyroid tissue is most commonly seen in a sublingual location. Thyroid hormone synthesis is possible in this location; therefore, the diagnosis of an ectopic sublingual gland may not be made until later in life. Most cases of TD are sporadic, and there is a female predominance with Hispanic and Asian populations more commonly affected than African Americans. Infants with TD have higher frequencies of cardiac, renal, and urinary tract anomalies [63, 64].

Monogenic forms of TD are uncommon, accounting for less than 10% of diagnoses. Monogenic causes include LOF mutations in genes involved in thyroid morphogenesis (*NKX2–1*, *PAX8*, *FOXE1*, and *NKX2–5*) and in thyroid responsiveness to TSH (*TSHR*) (Fig. 5.3) (Table 5.2) [65]. *NKX2–1* (also referred to as *TTF-1*) encodes a transcription factor critical for synthesis of TG, thyroid peroxidase (TPO), and the TSH receptor. It is also involved in the synthesis of surfactant protein B gene in epithelial lung cells and regulates neuronal migration in the brain. Haploinsufficiency in *NKX2–1* leads to TD, infant respiratory distress syndrome, and benign hereditary chorea [66]. *PAX8* is involved in early differentiation of thyrocytes and in maintenance of thyroid follicular cells. It also regulates expression of TG, TPO, and NIS. *PAX8* mutations may be sporadic or familial with an autosomal dominant inheritance pattern. A wide variability of clinical presentation has been described with familial *PAX8* mutations, leading to speculation that other genetic factors influence *PAX8* expression and function [65]. Although *PAX8* mutations are not associated with specific syndromic findings, it is expressed in the mesonephros and ureteric buds, which may account for the genitourinary abnormalities often seen in CH. Homozygous mutations in *FOXE1* are linked to Bamforth-Lazarus syndrome, characterized by athyreosis and other congenital malformations including cleft palate, bilateral choanal atresia, and spiky hair [67]. *NKX2–5* encodes a transcription factor found in the primitive pharynx and thyroid anlage. LOF mutations in *NKX2–5* have been described in patients with congenital heart disease and ectopic thyroid.

Thyroid unresponsiveness to TSH is also termed resistance to TSH (RTSH). The most common cause of RTSH is a LOF mutation in the *TSHR* gene, which encodes the G-protein-coupled TSH receptor. In normal states, the binding of TSH to its receptor results in activation of the cAMP (via Gsα) and phosphoinositol/calcium (via Gq) pathways. The Gsα is involved in iodide uptake, thyroid hormone synthesis, gland growth, and thyroid cell differentiation, while the Gq pathways regulates the organification of iodide. LOF mutations of *TSHR* result in insufficient TSH receptor presence on the thyroid follicular cell [68]. Affected patients have reduced thyroid hormone production, compensatory increase in TSH, and, notably, lack of

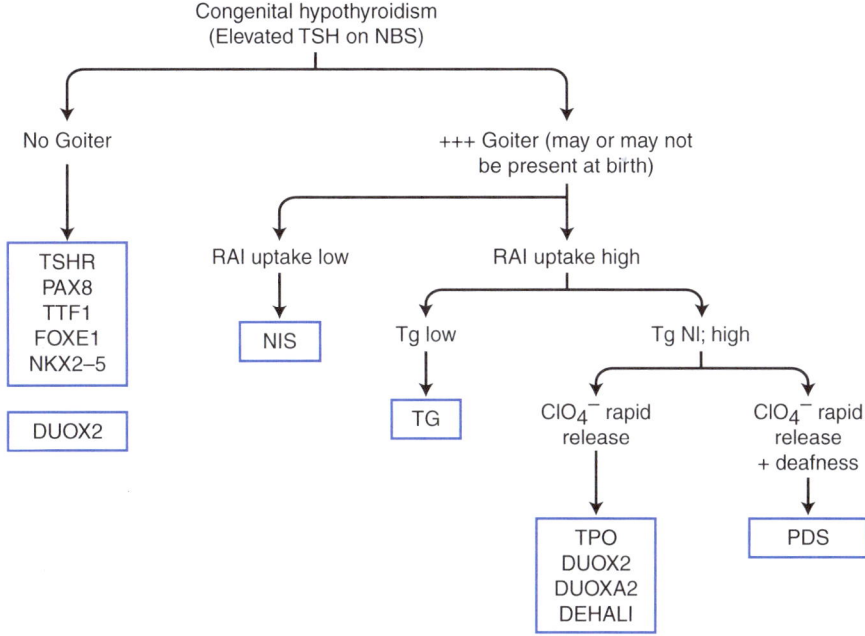

Fig. 5.3 Algorithm for genetic screening for disorders of thyroid hormone synthesis. TSH thyroid-stimulating hormone, NBS newborn screening, Nl normal, RAI radioactive iodine, Tg serum thyroglobulin, ClO_4^- perchlorate discharge. Genes: *TSHR* thyroid-stimulating hormone receptor, *PAX8* paired box gene 8, *TTF1* (*NKX2–1*) thyroid transcription factor 1, *FOXE1* Forkhead box protein E1, *NKX2–5* NK2 homeobox 5, *DUOX2* dual oxidase 2, *NIS* (*SLC5A5*) sodium iodine symporter, *TG* thyroglobulin, *TPO* thyroperoxidase, *DUOXA2* dual oxidase maturation factor 2, *DEHAL1* iodotyrosine deiodinase, *PDS* (*SLC26A4*) Pendrid syndrome. (Adapted with permission of Elsevier from Hannoush and Weiss [65])

Table 5.2 Causes of nongoitrous congenital hypothyroidism (dysgenesis)

Gene involved	TSH	Ft4	Tg	Comments
TSHR	Inc	Dec	Detectable	Normal-hypoplastic thyroid gland Does not trap pertechnetate
PAX8	Inc	Dec	Dec	Variable phenotype: partial to complete agenesis
TTF1 (*NKX2–1*)	Inc	Dec	Dec	Brain-thyroid-lung syndrome
FOXE1	Inc	Dec	Dec	Cleft palate, choanal atresia, spiky hair
NKX2–5	Inc	Dec	Dec	Congenital heart disease, ectopic thyroid

Adapted with permission of Elsevier from Hannoush and Weiss [65]
TSH thyroid-stimulating hormone, *fT4* free thyroxine, *Tg* serum thyroglobulin, *Dec* decreased, *N* normal, *Inc* increased, *DIT* diiodotyrosine, *MIT* monoiodotyrosine
Genes: *TSHR* thyroid-stimulating hormone receptor, *PAX8* paired box gene 8, *TTF1* (*NKX2–1*) thyroid transcription factor 1, *FOXE1* Forkhead box protein E1, *NKX2–5* NK2 homeobox 5

Table 5.3 Causes of goitrous congenital hypothyroidism (dyshormonogenesis)

Gene involved	TSH	fT4	Tg	Comments
NIS (SLC5A5)	Dec	Inc	Inc	Saliva/plasma I^{125} ratio < 20
PDS (SLC26A4)	N	N, Inc	Inc	Sensorineural hearing loss
TG	Dec	Inc	Dec	High uptake on scintigraphy
TPO	Dec	N, Inc	N, Inc	Positive perchlorate discharge test
DUOX2	Dec	Inc	N, Inc	May be transient or permanent hypothyroidism
DUOXA2	Dec	Inc	N, Inc	May be transient or permanent hypothyroidism
DEHAL1	Dec	Inc	N, Inc	Elevated urinary DIT and MIT levels

Adapted with permission of Elsevier from Hannoush and Weiss [65]
TSH thyroid-stimulating hormone, *fT4* free thyroxine, *Tg* serum thyroglobulin, *Dec* decreased, *N* normal, *Inc* increased, *DIT* diiodotyrosine, *MIT* monoiodotyrosine
Genes: *NIS (SLC5A5)* sodium iodine symporter, *PDS (SLC26A4)* Pendrid syndrome, *TG* thyroglobulin, *TPO* thyroperoxidase, *DUOX2* dual oxidase 2, *DUOXA2* dual oxidase maturation factor 2, *DEHAL1* iodotyrosine deiodinase

goiter. The phenotype and severity is highly variable in patients with RTSH depending on the mutation. Rare patients with RTSH have preserved Gsα activity and impaired Gq function, resulting in increased iodide uptake from deficient organification of iodide [68].

Thyroid Dyshormonogenesis

In contrast to CH caused by TD, defects in thyroid synthesis often have a known monogenic etiology, are generally inherited in an autosomal recessive manner, and are often associated with a goiter. CH resulting from defects in every step of thyroid hormone synthesis has been described (Table 5.3) [65].

Iodide Transport Defects

The *SLC5A5* gene encodes the NIS, which is responsible for iodide transport into the thyroid follicular cell and is present in many tissues including the salivary glands [69]. LOF mutation in NIS causes variable phenotypes of CH, ranging from compensated hypothyroidism to severe primary hypothyroidism. Imaging studies reveal minimal uptake of radioiodine and minimal discharge of iodine after perchlorate administration. Additionally, salivary measurement of radioiodine is decreased relative to serum and may aid in the diagnosis.

Iodide Organification Defects

The most common cause of thyroid dyshormonogenesis is defective TPO activity, which may result from a LOF mutation in *TPO* or from biallelic mutations in *DUOX2*, which is essential for TPO action. TPO catalyzes oxidation of iodide to iodine, organification of iodine to TG, and coupling of thyroid hormone precursors to form T4 and T3. Complete defects in TPO activity are most common and lead to total iodide organification defects (TIOD) and severe CH. TIOD is diagnosed when sodium perchlorate administration results in >90% release of thyroidal radioiodine. Less severe defects in TPO, DUOX2, and pendrin lead to partial iodide organificaton defects, which are diagnosed with a positive perchlorate discharge rate of 10–90% [51].

Pendred Syndrome

SLC264A (also referred to as *PDS*) encodes pendrin, a transmembrane chloride-iodide transporter expressed in the thyroid gland and the inner ear. In the thyroid, pendrin enables transport of iodide across the apex of the follicular cell into colloid, where oxidation occurs. In the inner ear, pendrin enables transport of bicarbonate and is necessary for normal development of the cochlea and vestibular aqueduct [70]. Pendred syndrome is characterized by a deficiency of pendrin and a triad of goiter, hypothyroidism, and sensorineural deafness. The majority of patients with Pendred syndrome are euthyroid, and goiter often develops despite normal thyroid studies. Pendred syndrome is the only form of dyshormonogenesis associated with a congenital malformation and is the most common cause of familial deafness [71].

Thyroglobulin Deficiency

TG plays a critical role in thyroid hormone synthesis as it houses thyroid precursors and fully formed thyroid hormone. Several mutations in TG have been described, including structural defects and defects in TG synthesis and transport. Structural defects lead to impaired coupling of mono- and di-iodotyrosines (MIT, DIT) within the TG molecule, and defects in TG synthesis and transport lead to reduced amount of the TG glycoprotein [72]. CH from TG deficiency is usually severe, and patients often develop a goiter in utero. Serum TG levels are markedly reduced with TG mutations, which can be used to differentiate these affected individuals from other forms of dyshormonogenesis.

Iodide Recycling Defects

Iodine is recycled from the thyroid precursors MIT and DIT through the actions of intracellular iodotyrosine deiodinase. This process provides a critical supply of iodine to the thyroid cell for new thyroid hormone synthesis. LOF of the gene encoding the iodotyrosine deiodinase enzyme, *DEHAL1*, leads to insufficient enzyme activity and hypothyroidism [73, 74]. Individuals with *DEHAL1* mutations have progressive hypothyroidism and goiter and often have profound intellectual disability. Diagnosis is confirmed with elevation of iodotyrosines in serum and urine. Importantly, NBS may fail to detect infants with *DEHAL1* mutations, possibly due to the protective effects of maternal iodine on fetal/neonatal thyroid synthesis.

Central Hypothyroidism

Central CH is characterized by low T4 and inappropriately low or normal TSH levels. The thyroid gland is eutopic but may be reduced in size due to a lack of stimulation by TSH [75]. Central CH is often milder than other causes of CH, and, thus, the diagnosis can be challenging. NBS programs use TSH only and may miss neonates with central CH. Additionally, THOP, non-thyroidal illness, and the use of pressors and/or glucocorticoids may mimic central CH. Features that can help distinguish central CH include signs of additional pituitary hormone deficits, such as hypoglycemia and micropenis, as well as midline defects, such as cleft lip and/or palate. Several gene mutations have been described with hypopituitarism, including *HESX1*, *LHX3*, *LHX4*, *PIT1*, and *PROP1* [75]. Although much less common, LOF mutations have been reported in the beta-subunit of TSH (*TSHB*) and in the TRH receptor (*TRHR*) genes in patients with isolated central CH.

Diagnosis of Congenital Hypothyroidism

CH is most often detected through NBS. Measurement of T4 and/or TSH is performed on a sample of dried whole blood collected on filter paper by skin puncture on day 2–4 of life. Most clinicians avoid drawing the sample on the first day of life to avoid false-positive results from the physiologic birth surge of TSH and T4. A diagnosis of primary hypothyroidism is made when the TSH value is elevated and the T4 value is low. Central hypothyroidism is characterized by low T4 and low or inappropriately normal TSH values. With any positive screening result for hypothyroidism on NBS, a confirmatory serum thyroid panel should be drawn. However, if severe primary hypothyroidism is suspected, therapy with levothyroxine should be initiated immediately upon receipt of the NBS results.

Imaging studies may be helpful when attempting to determine the cause of primary CH, although they should not delay treatment. Thyroid US is often the first-line study and in the hands of an experienced technician may differentiate between a normal gland, dysplastic or hypoplastic gland, or the absence of a gland. Scintigraphy can be useful in identifying ectopic thyroid tissue but must be performed within 7 days of therapy initiation. Iodine-123 (I^{123}) is preferred because it is organified and has better sensitivity than technetium-99 m (99mTc) [76]. When dyshormonogenesis is suspected, sodium perchlorate discharge testing may help the clinician to determine the etiology. Sodium perchlorate inhibits pendrin, the transport protein responsible for iodide transport across the apex of the thyroid follicular cell. In the test, perchlorate is administered 2 h after I^{123}, and thyroidal release of radiolabeled iodine is quantified. If CH is due to a defect in iodide transport or in iodine organification, there is increased radiotracer release from the thyroid after perchlorate administration.

Treatment of Congenital Hypothyroidism

The goal of therapy for CH is to normalize the thyroid studies as quickly as possible without causing hyperthyroidism. Because thyroid hormone is critical for neurodevelopment, treatment should not be delayed if CH is suspected. While recommendations vary regarding starting doses of levothyroxine, a typical dose endorsed by the American Academy of Pediatrics is 10–15 mcg/kg/day. The highest dosing is recommended for those infants suspected of having severe CH, defined by serum T4 < 5 mcg/dL [77].

Levothyroxine tablets can be crushed and mixed with a small amount of water or breast milk. Compounded liquid formulations of levothyroxine are not recommended due to concerns about accuracy of dosing. Levothyroxine should not be given with aluminum hydroxide (antacid), simethicone (infant colic drops), iron, calcium, soy, and/or fiber as these may prevent adequate absorption. T4 levels should rise to normal within a week of starting medication, while TSH may take up to a month to normalize. Close monitoring of thyroid studies is critical after starting therapy. Prolonged neonatal hypothyroidism has been associated with permanent neurocognitive delay, iatrogenic hyperthyroidism with increased anxiety, poor concentration, and social withdrawal [77].

Neonatal Hyperthyroidism

Neonatal hyperthyroidism is much less common than CH and is most often caused by maternal Graves' disease. Neonatal Graves' disease affects approximately 2% of infants born to mothers with Graves' disease with an incidence of 1 per 20,000 births. Maternal TRAbs can cross the placenta and bind the fetal/neonatal thyrotropin receptor, stimulating thyroid hormone synthesis (see section on Maternal Hyperthyroidism). Higher maternal TRAb levels have been associated with a greater risk of neonatal Graves' disease; thus, maternal TRAb titers should be monitored in mothers with Graves' disease during pregnancy. As TRAb titers may remain elevated despite successful Graves' disease treatment (surgery, radioiodine ablation), pregnant women with a history of Graves' disease should be included in this screening.

Neonatal Graves' disease is transient but can have severe manifestations if untreated including cardiac insufficiency, intrauterine growth retardation, prematurity, craniosynostosis, microcephaly, and psychomotor disabilities [78]. Importantly, maternally administered anti-thyroid drugs can cross the placenta, treat fetal hyperthyroidism, and persist in the neonate for the first week of life. Thus, infants may be minimally symptomatic at birth despite marked TRAb elevation. Careful monitoring of thyroid function after birth is essential to detect delayed hyperthyroidism in these infants. When neonatal hyperthyroidism does occur, infants are treated with MMI and, in some cases, beta-blockers. These medications are slowly weaned over a period of weeks to months based on the infant's thyroid labs, as the maternal antibodies are eliminated.

> **Clinical Case and Discussion**
>
> A 7-day-old male infant is referred to the pediatric endocrine clinic after his newborn screen returns positive for congenital hypothyroidism. He was born at term by spontaneous vaginal delivery, with a birth weight of 3.4 kg, and has been vigorous with breastfeeding. His newborn screen, drawn at 36 h of life, reveals TSH >100 mIU/L and T4 4.2 mcg/dL.
>
> The infant is alert and interactive with no dysmorphic features. No goiter is appreciated. Serum thyroid studies confirm primary hypothyroidism, with TSH 245 mIU/L, T4 3.6 mcg/dL, and fT4 0.58 ng/dL. Thyroid scintigraphy using iodine-123 (I^{123}) reveals no uptake of I^{123} by thyroid tissue. A thyroid ultrasound shows a thyroid gland in the normal location. What is the most likely explanation for this infant's findings? What is the expected course?
>
> The infant in this case has congenital primary hypothyroidism. Studies reveal a thyroid gland in the normal position that cannot take up radioiodine and does not produce sufficient thyroid hormone. This presentation is consistent with transient primary hypothyroidism due to transplacental passage of maternal thyroid-blocking antibodies (TBAb). Careful history would likely reveal a maternal history of Graves' disease. Thyroid labs would be expected to normalize over a several month period. The need for therapy with levothyroxine would depend on the severity of the hypothyroidism.

References

1. Pop VJ, Kuijpens JL, van Baar AL, Verkerk G, van Son MM, de Vijlder JJ, et al. Low maternal free thyroxine concentrations during early pregnancy are associated with impaired psychomotor development in infancy. Clin Endocrinol. 1999;50(2):149–55.
2. Haddow JE, Palomaki GE, Allan WC, Williams JR, Knight GJ, Gagnon J, et al. Maternal thyroid deficiency during pregnancy and subsequent neuropsychological development of the child. N Engl J Med. 1999;341(8):549–55.
3. DeLong GR, Leslie PW, Wang SH, Jiang XM, Zhang ML, Rakeman M, et al. Effect on infant mortality of iodination of irrigation water in a severely iodine-deficient area of China. Lancet. 1997;350(9080):771–3.
4. Besancon A, Beltrand J, Le Gac I, Luton D, Polak M. Management of neonates born to women with Graves' disease: a cohort study. Eur J Endocrinol. 2014;170(6):855–62.
5. Ford G, LaFranchi SH. Screening for congenital hypothyroidism: a worldwide view of strategies. Best Pract Res Clin Endocrinol Metab. 2014;28(2):175–87.
6. Fan X, Fu C, Shen Y, Li C, Luo S, Li Q, et al. Next-generation sequencing analysis of twelve known causative genes in congenital hypothyroidism. Clin Chim Acta. 2017;468:76–80.

7. Carre A, Stoupa A, Kariyawasam D, Gueriouz M, Ramond C, Monus T, et al. Mutations in BOREALIN cause thyroid dysgenesis. Hum Mol Genet. 2017;26(3):599–610.
8. Nicholas AK, Serra EG, Cangul H, Alyaarubi S, Ullah I, Schoenmakers E, et al. Comprehensive screening of eight known causative genes in congenital hypothyroidism with gland-in-situ. J Clin Endocrinol Metab. 2016;101(12):4521–31.
9. LaFranchi SH. Screening preterm infants for congenital hypothyroidism: better the second time around. J Pediatr. 2014;164(6):1259–61.
10. De Felice M, Di Lauro R. Thyroid development and its disorders: genetics and molecular mechanisms. Endocr Rev. 2004;25(5):722–46.
11. Fagman H, Nilsson M. Morphogenesis of the thyroid gland. Mol Cell Endocrinol. 2010;323(1):35–54.
12. Maenhaut C, Christophe D, Vassart G, Dumont J, Roger PP, Opitz R. Ontogeny, anatomy, metabolism and physiology of the thyroid. In: De Groot LJ, Chrousos G, Dungan K, Feingold KR, Grossman A, Hershman JM, et al. editors. Endotext [Internet]. South Dartmouth: MDText.com, Inc; 2000-. 2015 Jul 15.
13. Williams ED, Toyn CE, Harach HR. The ultimobranchial gland and congenital thyroid abnormalities in man. J Pathol. 1989;159(2):135–41.
14. Vandernoot I, Sartelet H, Abu-Khudir R, Chanoine JP, Deladoey J. Evidence for calcitonin-producing cells in human lingual thyroids. J Clin Endocrinol Metab. 2012;97(3):951–6.
15. Postiglione MP, Parlato R, Rodriguez-Mallon A, Rosica A, Mithbaokar P, Maresca M, et al. Role of the thyroid-stimulating hormone receptor signaling in development and differentiation of the thyroid gland. Proc Natl Acad Sci U S A. 2002;99(24):15462–7.
16. Bajoria R, Peek MJ, Fisk NM. Maternal-to-fetal transfer of thyrotropin-releasing hormone in vivo. Am J Obstet Gynecol. 1998;178(2):264–9.
17. Bajoria R, Fisk NM. Permeability of human placenta and fetal membranes to thyrotropin-stimulating hormone in vitro. Pediatr Res. 1998;43(5):621–8.
18. Loubiere LS, Vasilopoulou E, Bulmer JN, Taylor PM, Stieger B, Verrey F, et al. Expression of thyroid hormone transporters in the human placenta and changes associated with intrauterine growth restriction. Placenta. 2010;31(4):295–304.
19. Koopdonk-Kool JM, de Vijlder JJ, Veenboer GJ, Ris-Stalpers C, Kok JH, Vulsma T, et al. Type II and type III deiodinase activity in human placenta as a function of gestational age. J Clin Endocrinol Metab. 1996;81(6):2154–8.
20. Mortimer RH, Landers KA, Balakrishnan B, Li H, Mitchell MD, Patel J, et al. Secretion and transfer of the thyroid hormone binding protein transthyretin by human placenta. Placenta. 2012;33(4):252–6.
21. Vulsma T, Gons MH, de Vijlder JJ. Maternal-fetal transfer of thyroxine in congenital hypothyroidism due to a total organification defect or thyroid agenesis. N Engl J Med. 1989;321(1):13–6.
22. Mitchell AM, Manley SW, Morris JC, Powell KA, Bergert ER, Mortimer RH. Sodium iodide symporter (NIS) gene expression in human placenta. Placenta. 2001;22(2–3):256–8.
23. Thilly CH, Delange F, Lagasse R, Bourdoux P, Ramioul L, Berquist H, et al. Fetal hypothyroidism and maternal thyroid status in severe endemic goiter. J Clin Endocrinol Metab. 1978;47(2):354–60.
24. Thorpe-Beeston JG, Nicolaides KH, Felton CV, Butler J, McGregor AM. Maturation of the secretion of thyroid hormone and thyroid-stimulating hormone in the fetus. N Engl J Med. 1991;324(8):532–6.
25. Winters AJ, Eskay RL, Porter JC. Concentration and distribution of TRH and LRH in the human fetal brain. J Clin Endocrinol Metab. 1974;39(5):960–3.
26. Leduque P, Aratan-Spire S, Czernichow P, Dubois PM. Ontogenesis of thyrotropin-releasing hormone in the human fetal pancreas. A combined radioimmunological and immunocytochemical study. J Clin Invest. 1986;78(4):1028–34.
27. Shambaugh G 3rd, Kubek M, Wilber JF. Thyrotropin-releasing hormone activity in the human placenta. J Clin Endocrinol Metab. 1979;48(3):483–6.

28. Vliet GV, Deladoëy J. Chapter 7 - Disorders of the thyroid in the newborn and infant. In: Sperling MA, editor. Pediatric Endocrinology. 4th ed. Philadelphia: Elsevier; 2014. p. 186–208.
29. Neary JT, Nakamura C, Davies IJ, Soodak M, Maloof F. Lower levels of thyrotropin-releasing hormone-degrading activity in human cord and in maternal sera than in the serum of euthyroid, nonpregnant adults. J Clin Invest. 1978;62(1):1–5.
30. Thorpe-Beeston JG, Nicolaides KH, McGregor AM. Fetal thyroid function. Thyroid. 1992;2(3):207–17.
31. LaFranchi SH. Thyroid physiology and screening in preterm infants. In: Hoppin A, editor. UpToDate. Waltham: UpToDate. Accessed on 28 Nov 2017.
32. Dentice M, Salvatore D. Deiodinases: the balance of thyroid hormone: local impact of thyroid hormone inactivation. J Endocrinol. 2011;209(3):273–82.
33. Stanley EL, Hume R, Visser TJ, Coughtrie MW. Differential expression of sulfotransferase enzymes involved in thyroid hormone metabolism during human placental development. J Clin Endocrinol Metab. 2001;86(12):5944–55.
34. Kester MH, Martinez de Mena R, Obregon MJ, Marinkovic D, Howatson A, Visser TJ, et al. Iodothyronine levels in the human developing brain: major regulatory roles of iodothyronine deiodinases in different areas. J Clin Endocrinol Metab. 2004;89(7):3117–28.
35. Ribault V, Castanet M, Bertrand AM, Guibourdenche J, Vuillard E, Luton D, et al. Experience with intraamniotic thyroxine treatment in nonimmune fetal goitrous hypothyroidism in 12 cases. J Clin Endocrinol Metab. 2009;94(10):3731–9.
36. Guibourdenche J, Noel M, Chevenne D, Vuillard E, Volumenie JL, Polak M, et al. Biochemical investigation of foetal and neonatal thyroid function using the ACS-180SE analyser: clinical application. Ann Clin Biochem. 2001;38(Pt 5):520–6.
37. Ballard PL, Ballard RA, Creasy RK, Padbury J, Polk DH, Bracken M, et al. Plasma thyroid hormones and prolactin in premature infants and their mothers after prenatal treatment with thyrotropin-releasing hormone. Pediatr Res. 1992;32(6):673–8.
38. Kratzsch J, Pulzer F. Thyroid gland development and defects. Best Pract Res Clin Endocrinol Metab. 2008;22(1):57–75.
39. Roberts LM, Woodford K, Zhou M, Black DS, Haggerty JE, Tate EH, et al. Expression of the thyroid hormone transporters monocarboxylate transporter-8 (SLC16A2) and organic ion transporter-14 (SLCO1C1) at the blood-brain barrier. Endocrinology. 2008;149(12):6251–61.
40. Landers K, Richard K. Traversing barriers - How thyroid hormones pass placental, blood-brain and blood-cerebrospinal fluid barriers. Mol Cell Endocrinol. 2017;458:22–8.
41. Chan S, Kachilele S, McCabe CJ, Tannahill LA, Boelaert K, Gittoes NJ, et al. Early expression of thyroid hormone deiodinases and receptors in human fetal cerebral cortex. Brain Res Dev Brain Res. 2002;138(2):109–16.
42. Guadano-Ferraz A, Obregon MJ, St Germain DL, Bernal J. The type 2 iodothyronine deiodinase is expressed primarily in glial cells in the neonatal rat brain. Proc Natl Acad Sci U S A. 1997;94(19):10391–6.
43. Bernal J. Thyroid hormone regulated genes in cerebral cortex development. J Endocrinol. 2017;232(2):R83–97.
44. Bernal J, Pekonen F. Ontogenesis of the nuclear 3,5,3′-triiodothyronine receptor in the human fetal brain. Endocrinology. 1984;114(2):677–9.
45. Berbel P, Auso E, Garcia-Velasco JV, Molina ML, Camacho M. Role of thyroid hormones in the maturation and organisation of rat barrel cortex. Neuroscience. 2001;107(3):383–94.
46. Bernal J. Thyroid hormones in brain development and function. In: De Groot LJ, Chrousos G, Dungan K, Feingold KR, Grossman A, Hershman JM, et al. editors. Endotext [Internet]. South Dartmouth: MDText.com, Inc; 2000-. 2015 Sept 2.
47. Polak M, Luton D. Fetal thyroidology. Best Pract Res Clin Endocrinol Metab. 2014;28(2):161–73.
48. Hall JA, Ribich S, Christoffolete MA, Simovic G, Correa-Medina M, Patti ME, et al. Absence of thyroid hormone activation during development underlies a permanent defect in adaptive thermogenesis. Endocrinology. 2010;151(9):4573–82.

49. Wassner AJ, Brown RS. Hypothyroidism in the newborn period. Curr Opin Endocrinol Diabetes Obes. 2013;20(5):449–54.
50. Woo HC, Lizarda A, Tucker R, Mitchell ML, Vohr B, Oh W, et al. Congenital hypothyroidism with a delayed thyroid-stimulating hormone elevation in very premature infants: incidence and growth and developmental outcomes. J Pediatr. 2011;158(4):538–42.
51. Rastogi MV, LaFranchi SH. Congenital hypothyroidism. Orphanet J Rare Dis. 2010;5:17.
52. Delange F. Neonatal screening for congenital hypothyroidism: results and perspectives. Horm Res. 1997;48(2):51–61.
53. LaFranchi SH. Hypothyroidism. Pediatr Clin N Am. 1979;26(1):33–51.
54. Bhavani N. Transient congenital hypothyroidism. Indian J Endocr Metab. 2011;15(Suppl 2):S117–20.
55. Frassetto F, Tourneur Martel F, Barjhoux CE, Villier C, Bot BL, Vincent F. Goiter in a newborn exposed to lithium in utero. Ann Pharmacother. 2002;36(11):1745–8.
56. Koukkou EG, Roupas ND, Markou KB. Effect of excess iodine intake on thyroid on human health. Minerva Med. 2017;108(2):136–46.
57. Leung AM, Braverman LE. Consequences of excess iodine. Nat Rev Endocrinol. 2014;10(3):136–42.
58. Segni M. Disorders of the thyroid gland in infancy, childhood and adolescence. In: De Groot LJ, Chrousos G, Dungan K, Feingold KR, Grossman A, Hershman JM, et al. editors. Endotext [Internet]. South Dartmouth: MDText.com, Inc; 2000–2017 Mar 18.
59. Bucci I, Giuliani C, Napolitano G. Thyroid-stimulating hormone receptor antibodies in pregnancy: clinical relevance. Front Endocrinol (Lausanne). 2017;8:137.
60. Emir S, Ekici F, Ikiz MA, Vidinlisan S. The association of consumptive hypothyroidism secondary to hepatic hemangioma and severe heart failure in infancy. Turk Pediatri Ars. 2016;51(1):52–6.
61. Grasberger H. Defects of thyroidal hydrogen peroxide generation in congenital hypothyroidism. Mol Cell Endocrinol. 2010;322(1–2):99–106.
62. Grasberger H, Refetoff S. Identification of the maturation factor for dual oxidase. Evolution of an eukaryotic operon equivalent. J Biol Chem. 2006;281(27):18269–72.
63. Kumar J, Gordillo R, Kaskel FJ, Druschel CM, Woroniecki RP. Increased prevalence of renal and urinary tract anomalies in children with congenital hypothyroidism. J Pediatr. 2009;154(2):263–6.
64. Siebner R, Merlob P, Kaiserman I, Sack J. Congenital anomalies concomitant with persistent primary congenital hypothyroidism. Am J Med Genet. 1992;44(1):57–60.
65. Hannoush ZC, Weiss RE. Defects of thyroid hormone synthesis and action. Endocrinol Metab Clin N Am. 2017;46(2):375–88.
66. Hermanns P, Kumorowicz-Czoch M, Grasberger H, Refetoff S, Pohlenz J. Novel mutations in the NKX2.1 gene and the PAX8 gene in a Boy with Brain-Lung-Thyroid Syndrome. Exp Clin Endocrinol Diabetes. 2018 Feb;126(2):85–90.
67. Bamforth JS, Hughes IA, Lazarus JH, Weaver CM, Harper PS. Congenital hypothyroidism, spiky hair, and cleft palate. J Med Genet. 1989;26(1):49–51.
68. Grasberger H, Refetoff S. Resistance to thyrotropin. Best Pract Res Clin Endocrinol Metab. 2017;31(2):183–94.
69. Targovnik HM, Citterio CE, Rivolta CM. Iodide handling disorders (NIS, TPO, TG, IYD). Best Pract Res Clin Endocrinol Metab. 2017;31(2):195–212.
70. Wangemann P. Mouse models for pendrin-associated loss of cochlear and vestibular function. Cell Physiol Biochem. 2013;32(7):157–65.
71. Choi BY, Stewart AK, Madeo AC, Pryor SP, Lenhard S, Kittles R, et al. Hypo-functional SLC26A4 variants associated with nonsyndromic hearing loss and enlargement of the vestibular aqueduct: genotype-phenotype correlation or coincidental polymorphisms? Hum Mutat. 2009;30(4):599–608.
72. Citterio CE, Morales CM, Bouhours-Nouet N, Machiavelli GA, Bueno E, Gatelais F, et al. Novel compound heterozygous Thyroglobulin mutations c.745+1G>A/c.7036+2T>A associ-

ated with congenital goiter and hypothyroidism in a Vietnamese family. Identification of a new cryptic 5′ splice site in the exon 6. Mol Cell Endocrinol. 2015;404:102–12.
73. Iglesias A, Garcia-Nimo L, Cocho de Juan JA, Moreno JC. Towards the pre-clinical diagnosis of hypothyroidism caused by iodotyrosine deiodinase (DEHAL1) defects. Best Pract Res Clin Endocrinol Metab. 2014;28(2):151–9.
74. Moreno JC, Klootwijk W, van Toor H, Pinto G, D'Alessandro M, Leger A, et al. Mutations in the iodotyrosine deiodinase gene and hypothyroidism. N Engl J Med. 2008;358(17):1811–8.
75. Beck-Peccoz P, Rodari G, Giavoli C, Lania A. Central hypothyroidism – a neglected thyroid disorder. Nat Rev Endocrinol. 2017;13(10):588–98.
76. Keller-Petrot I, Leger J, Sergent-Alaoui A, de Labriolle-Vaylet C. Congenital hypothyroidism: role of nuclear medicine. Semin Nucl Med. 2017;47(2):135–42.
77. Rahmani K, Yarahmadi S, Etemad K, Koosha A, Mehrabi Y, Aghang N, et al. Congenital hypothyroidism: optimal initial dosage and time of initiation of treatment: a systematic review. Int J Endocrinol Metab. 2016;14(3):e36080.
78. Leger J. Management of fetal and neonatal Graves' disease. Horm Res Paediatr. 2017;87(1):1–6.

Chapter 6
Hypothyroidism in Pregnancy

Elizabeth N. Pearce

Abbreviations

ADHD	Attention deficit hyperactivity disorder
hCG	Human chorionic gonadotrophin
IQ	Intelligence quotient
T3	Triiodothyronine
T4	Thyroxine
TBG	Thyroxine binding globulin
TPO	Thyroperoxidase
TSH	Thyroid-stimulating hormone

> **Clinical Case**
> A 31-year-old woman presents for evaluation in the 8th week of her first pregnancy. She is feeling well, apart from mild nausea and new fatigue. She has no past medical history and is taking no medications other than a prenatal multivitamin. There is a history of Graves' hyperthyroidism in her maternal aunt and rheumatoid arthritis in her mother. A serum thyroid-stimulating hormone (TSH) value is 7.49 mIU/L, and her thyroperoxidase (TPO) antibodies are positive. She asks whether her mild hypothyroidism requires treatment.

E. N. Pearce
Boston Medical Center, Boston University School of Medicine, Section of Endocrinology, Diabetes, and Nutrition, Boston, MA, USA
e-mail: elizabeth.pearce@bmc.org

Introduction

Normally, thyroid hormone production increases by 50% during pregnancy, driven by thyroidal stimulation by human chorionic gonadotrophin (hCG), estrogen-mediated increases in thyroxine-binding globulin (TBG), and increased thyroid hormone metabolism due to the presence of placental deiodinase (Chap. 4). Women with iodine deficiency or underlying thyroid autoimmunity may be unable to meet the increased demands for thyroid hormone, and thus maternal thyroid hypofunction may manifest for the first time during gestation. Women with preexisting treated hypothyroidism prior to pregnancy require close monitoring during gestation, and most will need increased thyroid hormone doses in order to maintain euthyroidism.

Overt primary hypothyroidism is defined as an elevated serum thyroid-stimulating hormone (TSH) with low free thyroxine (T4) levels. Subclinical hypothyroidism has been variably defined in pregnancy, but the most commonly accepted definition is the presence of an elevated serum TSH with normal peripheral thyroid hormone values. Recommended reference ranges for TSH in pregnancy have varied over time, with prior clinical guidelines recommending upper TSH limits as low as 2.5 mIU/L in the first trimester [1, 2]. The most recent American Thyroid Association guidelines, however, recommend the use of a TSH upper limit of 4.0 mIU/L in the absence of appropriately derived assay-specific and trimester-specific reference ranges [3]. Isolated maternal hypothyroxinemia is most frequently defined as the lowest 2.5 to lowest 5th percentile of free T4 values for a given pregnancy cohort in the setting of normal TSH.

Maternal thyroid hypofunction is relatively common. Overt hypothyroidism occurs in approximately 0.3% of pregnancies [4]. The reported prevalence of subclinical hypothyroidism in pregnant women has varied substantially, depending on definitions employed, but TSH elevations are found in 2–3% of healthy women of childbearing age, with a higher prevalence in iodine-deficient regions [5]. The most frequent underlying etiology for hypothyroidism in iodine sufficient regions is chronic autoimmune thyroiditis, or Hashimoto's thyroiditis. Other causes include iodine deficiency, postablative and postsurgical hypothyroidism, and, rarely, secondary hypothyroidism caused by pituitary dysfunction. The causes of isolated maternal hypothyroxinemia are not well understood, but have been postulated to include iodine deficiency, iron deficiency, maternal obesity, and exposure to environmental endocrine disruptors [6].

Some of the classic symptoms of hypothyroidism are similar to those of normal pregnancy (Box 6.1). Studies in both pregnant and nonpregnant individuals have demonstrated substantial overlap between symptom scores in hypothyroid patients and euthyroid patients [7–9]. In pregnant women presenting with symptoms or signs suggestive of hypothyroidism, a serum TSH should be measured, since symptoms alone, in the absence of laboratory data, discriminate poorly between euthyroid and hypothyroid individuals.

> **Box 6.1 Signs and Symptoms of Hypothyroidism**
> Fatigue
> Constipation
> Cold intolerance
> Dry skin
> Weight gain
> Periorbital edema
> Hair loss
> Hoarseness
> Memory impairment
> Bradycardia
> Delayed relaxation of deep tendon reflexes

Overt Hypothyroidism in Pregnancy

Adverse Obstetric Outcomes of Overt Hypothyroidism

Overt hypothyroidism has been associated with multiple adverse pregnancy outcomes. In 1969, Jones and Man were the first to demonstrate that pregnant women with low serum thyroxine (assessed at that time using serum butanol-extractable iodine) had substantially increased rates of fetal death and preterm delivery [10]. In a retrospective cohort of 14 overtly hypothyroid pregnant women, reported complications included anemia in 31%, preeclampsia in 44%, placental abruption in 19%, postpartum hemorrhage in 19%, low birth weight in 31%, and fetal death in 12% [11]. In another retrospective analysis which included 23 overtly hypothyroid women, overt hypothyroidism was associated with increased risk for gestational hypertension, preeclampsia, and low birth weight [12]. Conversely, in the Northern Finland Birth Cohort, maternal overt hypothyroidism was associated with increased placental weight, birth weight, and risk for large-for-gestational-age infants [13]. Among Indian women, overt hypothyroidism in the second trimester was associated with increased rates of pregnancy-induced hypertension, intrauterine growth restriction, and fetal demise [14]. Abalovich and colleagues similarly found that inadequately treated overt maternal hypothyroidism was associated with increased risk of fetal loss and preterm delivery [15], and Allan and colleagues reported that fetal death rates were fourfold higher in women with a serum TSH ≥ 6 mIU/L compared with women who were euthyroid [5].

Adverse Effects of Maternal Overt Hypothyroidism on Child Outcomes

Adequate thyroid hormone is required in utero for normal development and maturation of the fetal nervous system [16]. Severe iodine deficiency, which can result in both maternal and fetal hypothyroidism in gestation, has long been known to cause impaired intellectual development in offspring [17]. Man and Jones in 1969 reported that low maternal thyroid function in pregnancy was associated with abnormal neurodevelopmental testing in over half of the infants studied at age 8 months [18]. In a case-control study, 7–9-year-old children of women with a history of untreated hypothyroidism in gestation were more likely to have an intelligence quotient (IQ) ≤85 and had an average IQ 7 points lower than that of matched controls [19].

Evidence for Treatment Benefit in Overt Hypothyroidism

No randomized clinical trials have been performed to demonstrate treatment benefits in pregnancy, and it would be considered unethical to conduct a placebo-controlled trial in overtly hypothyroid women. However, in retrospective analyses, adequate levothyroxine treatment decreases rates of preterm delivery and miscarriage [15], and animal studies strongly suggest that treatment of overtly hypothyroid pregnant women is likely to improve child neurodevelopment [16]. There is universal agreement that overt hypothyroidism in pregnancy should be treated with thyroid hormone replacement [2, 3, 20].

Subclinical Hypothyroidism in Pregnancy

Adverse Effects of Subclinical Hypothyroidism on Obstetric and Neonatal Outcomes

There is now a large literature describing associations between maternal subclinical hypothyroidism and adverse obstetric and neonatal outcomes in observational studies. Although associations of subclinical hypothyroidism with outcomes such as miscarriage, premature delivery gestational hypertension, gestational diabetes, and placental abruption have been reported, associations have differed across studies, and some large cohorts [21, 22] have not reported any adverse effects at all. The heterogeneity of study results is likely due to differences in the definitions of subclinical hypothyroidism used, in the size of studies (and thus the adequacy of power to examine rare outcomes), and in the timing of maternal thyroid function testing during gestation. Whether or not studies excluded women with positive thyroid autoantibodies may also have influenced results; evidence suggests that women with thyroid autoimmunity may experience a higher risk for miscarriage at lower TSH thresholds [23].

Recently, several systematic reviews and meta-analyses have examined associations between maternal subclinical hypothyroidism and adverse obstetric outcomes. A 2011 meta-analysis of three studies, including 1010 subclinically hypothyroid women, demonstrated an increased risk of perinatal mortality in women with subclinical hypothyroidism compared to euthyroid controls (OR 2.7, 95% CI 1.6–4.7) [24]. However, in the same systematic review, meta-analyses did not show associations between subclinical hypothyroidism and either pregnancy-induced hypertension or preterm delivery. In a 2015 meta-analysis which included 16 observational studies, Chan and Boelaert found that maternal subclinical hypothyroidism was associated with increased risks for pregnancy loss, preterm delivery, placental abruption, and breech presentation [25]. In a 2016 meta-analysis of seven studies, Gong and co-authors reported that risk for gestational diabetes was increased in subclinically hypothyroid women (OR 1.558; 95% CI 1.292–1.877) [26]. In 2016 Tong and colleagues performed a meta-analysis of seven studies and reported a significant association of subclinical hypothyroidism with intrauterine growth restriction (OR 1.54, 95% CI 1.06–2.25) [27]. In 2016 Maraka and colleagues completed a systematic review including 18 studies, which together incorporated 3995 pregnant women with subclinical hypothyroidism [28]. Although significant associations between subclinical hypothyroidism and pregnancy loss, placental abruption, premature rupture of membranes, and neonatal death were seen in the pooled analyses, there were no significant associations with other outcomes such as premature delivery, preeclampsia, gestational hypertension, and low birth weight. Most recently, in 2017, Zhang and colleagues performed a meta-analysis of 7 studies which included 3137 untreated subclinically hypothyroid women and found that women with subclinical hypothyroidism had a higher prevalence of miscarriage (RR = 1.90, 95% CI1.59–2.27) than women who were euthyroid [29]. Taken together, these data strongly suggest that maternal subclinical hypothyroidism is associated with multiple adverse obstetric outcomes, although the underlying mechanisms remain unclear.

Adverse Effects of Subclinical Hypothyroidism on Child Outcomes

In contrast to the large evidence base for associations between maternal subclinical hypothyroidism and adverse obstetric outcomes, data suggesting a link between subclinical hypothyroidism and adverse child neurodevelopmental outcomes are relatively sparse. In a small prospective study, maternal thyroid function was assessed at 17 weeks gestation and child neurodevelopment at 8 years of age. Child IQ was significantly higher in children of 124 euthyroid women (107) than in 28 children whose mother's TSH values were between the 98th and 99.85th percentiles (102) or among 20 children of untreated hypothyroid women whose TSH was ≥99.85th percentile (97; $p = 0.003$) [30]. In a Chinese cohort study, Li and colleagues found that children of women with gestational subclinical hypothyroidism had mean intelligence scores 8.88 points lower ($P = 0.008$) and mean motor scores 9.98 lower ($p < 0.001$) than children of euthyroid women

[31]. In another Chinese cohort study which included 31 subclinically hypothyroid women, Su and co-authors reported that maternal subclinical hypothyroidism was associated with increased risk for neurodevelopmental delay in infants at up to 6 months of age (OR 10.49, 95% CI1.01–119.19) [32]. However, these findings have not been universal. In a small prospective study including only seven subclinically hypothyroid pregnant women, mean mental developmental index scores were lower in infants of the subclinically hypothyroid mothers than in infants of euthyroid mothers at 6 and 12 months of age, but by 24 months, the difference was no longer significant, and psychomotor development scores did not differ at any time point [33]. Among 3659 mother-child pairs from the Generation R cohort, maternal TSH levels at 13 weeks gestation were not associated with verbal or nonverbal cognitive functioning in children at 30 months of age [34]. Similarly, in a Boston-area cohort of 500 children, cognitive testing at 6 months and 3 years of age was not associated with maternal thyroid function at a mean of 10 weeks gestation [35].

Evidence for Treatment Benefit in Subclinical Hypothyroidism

Although observational data strongly suggest adverse effects of maternal subclinical hypothyroidism on obstetric outcomes, and possibly on adverse child cognitive outcomes, evidence for a benefit of levothyroxine treatment is sparse. A retrospective US study which included 5405 subclinically hypothyroid women found that women with a pretreatment TSH value of 4.1–10.0 mIU/L who received levothyroxine had a reduced risk for pregnancy loss (odds ratio 0.45, 95% CI 0.30–0.65), but treatment was associated with higher risks for preterm delivery, gestational diabetes, and preeclampsia [36].

Negro and colleagues randomized first-trimester pregnant women to a case-finding vs. a universal screening strategy [37]. Women with TSH >2.5 mIU/L who were TPO antibody positive were treated with levothyroxine. The primary outcome was a composite of adverse obstetric outcomes that have been associated with subclinical hypothyroidism in the literature, including some subjective outcomes such as need for Cesarean section. The study overall did not find any difference in the composite outcome between the case-finding and universal screening groups. In secondary analyses, among women initially classified as being at low risk for having thyroid dysfunction who had TSH elevations, treatment with levothyroxine appeared to reduce the risk of adverse outcomes. Azizi and co-authors randomized TPO antibody-positive women with a TSH up to 10.0 mIU/L to levothyroxine vs. no treatment early in gestation [38]. Treatment was associated with a decrease in risk for premature delivery; in secondary analyses, this treatment benefit was only seen in women with TSH >4.0 mIU/L at baseline.

Two randomized clinical trials have examined the effects of levothyroxine treatment in subclinically hypothyroid pregnant women on child cognitive outcomes. In the Controlled Antenatal Thyroid Screening (CATS) trial, conducted in the United

Kingdom and in Italy, pregnant women were randomized to either screening with initiation of 150 μg/day levothyroxine treatment for those with TSH in the highest 2.5th percentile or free T4 in the lowest 2.5th percentile or a strategy in which blood was drawn in early gestation but thyroid function only measured after delivery [39]. Children of 390 treated and 404 untreated women were followed until age 3, when IQ tests were administered. Mean IQ scores and the likelihood of having IQ <85 did not differ by group. More recently, Casey and co-authors conducted a similar multicenter trial in the United States in which women were screened for two parallel randomized clinical trials: one assessing levothyroxine therapy for subclinical hypothyroidism (defined for most of the study as a TSH > 4.0 mIU/L with normal free T4) and the other assessing the effects of levothyroxine treatment for maternal hypothyroxinemia [40]. This trial found no treatment effect on the primary outcome, which was child IQ assessed at 5 years of age. Multiple obstetric and neonatal adverse outcomes were assessed in secondary analyses, and no difference was found by treatment group. Both the CATS trial and the Casey study have been criticized for late gestational ages at treatment initiation: a mean 13 weeks 3 days in CATS and 16.7 weeks for the subclinically hypothyroid women in the Casey study. Additional trials are needed to determine whether earlier intervention improves child outcomes.

In the absence of definitive data for treatment benefit, recommendations vary. The American Congress of Obstetricians and Gynecologists states that "currently, there is no evidence that identification and treatment of subclinical hypothyroidism during pregnancy improves…outcomes." [41] By contrast, the European Thyroid Association recommends levothyroxine treatment of subclinical hypothyroidism when detected either preconception or during gestation [42]. The American Thyroid Association currently recommends a stepwise approach, taking into account both the TSH level and the TPO antibody status (Table 6.1) [3].

Table 6.1 American Thyroid Association recommendations for the management of subclinical hypothyroidism and hypothyroxinemia in pregnancy

Laboratory data	Levothyroxine therapy	Recommendation strength	Evidence quality
Anti-TPO-positive and TSH level > pregnancy-specific reference range	Yes	Strong	Moderate
Anti-TPO-negative and TSH level >10 mIU/L	Yes	Strong	Low
Anti-TPO-positive and TSH level >2.5 mIU/L and < upper limit of the reference range	Consider	Weak	Moderate
Anti-TPO-negative and TSH level > upper limit of the reference range and <10 mIU/L	Consider	Weak	Low
Isolated maternal hypothyroxinemia	No	Weak	Low

Adapted with permission from Cooper and Pearce [65]. Copyright © (2017) Massachusetts Medical Society

Isolated Maternal Hypothyroxinemia

Adverse Obstetric Outcomes in Maternal Hypothyroxinemia

The results of cohort studies examining the effects of isolated maternal hypothyroxinemia on obstetric and neonatal outcomes have been variable [6]. Differences in findings across studies may be due in part to a lack of power to detect rare outcomes in many of the cohorts, as well as to the use of differing thresholds to define maternal hypothyroxinemia. In a large US pregnancy cohort which included 233 women with isolated maternal hypothyroxinemia, risk for gestational hypertension, diabetes, placental abruption, and premature or Cesarean deliveries did not differ in the women with hypothyroxinemia compared to euthyroid controls [43]. By contrast, in another US cohort which included 232 women with hypothyroxinemia in the first trimester and 247 in the second trimester, Cleary-Goldman found that first-trimester hypothyroxinemia was associated with increased risk for preterm labor and macrosomia, while in the second trimester, there was an association with increased risk for gestational diabetes [21]. In the Generation R cohort in the Netherlands, isolated maternal hypothyroxinemia was associated with an increased risk for premature delivery [44], and higher maternal FT4 levels among euthyroid women were associated with lower birth weights [45]. Similarly, in a Spanish cohort, isolated maternal hypothyroxinemia was associated with higher birth weights [46]. A recent meta-analysis examining the effects of isolated maternal hypothyroxinemia in observational studies found an increased placental abruption (OR 2.30; 95% CI: 1.10–4.80), but no differences in risks for other outcomes including pregnancy loss, gestational diabetes, gestational hypertension, or birth weights [25].

Adverse Effects of Maternal Hypothyroxinemia on Child Outcomes

Multiple studies have examined associations between isolated maternal hypothyroxinemia and child cognition. In 2003, Pop and co-authors assessed maternal thyroid function at 12 weeks gestation and then assessed child neurocognition at ages 1 and 2 years [47]. Children of hypothyroxinemic mothers had delays in mental and motor function compared to children of euthyroid controls at both time points. In a Chinese cohort study, children of mothers with hypothyroxinemia at weeks 16–20 of gestation, when assessed at 25–30 months of age, had a mean IQ score 9.30 points lower than that of the controls and also had lower mean motor scores [31]. In the Generation R cohort, maternal hypothyroxinemia was associated with a higher risk of child expressive language delay at 18 and 30 months of age, a higher risk of nonverbal cognitive delay at 30 months, and a mean IQ at 8 years of age that was

4.3 points lower than the children of mothers with normal gestational thyroid function [34, 48]. In that cohort, however, brain MRI revealed no differences in brain volumetric measures, cortical thickness, or surface area between children of mothers with gestational hypothyroxinemia and controls [48]. Interestingly, however, subsequent analyses from the same cohort have demonstrated that maternal free thyroxine concentrations had an inverted U-shaped association with child IQ at age 6 years ($p = 0.0044$), with child gray matter volume ($p = 0.0062$), and with cortex volume ($p = 0.0011$) as assessed by MRI at age 8 years [49]. In a small cohort of 147 mother-child pairs from Spain, maternal hypothyroxinemia in late gestation (37 weeks) was associated with lower child development scores at 38 and 60 months of age [50].

Importantly, several studies have failed to show associations between maternal hypothyroxinemia and child cognitive development. Among 1017 mother-child pairs in the China-Anhui Birth Defects and Child Development study, maternal hypothyroxinemia before 20 weeks gestation was not associated with child developmental delay at up to 9 months of age [32]. In a Boston-area cohort of 500 infants, first-trimester maternal thyroid total T4 levels were not associated with child cognitive function at either 6 months or 3 years of age [35]. In a matched case-control study, Craig and colleagues noted that unadjusted cognitive, language, and motor scores were 3% lower at 2 years of age among offspring of 98 hypothyroxinemic women compared to children of controls but that the difference was not significant after adjustment for potential confounders [51]. In a California birth cohort of primarily Latino children, maternal free T4 levels in the second half of gestation were not associated with child cognitive measures at 6, 12, 24, or 60 months of age [52]. Finally, Grau and colleagues assessed 455 children from a Spanish birth cohort at 1 year of age and reevaluated 289 of them at 6–8 years [53]. There was no difference in cognitive scores between children of hypothyroxinemic and euthyroid mothers. Overall, current observational data strongly suggest a link between maternal hypothyroxinemia and lower child cognition, but the evidence is not conclusive.

Limited data suggest a possible association between maternal hypothyroxinemia and child neurobehavioral disorders. In the Generation R cohort, isolated maternal hypothyroxinemia at a mean 13.6 weeks gestation was associated with higher attention deficit hyperactivity disorder (ADHD) symptom scores in children at the age of 8 years [54]. Similarly, in a separate cohort from the Netherlands which included 2000 mother-child pairs, maternal hypothyroxinemia at a median gestational age of 12.9 weeks was associated with a higher risk (OR 1.70; 95% CI 1.01–2.86) for teacher-reported hyperactivity/inattention in children at age 5–6 years [55]. In the Generation R study, maternal hypothyroxinemia has also been linked to a fourfold risk for having children with autistic symptoms [56]. A case-control study nested within a national Finnish birth registry reported that isolated maternal hypothyroxinemia was associated with increased odds for schizophrenia in children (OR 1.75, 95% CI 1.22–2.50) [57]. Additional studies are required to confirm these results and to better understand underlying mechanisms for these associations.

Evidence for Treatment Benefit in Maternal Hypothyroxinemia

The only two randomized clinical trials to date both failed to show a benefit of treatment of isolated maternal hypothyroxinemia for child developmental outcomes [39, 40]. In addition, the poor accuracy of free T4 assays in pregnancy [58] and different laboratory thresholds for defining hypothyroxinemia across studies would make it challenging to define either thresholds for treatment initiation or targets for therapy. Most current guidelines recommend against screening for or treatment of isolated maternal hypothyroxinemia (Table 6.1) [3].

Treatment of Hypothyroidism in Pregnancy

For all women with overt hypothyroidism, and for those women with subclinical hypothyroidism in whom therapy is elected, the recommended treatment is levothyroxine [3]. Thyroid replacement with desiccated thyroid, or with liothyronine alone or in combination with levothyroxine, is not recommended in pregnancy because it is primarily T4, rather than T3, that crosses the placenta in early pregnancy and thus these treatments confer a risk of selective fetal hypothyroidism even when the maternal TSH is normal [59]. It is recommended that levothyroxine therapy should be titrated in order to maintain a maternal serum TSH <2.5 mIU/L both preconception and during gestation [3]. A retrospective study has demonstrated that levothyroxine-treated women with first-trimester TSH values >2.5 mU/L had a higher risk of miscarriage compared to women with TSH values of 0.2–2.5 mU/L [60].

Preconception counseling is important for all women with known hypothyroidism. The majority of women on levothyroxine, even if adequately treated prior to conception, will need dose increases to maintain euthyroidism throughout gestation [61]. Thyroid hormone requirements increase starting in weeks 4–6 of gestation and gradually increase until about weeks 16–20 [62]. Levothyroxine requirements are dependent in part on the underlying cause of hypothyroidism, with women who are athyreotic due to thyroidectomy or radioactive iodine ablation most likely to require increased doses during gestation [63]. It is recommended that levothyroxine doses be empirically increased by 25–30% as soon as pregnancy is diagnosed [3, 64]. One way to achieve this is by instructing women to increase from seven to nine levothyroxine tablets per week as soon as pregnancy is confirmed. In all levothyroxine-treated women, serum TSH should be assessed every 4 weeks during the first half of gestation and at least once around week 30 [3]. Following delivery, levothyroxine doses can be decreased to preconception levels, with serum TSH testing performed at approximately 6 weeks postpartum.

Clinical Case and Discussion

A 31-year-old woman presents for evaluation in the 8th week of her first pregnancy. She is feeling well, apart from mild nausea and new fatigue. She has no past medical history and is taking no medications other than a prenatal multivitamin. There is a history of Graves' hyperthyroidism in her maternal aunt and rheumatoid arthritis in her mother. A serum thyroid-stimulating hormone (TSH) value is 7.49 mIU/L, and her thyroperoxidase (TPO) antibodies are positive. She asks whether her mild hypothyroidism requires treatment.

Overt hypothyroidism during gestation is unequivocally associated with adverse obstetric and child developmental outcomes and always requires treatment with levothyroxine. Maternal subclinical hypothyroidism, as seen in this patient, has been associated with several adverse obstetric outcomes, including pregnancy loss, placental abruption, premature rupture of membranes, and neonatal death, and may also be linked to adverse effects on child development, although this is not definitively established. Positive TPO antibodies appear to confer an increased risk for adverse obstetric outcomes in subclinically hypothyroid women. The American Thyroid Association recommends a stepwise approach for the consideration of treatment for subclinically hypothyroid pregnant women, taking into account both the degree of TSH elevation and the TPO antibody status.

Additional studies are needed to definitively determine whether treatment of subclinical hypothyroidism, started early in gestation, improves child or pregnancy outcomes. In this patient, however, with both subclinical hypothyroidism and positive TPO antibodies, current guidelines recommend initiation of levothyroxine treatment.

For women who are treated with levothyroxine during pregnancy, close TSH monitoring is essential.

References

1. Stagnaro-Green A, Abalovich M, Alexander E, Azizi F, Mestman J, Negro R, Nixon A, Pearce EN, Soldin OP, Sullivan S, Wiersinga W, American Thyroid Association Taskforce on Thyroid Disease During Pregnancy and Postpartum. Guidelines of the American Thyroid Association for the diagnosis and management of thyroid disease during pregnancy and postpartum. Thyroid. 2011;21(10):1081–125.
2. De Groot L, Abalovich M, Alexander EK, Amino N, Barbour L, Cobin RH, Eastman CJ, Lazarus JH, Luton D, Mandel SJ, Mestman J, Rovet J, Sullivan S. Management of thyroid dysfunction during pregnancy and postpartum: an Endocrine Society clinical practice guideline. J Clin Endocrinol Metab. 2012;97(8):2543–65.

3. Alexander EK, Pearce EN, Brent GA, Brown RS, Chen H, Dosiou C, Grobman WA, Laurberg P, Lazarus JH, Mandel SJ, Peeters RP, Sullivan S. 2017 guidelines of the American Thyroid Association for the diagnosis and management of thyroid disease during pregnancy and the postpartum. Thyroid. 2017;27(3):315–89.
4. Stagnaro-Green A. Overt hyperthyroidism and hypothyroidism during pregnancy. Clin Obstet Gynecol. 2011;54(3):478–87.
5. Allan WC, Haddow JE, Palomaki GE, Williams JR, Mitchell ML, Hermos RJ, Faix JD, Klein RZ. Maternal thyroid deficiency and pregnancy complications: implications for population screening. J Med Screen. 2000;7(3):127–30.
6. Dosiou C, Medici M. Management of endocrine disease: isolated maternal hypothyroxinemia during pregnancy: knowns and unknowns. Eur J Endocrinol. 2017;176(1):R21–38.
7. Pop VJ, Broeren MA, Wiersinga WM, Stagnaro-Green A. Thyroid disease symptoms during early pregnancy do not identify women with thyroid hypofunction that should be treated. Clin Endocrinol. 2017;87(6):838–43.
8. Canaris GJ, Manowitz NR, Mayor G, Ridgway EC. The Colorado thyroid disease prevalence stud. Arch Intern Med. 2000;160(4):526–34.
9. Carlé A, Pedersen IB, Knudsen N, Perrild H, Ovesen L, Laurberg P. Hypothyroid symptoms and the likelihood of overt thyroid failure: a population-based case-control study. Eur J Endocrinol. 2014;171(5):593–602.
10. Jones WS, Man EB. Thyroid function in human pregnancy. VI. Premature deliveries and reproductive failures of pregnant women with low serum butanol-extractable iodines. Maternal serum TBG and TBPA capacities. Am J Obstet Gynecol. 1969;104(6):909–14.
11. Davis LE, Leveno KJ, Cunningham FG. Hypothyroidism complicating pregnancy. Obstet Gynecol. 1988;72(1):108–12.
12. Leung AS, Millar LK, Koonings PP, Montoro M, Mestman JH. Perinatal outcome in hypothyroid pregnancies. Obstet Gynecol. 1993;81(3):349–53.
13. Männistö T, Vääräsmäki M, Pouta A, Hartikainen AL, Ruokonen A, Surcel HM, Bloigu A, Järvelin MR, Suvanto-Luukkonen E. Perinatal outcome of children born to mothers with thyroid dysfunction or antibodies: a prospective population-based cohort study. J Clin Endocrinol Metab. 2009;94(3):772–9.
14. Sahu MT, Das V, Mittal S, Agarwal A, Sahu M. Overt and subclinical thyroid dysfunction among Indian pregnant women and its effect on maternal and fetal outcome. Arch Gynecol Obstet. 2010;281(2):215–20.
15. Abalovich M, Gutierrez S, Alcaraz G, Maccallini G, Garcia A, Levalle O. Overt and subclinical hypothyroidism complicating pregnancy. Thyroid. 2002;12(1):63–8.
16. de Escobar GM, Obregón MJ, del Rey FE. Iodine deficiency and brain development in the first half of pregnancy. Public Health Nutr. 2007;10(12A):1554–70.
17. Zimmermann MB. Iodine deficiency. Endocr Rev. 2009;30(4):376–408.
18. Man EB, Jones WS. Thyroid function in human pregnancy. V. Incidence of maternal serum low butanol-extractable iodines and of normal gestational TBG and TBPA capacities; retardation of 8-month-old infants. Am J Obstet Gynecol. 1969;104(6):898–908.
19. Haddow JE, Palomaki GE, Allan WC, Williams JR, Knight GJ, Gagnon J, O'Heir CE, Mitchell ML, Hermos RJ, Waisbren SE, Faix JD, Klein RZ. Maternal thyroid deficiency during pregnancy and subsequent neuropsychological development of the child. N Engl J Med. 1999;341(8):549–55.
20. Garber JR, Cobin RH, Gharib H, Hennessey JV, Klein I, Mechanick JI, Pessah-Pollack R, Singer PA, Woeber KA, American Association of Clinical Endocrinologists and American Thyroid Association Taskforce on Hypothyroidism in Adults. Clinical practice guidelines for hypothyroidism in adults: cosponsored by the American Association of Clinical Endocrinologists and the American Thyroid Association. Thyroid. 2012;22(12):1200–35.
21. Cleary-Goldman J, Malone FD, Lambert-Messerlian G, Sullivan L, Canick J, Porter TF, Luthy D, Gross S, Bianchi DW, D'Alton ME. Maternal thyroid hypofunction and pregnancy outcome. Obstet Gynecol. 2008;112(1):85–92.

22. Männistö T, Vääräsmäki M, Pouta A, Hartikainen AL, Ruokonen A, Surcel HM, Bloigu A, Järvelin MR, Suvanto E. Thyroid dysfunction and autoantibodies during pregnancy as predictive factors of pregnancy complications and maternal morbidity in later life. J Clin Endocrinol Metab. 2010;95(3):1084–94.
23. Liu H, Shan Z, Li C, Mao J, Xie X, Wang W, Fan C, Wang H, Zhang H, Han C, Wang X, Liu X, Fan Y, Bao S, Teng W. Maternal subclinical hypothyroidism, thyroid autoimmunity, and the risk of miscarriage: a prospective cohort study. Thyroid. 2014;24(11):1642–9.
24. van den Boogaard E, Vissenberg R, Land JA, van Wely M, van der Post JA, Goddijn M, Bisschop PH. Significance of (sub)clinical thyroid dysfunction and thyroid autoimmunity before conception and in early pregnancy: a systematic review. Hum Reprod Update. 2011;17(5):605–19.
25. Chan S, Boelaert K. Optimal management of hypothyroidism, hypothyroxinaemia and euthyroid TPO antibody positivity preconception and in pregnancy. Clin Endocrinol. 2015;82(3):313–26.
26. Gong LL, Liu H, Liu LH. Relationship between hypothyroidism and the incidence of gestational diabetes: a meta-analysis. Taiwan J Obstet Gynecol. 2016;55(2):171–5.
27. Tong Z, Xiaowen Z, Baomin C, Aihua L, Yingying Z, Weiping T, Zhongyan S. The effect of subclinical maternal thyroid dysfunction and autoimmunity on intrauterine growth restriction: a systematic review and meta-analysis. Medicine (Baltimore). 2016;95(19):e3677.
28. Maraka S, Ospina NM, O'Keeffe DT, Espinosa De Ycaza AE, Gionfriddo MR, Erwin PJ, Coddington CC 3rd, Stan MN, Murad MH, Montori VM. Subclinical hypothyroidism in pregnancy: a systematic review and meta-analysis. Thyroid. 2016;26(4):580–90.
29. Zhang Y, Wang H, Pan X, Teng W, Shan Z. Patients with subclinical hypothyroidism before 20 weeks of pregnancy have a higher risk of miscarriage: a systematic review and meta-analysis. PLoS One. 2017;12(4):e0175708.
30. Klein RZ, Sargent JD, Larsen PR, Waisbren SE, Haddow JE, Mitchell ML. Relation of severity of maternal hypothyroidism to cognitive development of offspring. J Med Screen. 2001;8(1):18–20.
31. Li Y, Shan Z, Teng W, Yu X, Li Y, Fan C, Teng X, Guo R, Wang H, Li J, Chen Y, Wang W, Chawinga M, Zhang L, Yang L, Zhao Y, Hua T. Abnormalities of maternal thyroid function during pregnancy affect neuropsychological development of their children at 25–30 months. Clin Endocrinol. 2010;72(6):825–9.
32. Su PY, Huang K, Hao JH, Xu YQ, Yan SQ, Li T, Xu YH, Tao FB. Maternal thyroid function in the first twenty weeks of pregnancy and subsequent fetal and infant development: a prospective population-based cohort study in China. J Clin Endocrinol Metab. 2011;96(10):3234–41.
33. Smit BJ, Kok JH, Vulsma T, Briët JM, Boer K, Wiersinga WM. Neurologic development of the newborn and young child in relation to maternal thyroid function. Acta Paediatr. 2000;89(3):291–5.
34. Henrichs J, Bongers-Schokking JJ, Schenk JJ, Ghassabian A, Schmidt HG, Visser TJ, Hooijkaas H, de Muinck Keizer-Schrama SM, Hofman A, Jaddoe VV, Visser W, Steegers EA, Verhulst FC, de Rijke YB, Tiemeier H. Maternal thyroid function during early pregnancy and cognitive functioning in early childhood: the generation R study. J Clin Endocrinol Metab. 2010;95(9):4227–34.
35. Oken E, Braverman LE, Platek D, Mitchell ML, Lee SL, Pearce EN. Neonatal thyroxine, maternal thyroid function, and child cognition. J Clin Endocrinol Metab. 2009;94(2):497–503.
36. Maraka S, Mwangi R, McCoy RG, Yao X, Sangaralingham LR, Singh Ospina NM, O'Keeffe DT, De Ycaza AE, Rodriguez-Gutierrez R, Coddington CC 3rd, Stan MN, Brito JP, Montori VM. Thyroid hormone treatment among pregnant women with subclinical hypothyroidism: US national assessment. BMJ. 2017;356:i6865.
37. Negro R, Schwartz A, Gismondi R, Tinelli A, Mangieri T, Stagnaro-Green A. Universal screening versus case finding for detection and treatment of thyroid hormonal dysfunction during pregnancy. J Clin Endocrinol Metab. 2010;95(4):1699–707.

38. Nazarpour S, Ramezani Tehrani F, Simbar M, Tohidi M, Alavi Majd H, Azizi F. Effects of levothyroxine treatment on pregnancy outcomes in pregnant women with autoimmune thyroid disease. Eur J Endocrinol. 2017;176(2):253–65.
39. Lazarus JH, Bestwick JP, Channon S, Paradice R, Maina A, Rees R, Chiusano E, John R, Guaraldo V, George LM, Perona M, Dall'Amico D, Parkes AB, Joomun M, Wald NJ. Antenatal thyroid screening and childhood cognitive function. N Engl J Med. 2012;366(6):493–501.
40. Casey BM, Thom EA, Peaceman AM, Varner MW, Sorokin Y, Hirtz DG, Reddy UM, Wapner RJ, Thorp JM Jr, Saade G, Tita AT, Rouse DJ, Sibai B, Iams JD, Mercer BM, Tolosa J, Caritis SN, Van Dorsten JP, Eunice Kennedy Shriver National Institute of Child Health and Human Development Maternal–Fetal Medicine Units Network. Treatment of subclinical hypothyroidism or hypothyroxinemia in pregnancy. N Engl J Med. 2017;376(9):815–25.
41. ACOG. Practice Bulletin Number 148: thyroid disease in pregnancy, April 2015. Obstet Gynecol. 2015;125:996–1005.
42. Lazarus J, Brown RS, Daumerie C, Hubalewska-Dydejczyk A, Negro R, Vaidya B. 2014 European thyroid association guidelines for the management of subclinical hypothyroidism in pregnancy and in children. Eur Thyroid J. 2014;3(2):76–94.
43. Casey BM, Dashe JS, Spong CY, McIntire DD, Leveno KJ, Cunningham GF. Perinatal significance of isolated maternal hypothyroxinemia identified in the first half of pregnancy. Obstet Gynecol. 2007;109(5):1129–35.
44. Korevaar TI, Schalekamp-Timmermans S, de Rijke YB, Visser WE, Visser W, de Muinck Keizer-Schrama SM, Hofman A, Ross HA, Hooijkaas H, Tiemeier H, Bongers-Schokking JJ, Jaddoe VW, Visser TJ, Steegers EA, Medici M, Peeters RP. Hypothyroxinemia and TPO-antibody positivity are risk factors for premature delivery: the Generation R study. J Clin Endocrinol Metab. 2013;98(11):4382–90.
45. Medici M, Timmermans S, Visser W, de Muinck Keizer-Schrama SM, Jaddoe VW, Hofman A, Hooijkaas H, de Rijke YB, Tiemeier H, Bongers-Schokking JJ, Visser TJ, Peeters RP, Steegers EA. Maternal thyroid hormone parameters during early pregnancy and birth weight: the Generation R Study. J Clin Endocrinol Metab. 2013;98(1):59–66.
46. León G, Murcia M, Rebagliato M, Álvarez-Pedrerol M, Castilla AM, Basterrechea M, Iñiguez C, Fernández-Somoano A, Blarduni E, Foradada CM, Tardón A, Vioque J. Maternal thyroid dysfunction during gestation, preterm delivery, and birthweight. The Infancia y Medio Ambiente Cohort, Spain. Paediatr Perinat Epidemiol. 2015;29(2):113–22.
47. Pop VJ, Brouwers EP, Vader HL, Vulsma T, van Baar AL, de Vijlder JJ. Maternal hypothyroxinaemia during early pregnancy and subsequent child development: a 3-year follow-up study. Clin Endocrinol. 2003;59(3):282–8.
48. Ghassabian A, El Marroun H, Peeters RP, Jaddoe VW, Hofman A, Verhulst FC, Tiemeier H, White T. Downstream effects of maternal hypothyroxinemia in early pregnancy: nonverbal IQ and brain morphology in school-age children. J Clin Endocrinol Metab. 2014;99(7):2383–90.
49. Korevaar TI, Muetzel R, Medici M, Chaker L, Jaddoe VW, de Rijke YB, Steegers EA, Visser TJ, White T, Tiemeier H, Peeters RP. Association of maternal thyroid function during early pregnancy with offspring IQ and brain morphology in childhood: a population-based prospective cohort study. Lancet Diabetes Endocrinol. 2016;4(1):35–43.
50. Suárez-Rodríguez M, Azcona-San Julián C, Alzina de Aguilar V. Hypothyroxinemia during pregnancy: the effect on neurodevelopment in the child. Int J Dev Neurosci. 2012;30(6):435–8.
51. Craig WY, Allan WC, Kloza EM, Pulkkinen AJ, Waisbren S, Spratt DI, Palomaki GE, Neveux LM, Haddow JE. Mid-gestational maternal free thyroxine concentration and offspring neurocognitive development at age two years. J Clin Endocrinol Metab. 2012;97(1):E22–8.
52. Chevrier J, Harley KG, Kogut K, Holland N, Johnson C, Eskenazi B. Maternal thyroid function during the second half of pregnancy and child neurodevelopment at 6, 12, 24, and 60 months of age. J Thyroid Res. 2011;2011:426427.
53. Grau G, Aguayo A, Vela A, Aniel-Quiroga A, Espada M, Miranda G, Martinez-Indart L, Martul P, Castaño L, Rica I. Normal intellectual development in children born from women with hypothyroxinemia during their pregnancy. J Trace Elem Med Biol. 2015;31:18–24.

54. Modesto T, Tiemeier H, Peeters RP, Jaddoe VW, Hofman A, Verhulst FC, Ghassabian A. Maternal mild thyroid hormone insufficiency in early pregnancy and attention-deficit/hyperactivity disorder symptoms in children. JAMA Pediatr. 2015;169(9):838–45.
55. Oostenbroek MHW, Kersten RHJ, Tros B, Kunst AE, Vrijkotte TGM, Finken MJJ. Maternal hypothyroxinaemia in early pregnancy and problem behavior in 5-year-old offspring. Psychoneuroendocrinology. 2017;81:29–35.
56. Román GC, Ghassabian A, Bongers-Schokking JJ, Jaddoe VW, Hofman A, de Rijke YB, Verhulst FC, Tiemeier H. Association of gestational maternal hypothyroxinemia and increased autism risk. Ann Neurol. 2013;74(5):733–42.
57. Gyllenberg D, Sourander A, Surcel HM, Hinkka-Yli-Salomäki S, McKeague IW, Brown AS. Hypothyroxinemia during gestation and offspring schizophrenia in a national birth cohort. Biol Psychiatry. 2016;79(12):962–70.
58. Lee RH, Spencer CA, Mestman JH, Miller EA, Petrovic I, Braverman LE, Goodwin TM. Free T4 immunoassays are flawed during pregnancy. Am J Obstet Gynecol. 2009;200(3):260.e1–6.
59. Calvo RM, Jauniaux E, Gulbis B, Asunción M, Gervy C, Contempré B, Morreale de Escobar G. Fetal tissues are exposed to biologically relevant free thyroxine concentrations during early phases of development. J Clin Endocrinol Metab. 2002;87(4):1768–77.
60. Taylor PN, Minassian C, Rehman A, Iqbal A, Draman MS, Hamilton W, Dunlop D, Robinson A, Vaidya B, Lazarus JH, Thomas S, Dayan CM, Okosieme OE. TSH levels and risk of miscarriage in women on long-term levothyroxine: a community-based study. J Clin Endocrinol Metab. 2014;99(10):3895–902.
61. Mandel SJ, Larsen PR, Seely EW, Brent GA. Increased need for thyroxine during pregnancy in women with primary hypothyroidism. N Engl J Med. 1990;323(2):91–6.
62. Alexander EK, Marqusee E, Lawrence J, Jarolim P, Fischer GA, Larsen PR. Timing and magnitude of increases in levothyroxine requirements during pregnancy in women with hypothyroidism. N Engl J Med. 2004;351(3):241–9.
63. Loh JA, Wartofsky L, Jonklaas J, Burman KD. The magnitude of increased levothyroxine requirements in hypothyroid pregnant women depends upon the etiology of the hypothyroidism. Thyroid. 2009;19(3):269–75.
64. Yassa L, Marqusee E, Fawcett R, Alexander EK. Thyroid hormone early adjustment in pregnancy (the THERAPY) trial. J Clin Endocrinol Metab. 2010;95(7):3234–41.
65. Cooper DS, Pearce EN. Subclinical hypothyroidism and hypothyroxinemia in pregnancy – still no answers. N Engl J Med. 2017;376(9):876–7.

Chapter 7
Thyrotoxicosis in Pregnancy

Wilburn D. Bolton III and Jennifer M. Perkins

Clinical Case

A 25-year-old G2P1 female is referred to endocrinology for abnormal thyroid levels in pregnancy. She is currently 13 weeks gestational age. Upon review of records, her TSH (thyroid-stimulating hormone) was 0.1 mIU/L about 4 weeks prior with a free T4 within normal reference range at the upper range of normal. She denies a history of known thyroid disease and had no known thyroid problems in her first pregnancy. She denies recent iodine exposure, thyroid pain, or recent viral illness. She has had a confirmed viable singleton intrauterine pregnancy at her obstetrician's office via ultrasound. Upon interview, she denies weight loss, diarrhea, or tremor. She has noted some heat intolerance, racing heart, and insomnia. She is taking only a prenatal vitamin. She does not use tobacco products and does not drink alcohol. She reports her mother has Hashimoto's thyroiditis and takes levothyroxine supplementation. She has no other family history of thyroid disease.

Upon examination, her heart rate is 102 beats per minute. Her blood pressure is normal at 112/72 mmHG. She weighs 134 pounds and is five feet, three inches tall. Her temperature is normal. She has no obvious exophthalmos, lid lag, stare, scleral injection, or chemosis. Her skin is mildly warm and a bit smooth but dry. No tremor of the outstretched hands is noted and her reflexes are normal with a normal relaxation phase. Abdomen is soft non-tender and non-distended. Normal bowel sounds are appreciated. Her hair has a normal distribution and there are no skin rashes. Her thyroid is about 20% above normal size, smooth, and without masses or bruit. What is your differential diagnosis? What tests will you order?

W. D. Bolton III · J. M. Perkins (✉)
Duke University Medical Center, Division of Endocrinology, Metabolism, and Nutrition, Department of Medicine, Durham, NC, USA
e-mail: jen.perkins@duke.edu

Introduction and Epidemiology

Thyroid disorders constitute one of the most common endocrine disorders in pregnancy [1] and occur in about 4% of all pregnancies, with primary hypothyroidism being the most common [2]. Hyperthyroidism in women of reproductive age is most often due to Graves' disease, an autoimmune disorder in which antibodies are formed against the TSH receptor. Graves' disease has an incidence of roughly 55–80 cases per 100,000 per year in women older than 30 years. In women aged 20–29 years, the incidence is 35–50 cases per 100,000 per year; for women younger than 20 years, the incidence is much lower [3, 4] Other rarer causes of hyperthyroidism in pregnancy include toxic nodular goiter comprised of an autonomously functioning nodule or nodules, but this is uncommon in women <40 years of age (<1–2 cases per 100,000 year) [4]. Of note, toxic nodular goiter is more prevalent in areas of dietary iodine deficiency [5].

Multiple studies have utilized the Danish National Birth Cohort to examine the prevalence of thyroid disease in pregnancy [6, 7]. In one study, the reported prevalence of hyperthyroidism in pregnancy was 1.6%, whereby 0.8% of the population was diagnosed prior to pregnancy, 0.04% in early pregnancy, 0.02% in late pregnancy, and 0.7% after pregnancy [6]. These authors also concluded that in general, women with thyroid disease were older with a higher parity. Additional risk factors for hyperthyroidism included smoking during pregnancy and moderate iodine deficiency. Prepregnancy alcohol intake had a protective effect [6]. Another study reported a prevalence of hyperthyroidism of 0.9% at a median age of 31.9 years (interquartile range of 27.7–36.1 years) [7]. The incidence rate of hyperthyroidism in and around pregnancy was high in the first trimester of pregnancy, very low in the third trimester, and highest at 7–9 months postpartum [7].

It is also important to consider that detection of underlying hyperthyroidism, either subclinical or overt, is more likely to occur in early pregnancy when clinical symptoms emerge due to thyroid stimulation by hCG. Most commonly, emesis leads to first-time thyroid function testing. Gestational transient thyrotoxicosis, caused by elevated serum hCG concentrations, is most often observed in women with hyperemesis gravidarum, as discussed later [8].

Maternal and Fetal Effects of Thyrotoxicosis

Untreated thyrotoxicosis in pregnancy can have severe consequences for the pregnant female and the fetus [8]. For example, pregnant women are at increased risk of developing heart failure due to thyrotoxicosis. Excessive thyroid hormone levels increase cardiac contractility indirectly, by diminishing systemic vascular resistance with resultant increased heart rate and cardiac output. Without intervention, these two mechanisms can result in increased left ventricular mass and a high-output state [9]. In turn, this baseline high-output state can result in heart failure due to increased cardiac burden. Nonpregnant patients with overt thyrotoxicosis rarely develop heart failure [10], but by contrast, nearly 10% of women with untreated thyrotoxicosis develop heart failure during pregnancy [11].

Sheffield and Cunningham identified 13 cases of high-output heart failure in 150 hyperthyroid pregnant women [12]. All 13 women were either noncompliant with their antithyroidal therapy or had no medical care during pregnancy. Six of the 13 women had heart failure prior to fetal viability and decompensation was precipitated by either hemorrhage, sepsis, or both. The remaining seven women were in their final trimester when the heart failure developed. Four of the seven were precipitated by severe preeclampsia or eclampsia; two were precipitated by sepsis [12].

Obstetrical complications are also more common among women with thyrotoxicosis. Several studies have shown that poorly controlled thyrotoxicosis during pregnancy is associated with an increased risk of miscarriage, stillbirth, gestational hypertension, preeclampsia, preterm birth, IUGR, and thyroid storm [13, 14]. A retrospective study of 223,512 pregnant women found that hyperthyroidism was associated with increased odds of induction, but not of cesarean section [14]. It was also associated with a 1.8-fold odds of preeclampsia, 3.6-fold odds of superimposed preeclampsia, 3.7-fold odds of intensive care unit admission, and 2.1- and 1.8-fold odds of threatened and observed preterm birth, respectively [14].

Some studies have reported that obstetric outcomes are directly related to control of hyperthyroidism and duration of euthyroidism in pregnancy [13, 15]. Aggarawal and colleagues conducted a retrospective study over 28 years of 208 hyperthyroid pregnant women compared to 403 healthy controls [16]. Women with hyperthyroidism were at increased risk of preeclampsia (odds ratio (OR): 3.94), spontaneous preterm labor (OR: 1.73), preterm birth (OR: 1.7), gestational diabetes mellitus (OR: 1.8), and cesarean delivery (OR: 1.47). They also found that hyperthyroid women required induction of labor more frequently (OR: 3.61). Outcomes were worsened by uncontrolled disease [16]. Compared to women with controlled hyperthyroidism, women with uncontrolled hyperthyroidism had a significantly increased incidence of preterm birth (49 vs 23%), preterm labor (42% vs 20%), and abruption placentae (6.7 vs 0%) [16]. The authors also compared outcomes between women with pregestational hyperthyroidism and those diagnosed during pregnancy. Overall, the incidence of obstetrical complications was similar between groups (65.1% vs 63.6%, $p = 0.89$). However, women diagnosed during pregnancy had increased risks of intrauterine growth restriction and abruptio placentae [16].

Additional adverse outcomes associated with hyperthyroidism include intrauterine growth restriction (IUGR), low birth weight, neurocognitive development, and fetal thyrotoxicosis/Graves' disease as well as fetal goiter [17, 18]. In the aforementioned study by Aggarawal, women with hyperthyroidism had 2.16 times the odds of intrauterine growth restriction compared to the control group [16]. The mean birth weight of the newborns born to hyperthyroid mothers was significantly lower than controls (2.5 vs 2.7 kg, $p = 0.0001$) [16]. Additionally, the risk of IUGR was higher in women diagnosed with hyperthyroidism during pregnancy than in those diagnosed before pregnancy (OR: 2.75). The authors also showed that poorly controlled disease increased the rate of IUGR (38% with poorly controlled hyperthyroidism vs 21.5% in women with adequate control) [16].

Finally, hyperthyroidism may also influence neurocognitive development [19]. In a population-based prospective cohort study of 7069 women, the authors demonstrated that both low and high maternal free thyroxine concentrations were associated with lower child IQ, lower gray matter, and cortex volume. The mean point reduction in child IQ was 1.4–3.8 points [20].

Special Considerations for the Fetus and Neonate in Graves' Disease: Evaluating TSH Receptor Antibody Status

Neonates born to mothers with active or treated Graves' disease are at risk for significant morbidity and mortality. The causative antibody in Graves' disease belongs to the immunoglobulin G class and freely crosses the placenta, particularly during the second half of pregnancy [21]. Placental transfer of the stimulating TSH receptor antibody (TRAb) to the fetus can lead to in utero or postnatal hyperthyroidism and goiter [22]. When fetal hyperthyroidism develops, it most commonly does so in the third trimester and can cause fetal tachycardia, heart failure, nonimmune hydrops, IUGR, preterm birth, advanced skeletal maturation, and craniosynostosis [23]. Signs and symptoms of neonatal Graves' disease can vary and may include goiter with tracheal compression, stare, ophthalmological findings, hyperthermia, irritability, heart failure, hepatomegaly, splenomegaly, tachycardia, and others [15]. Additionally, development of fetal hyper- or hypothyroidism, as well as neonatal hyper- or hypothyroidism, can occur [17]. Without proper recognition and therapy, mortality may reach 20% [24]. Given this, consensus guidelines from the American Thyroid Association (ATA) and Endocrine Society recommend determining maternal TRAb levels in women with active or a past history of Graves' disease or a previous infant affected by neonatal Graves' disease [17, 25]. If the patient has a past history of Graves' disease treated with ablation, medical therapy, or surgery, a maternal serum TRAb is recommended at initial thyroid testing in early pregnancy. If the maternal TRAb level is elevated in early pregnancy, repeat testing should be undertaken between weeks 18–22. If maternal TRAb is undetectable or low in early pregnancy, then no further TRAb testing is needed [17].

In contrast, if a patient is taking antithyroidal agents for Graves' disease when pregnancy is confirmed, a maternal serum TRAb should be obtained at baseline and again at 18–22 weeks gestation. If TRAbs are elevated at weeks 18–22 or the mother is taking antithyroidals in the third trimester, a TRAb measurement should again be performed in late pregnancy (30–34 weeks) to evaluate the need for neonatal and postnatal monitoring [17].

Per the American Thyroid Association guidelines, fetal surveillance should be performed in women who have uncontrolled hyperthyroidism in the second half of pregnancy or in women with TRAb levels detected at any time during pregnancy (greater than 3 times the upper limit of normal). A consultation with an experienced obstetrician or maternal-fetal medicine specialist is recommended. Monitoring may include ultrasound to assess heart rate, volume of amniotic fluid, and for fetal goiter, which could precipitate the need for cesarean delivery to avoid asphyxiation in the birth canal [17]. Cordocentesis is not routinely recommended but should be used in rare circumstances such as when there is fetal goiter present in women taking antithyroidals [17].

Diagnostic Evaluation

The diagnosis of thyrotoxicosis in pregnancy requires knowledge of both clinical signs and symptoms of thyrotoxicosis as well as the expected changes in thyroid hormone levels with pregnancy. The vast majority of cases of endogenous hyperthyroidism in pregnancy are due to one of two conditions, gestational transient thyrotoxicosis and Graves' disease. Other causes of thyrotoxicosis in pregnancy are rare (Box 7.1).

Box 7.1 Differential Diagnosis of Hyperthyroidism in Pregnancy
Disorders of Excessive TSH Receptor Stimulation

- Graves' disease via TSH receptor autoantibodies
- Gestational transient thyrotoxicosis (hCG induced)
- Familial gestational hyperthyroidism (TSH receptor mutation) *rare
- Trophoblastic disease (hCG induced)
- TSH-producing pituitary adenoma

Disorders of Autonomous Thyroid Hormone Secretion

- Toxic adenoma or toxic multinodular goiter
- Activating TSH receptor mutation

Extrathyroidal Sources of Thyroid Hormone

- Overtreatment with thyroid hormone
- Factitious intake of thyroid hormone
- Functioning struma ovarii
- Functional thyroid cancer metastases

Destruction of Thyroid Follicles with Subsequent Release of Preformed Thyroid Hormone

- Subacute thyroiditis
- Painless thyroiditis
- Acute thyroiditis

Adapted with permission of Elsevier from Cooper and Laurberg [70]

Hyperthyroidism is divided into overt or subclinical, depending on the biochemical severity of the hyperthyroidism. Overt hyperthyroidism is defined as a subnormal serum thyrotropin (TSH) with elevated serum levels of thyroid hormone. Subclinical hyperthyroidism is defined as a low or undetectable serum TSH with hormonal values within the normal reference range [26].

Initial Evaluation of a Suppressed TSH in Pregnancy

A normal pregnancy is associated with a number of physiological changes in the thyroid axis. Knowledge of these changes is essential to accurately interpreting thyroid test results. When evaluating a pregnant patient for thyrotoxicosis, it is important to recognize that the standard values of TSH are shifted downward in pregnancy. While there are numerous studies establishing normative values for TSH in pregnancy, we will highlight just a few. In a study of 1126 Caucasian women with viable pregnancies, the first trimester 5th percentile TSH was 0.1 mIU/L and the second trimester was 0.39 mIU/L [27]. Another study assessed gestational age-specific TSH levels in 4800 healthy Chinese women between 7 and 12 weeks gestation [28]. In that study, the 2.5 percentile was 0.1mIU/L, and the 98th percentile was 4 mIU/L. When TSH ranges were stratified by gestational week, TSH values were lowest in week 10 where the 2.5 percentile for TSH was between 0.02 and 0.06mIU/L. These lower values correspond with the peak hCG levels that occur between weeks 8–11 [28].

The American Thyroid Association recommends the use of population- and trimester-specific TSH reference ranges. In the absence of these, however, the lower reference limit for TSH can be reduced by 0.4 mU/L in the first trimester and the upper reference limit can be reduced by approximately 0.5 mU/L. Of the 19 studies included in the ATA guideline, the first trimester TSH lower limit was 0.02–0.41 with 17/19 studies demonstrating a TSH lower limit of 0.2 mU/L or less and 11 of 19 studies with a TSH limit of 0.1 mU/L or less [17].

As discussed in Chap. 4, the decrease in the lower reference limit of TSH in the first trimester is due to human chorionic gonadotropin, which is structurally similar to TSH and is weakly capable of stimulating the TSH receptor, leading to reduced TSH levels [29] (Fig. 7.1).

In contrast to TSH, thyroxine-binding globulin (TBG) levels increase during pregnancy and peak at approximately 16–20 weeks. With the rise in TBG, total hormone levels also increase [30]. TBG has a 20-fold greater affinity for T4 than T3, so the rise in T4 parallels the rise in TBG more closely [30]. The magnitude of the increase in TBG is greater than the increase in T4, resulting in a progressively decreasing T4/TBG ratio. This leads to a 10–15% decrease in free hormone values in the latter part of pregnancy [31].

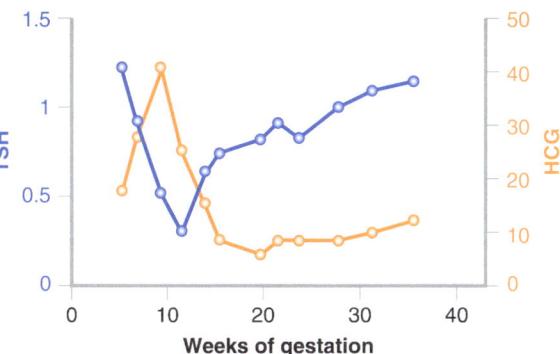

Fig. 7.1 Relationship between hCG and TSH in early pregnancy. (Reproduced with permission of Oxford University Press from Glinoer and de Nayer [71])

Determination of Maternal Thyroid Hormone Levels

An abnormal TSH level warrants measurement of maternal thyroid hormone levels. As discussed in earlier chapters, thyroid hormones (T4 and T3) are carried in the bloodstream by three different serum proteins: thyroid-binding globulin, transthyretin, and albumin. Free hormones are those that are unbound from any transport proteins, and it is these that are biologically active. However, the free component is a tiny fraction of the total hormone stores, representing just 0.4% of the total T4 and 0.5% of T3 [30]. In pregnancy, thyroid hormone levels are typically assessed with total hormone levels (total T4) and a calculation known as the free T4 index (FT4I) to derive estimated free hormone levels. Alternatively, the free hormones themselves are measured directly. There is debate over whether it is better to use free T4 (FT4) or TT4/FT4I in pregnancy. This is because the automated immunoassays used by most laboratories can be affected by the rise in TBG and decrease in albumin in pregnancy. Measurement techniques such as equilibrium dialysis and ultrafiltration are not influenced by changes in binding protein concentrations, but they are time-consuming, not widely available, and expensive. Free T4 immunoassays tend to show a reduction in FT4 values in the third trimester that is greater than is seen with more precise methods [17].

The concerns over the use of FT4 are highlighted by Lee and colleagues, who compared TT4 and FT4 index values versus two currently available FT4 commercial assays. The investigators reported that no patient in the study was found to be hypothyroxinemic with the use of TT4 or FT4I; however, when the same samples were run on the automated FT4 assays, between 57 and 67% of subjects were found to have FT4 values below the manufacturer's lower reference limit. Given the good correlation of TT4 and FT4I, they recommended against commonly used FT4 assays in pregnancy [32].

In contrast, others have argued that FT4 more accurately reflects thyroid status than TT4. In one study, FT4 correlated much better with change in the hypothalamic-pituitary-thyroid (HPT) axis than TT4. Moreover, TT4 had no correlation with adverse pregnancy or child outcomes while the FT4 did [33]. Finally, an analysis of over 17,000 women demonstrated that FT4 had a higher sensitivity than total T4 in identifying adverse outcomes associated with the diagnosis of subclinical hypothyroidism [34].

The European Thyroid Association states that either the FT4 or TT4 can be used to assess maternal thyroid hormone content [35]. The American Thyroid Association suggests that if FT4 assays are used in pregnancy, trimester-specific reference ranges for the assay must be utilized. Next, they recommend that TT4 be used as the standard in the last half of pregnancy [17]. Following week 16 of gestation, the total T4 should be about 1.5 times the upper reference range due to elevated thyroid-binding globulin [17].

Etiologies of Thyrotoxicosis in Pregnancy

The main two conditions in the differential diagnosis are gestational transient thyrotoxicosis (GTT), which is seen in first half of pregnancy, and Graves' disease. Other less common etiologies include toxic adenoma, multinodular goiter, or thyroiditis. If a cause of thyrotoxicosis other than GTT is suspected, TRAb levels, thyroid ultrasonography, or the TT3/TT4 ratio may be helpful. The TT3/TT4 ratio is typically >20 in cases of overproduction such as Graves' disease and <20 in cases such as thyroiditis. Thyroid ultrasonography has not been shown to be helpful in differentiating Graves' disease from GTT but is indicated if the physical exam suggests thyroid nodules. Of note, the thyroid gland increases in size by about 30% between the first and third trimester [36]. The differences between GTT and Graves' disease are detailed below.

Gestational Transient Thyrotoxicosis (GTT)

While this is the most current nomenclature, differing terms have been used to describe this phenomenon: transient non-autoimmune hyperthyroidism of early pregnancy or transient hyperthyroidism of hyperemesis gravidarum. The clinical features of GTT are biochemical hyperthyroidism that is self-limited, without evidence of thyroid autoimmunity, diagnosed in the first trimester of pregnancy, typically associated with vomiting. It is caused by the stimulating effect of high concentrations of human chorionic gonadotropin (hCG) on the TSH receptor during the first trimester. Gestational transient thyrotoxicosis is thought to have an incidence of 2–3% of all pregnancies but has been reported to be as high as 5.5% in Japan and 11% in Singapore [37]. It is seen most commonly in women diagnosed with hyperemesis gravidarum, in whom transient hyperthyroidism is seen in up to 67% [38]. Familial gestational hyperthyroidism is due to rare variants of the TSH receptor that are very sensitive to hCG and have been reported to cause hyperthyroidism in pregnancy in the absence of hyperemesis gravidarum [17].

Clues from the patient's clinical history that favor GTT over Graves' disease are as follows: no symptoms of hyperthyroidism prior to pregnancy, symptom onset in the first trimester, no family history of Graves' disease, minimal or absent signs of hyperthyroidism, hyperemesis, similar vomiting in prior pregnancy, and a family history of hyperemesis gravidarum. During the physical exam, there is no evidence of ophthalmopathy, dermopathy (pretibial myxedema), goiter, or Graves' acropachy. Biochemically, GTT is associated with a low or suppressed TSH, elevated free T4 or TT4/FT4I, negative antibodies for thyroid autoimmunity (TRAb and TPO), and a TT3/TT4 ratio of <20 [8, 38].

In a prospective observational study of 87 women admitted with hyperemesis gravidarum, 53 (61%) were diagnosed with hyperthyroidism defined as a TSH less than 0.1 mU/L and a free T4 > 26 pmol/L. Nine of these women were excluded due to incomplete follow-up, leaving 44 patients for evaluation. Five of these 44 women were subsequently diagnosed with Graves' disease [38].

Gestational transient thyrotoxicosis and subclinical hyperthyroidism are not associated with adverse pregnancy [39] outcomes; therefore, supportive care is all that is typically needed. As it is a self-limited condition, the risk of birth defects due to antithyroidal drugs outweighs the clinical benefits. Short courses of beta-blockers can be used for symptomatic relief if needed [17]. Generally, beta-blockers are regarded as safe in pregnancy although long-term use has been associated with low birth weight [8]. As with many drugs in used in pregnancy, these drugs should be discontinued as soon as they are no longer needed. It is reasonable to repeat thyroid levels in 4 weeks.

Graves' Disease (GD)

Graves' disease is the most common cause of hyperthyroidism in all populations, with the highest incidence seen in women between 40–60 years of age [40]. The immunopathogenesis is related to TSH receptor antibodies (TRAb) that lead to continuous stimulation of thyroid hormone production. Graves' disease in pregnancy can be divided into two categories: Graves' disease diagnosed during pregnancy and Graves' disease diagnosed before pregnancy, with the latter being the far more common. Graves' disease during pregnancy may be missed due to symptomatic overlap with normal pregnancy-related changes [8, 30]. The course of hyperthyroidism due to Graves' disease tends to improve during pregnancy because of three independent factors: (1) immunosuppression related to pregnancy tends to decrease production of TRAbs; (2) increased TBG and reduced free thyroid hormone concentrations tend to blunt the effect of excessive thyroid hormone production; and (3) in iodine restricted areas, increased iodine demand along with decreased supply blunts excessive production. This being said, not everyone is protected from hyperthyroidism by these changes [30].

Table 7.1 Differentiating between gestational transient thyrotoxicosis and Graves' hyperthyroidism

Graves' hyperthyroidism	Gestational transient thyrotoxicosis
Family history might be present	No suggestive family history
Diagnosed anytime in pregnancy, typically in the first trimester	Diagnosis in the first trimester
Symptoms prior to pregnancy	No prior symptoms before pregnancy
No relation to hyperemesis or multiple gestation	Seen more commonly in hyperemesis and multiple gestation pregnancy
Clinical findings suggestive of Graves' orbitopathy, diffuse goiter, dermopathy	No Graves' associated manifestations
Any grade of hyperthyroidism present	Minimal or lack of signs of hyperthyroidism
Likely to have positive thyroid antibodies	Negative thyroid antibodies
Course of disease unpredictable	Usually a self-limited course

Adapted with permission of Elsevier from Cooper and Laurberg [70]

In differentiating Graves' disease from GTT or other causes of hyperthyroidism, the history and physical exam can be especially helpful. The clinical features unique to Graves' disease include ophthalmopathy, dermopathy, and acropachy [41]. Graves' ophthalmopathy includes both eyelid lag and retraction, proptosis, double vision due to extraocular muscle dysfunction, periorbital edema, chemosis, scleral injection, exposure keratitis, and optic neuropathy. About 50% of patients with Graves' disease report symptoms of ophthalmopathy, but only 3–5% of patients with ophthalmopathy have severe disease. Of note, mild lid lag due to sympathetic stimulation of the levator palpebrae may occur in hyperthyroidism of other causes as well. Thyroid dermopathy is seen in only a small proportion of patients with Graves' disease (1–4%) and is mostly seen in those with concomitant ophthalmopathy. Graves' acropachy (clubbing) is also typically only seen in those with dermopathy [42, 43].

The other types of hyperthyroidism are extremely rare in pregnancy. Overproduction of thyroid hormone by a single or multiple autonomous thyroid nodules has an incidence of <1–2 case per 100,000 per year and is typically only seen in areas of iodine deficiency or older adults [8]. The management of these conditions is similar to that of Graves' disease as both are overproduction of thyroid hormone. See Table 7.1 for a comparison of Graves' disease and GTT.

Management Options for Patients with Graves' Disease in Pregnancy

For patients with Graves' disease, the three established treatment modalities are antithyroid drugs (methimazole, propylthiouracil), ablation with radioactive iodine, or surgery. During pregnancy, radioactive iodine for treatment or diagnostics is absolutely contraindicated due to its accumulation and damage to the fetal thyroid gland [44]. Antithyroid drugs (ATDs) are used most commonly, with surgery being reserved for special cases which will be reviewed in detail later in the chapter.

Antithyroid Drugs

The antithyroidal drugs (ATDs), methimazole (MMI), its prodrug carbimazole, and propylthiouracil (PTU) are the primary drugs for the management of Graves' disease in pregnancy. In a nonpregnant patient, methimazole is preferred because it has a lower risk of hepatotoxicity and the convenience of once or twice daily dosing versus three times daily for PTU. Both methimazole and PTU work by inhibiting the oxidation and organic binding of thyroid iodide, leading to an intrathyroidal iodine deficiency and decreasing output of thyroid hormone. PTU also has the ability to block type 1 deiodinase (D1) which is the major source of peripheral conversion of T4 to T3.

While these medications are generally well tolerated, they do have the potential for both minor and major side effects. The minor side effects occur in 5–10% of patients in the first few weeks of therapy and include rash, pruritus, nausea, and fever [8]. Patients with a mild rash may experience resolution with continuation of therapy or an antihistamine, but others will require discontinuation of the drug. Unfortunately, 30–50% of patients with a rash or pruritus from MMI will have a similar reaction to PTU [45].

The two most serious side effects – agranulocytosis and hepatotoxicity – are quite rare. Each patient prescribed these medications should be informed about the typical presentations of these conditions and when to call or seek help. The most common symptoms of agranulocytosis are fever and sore throat. Patients who develop these symptoms should be clearly instructed to stop the medication and seek medical attention urgently, as agranulocytosis can be life-threatening. While dangerous, this adverse drug reaction is quite rare. In a large retrospective cohort analysis of over 50,000 Japanese patients with Graves' disease, there were only 55 cases of agranulocytosis, yielding an estimated incidence of 0.3% at 100 days. 77.7% of these patients were administered an ATD, predominantly methimazole [46]. Another retrospective cohort analysis of 30,798 patients with Graves' disease reported agranulocytosis in 0.37% of patients on PTU and 0.35% of patients on MMI [47, 48]. The risk of agranulocytosis with MMI is dose-related. In one study, the incidence was 0.814% with a starting dose of 30 mg, compared to 0.219% with a starting dose of 15 mg [48]. Agranulocytosis associated with PTU, however, is dose independent [49]. In a review of 29,000 patients taking ATDs, the incidence of agranulocytosis was 0.11% with MMI compared to 0.27% with PTU [50].

Hepatotoxicity is another potential serious adverse drug reaction. MMI-associated hepatotoxicity has typically been described as cholestatic but can also be hepatocellular in nature. PTU, on the other hand, can cause fulminant hepatic necrosis that can be fatal or require liver transplantation. The FDA issued a medication alert for this reaction to PTU in 2010 and further review of data noted children to be at higher risk of this reaction. In a review of over 70,000 ATD users in Taiwan, the rates of noninfectious hepatitis were 0.25% for MMI and 0.08% for PTU. The rates of liver failure, however, were higher with PTU than with MMI, 0.048% vs 0.026%, respectively [51]. Another review over 29,000 individuals reported that liver failure rates were 0.03% with MMI and 0.05% with PTU [50].

Because Graves' disease is associated with leukopenia and elevated liver enzymes, a complete blood count and liver function tests should be obtained before starting ATD therapy. These medications should be avoided when the absolute neutrophil count is less than 1500 or when liver function tests are greater than three times the upper limit of normal [45]. Serious adverse events from MMI/PTU typically occur within 90–120 days of initiating therapy. While many physicians do routinely monitor the complete blood count and liver function, it is not clear that monitoring prevents adverse events [26]. Agranulocytosis generally occurs within the first 90 days of exposure; therefore, this is the period of maximum benefit from monitoring the white blood cell count. Likewise, the benefit of monitoring for hepatotoxicity would be in the first 120 days [26]. The American Thyroid Association and others do recommend obtaining a CBC with any febrile illness and at the onset of pharyngitis in all patients on ATD. They also recommend that liver function and associated enzymes be assessed in any patient with a pruritic rash, jaundice, light-colored stool or dark urine, joint pain, abdominal pain or bloating, anorexia, nausea, or fatigue [17].

The third and least common major side effect of ATDs is antineutrophil cytoplasmic antibody-mediated vasculitis (ANCA). This condition is seen predominantly in Asian patients treated with PTU but can rarely be seen with MMI. It is rare, with an estimated annual incidence between 0.47 and 0.71 patients per 10,000 patients on PTU and between 0.057 and 0.085 patients per 10,000 patients on MMI [52]. The target antigen is typically myeloperoxidase, but it can alternatively be other proteins. The incidence of this condition is higher in children. The clinical features of drug-induced ANCA-positive vasculitis can vary from mild constitutional symptoms such as fatigue, fever, weight loss, and arthralgias to more severe symptoms such as renal dysfunction, ulceration, and upper and lower respiratory tract symptoms including hemorrhage. It typically resolves with drug discontinuation, but sometimes it requires immunosuppressive therapy [53, 54].

Antithyroid Drugs: Special Considerations in Pregnancy

In the pregnant patient, considerations of both maternal health and teratogenicity are taken into consideration in deciding appropriate medications for treatment. PTU is preferred over MMI in the first 16 weeks due to increased risk of birth defects with methimazole, about 1/30 pregnancies exposed during the first trimester. The defects that comprise what is known as methimazole embryopathy include choanal atresia, omphalocele, esophageal atresia, omphalomesenteric duct anomalies, and aplasia cutis [55]. Although lower risk than MMI, PTU has also been linked to birth defects in some studies. For example, a Danish national registry study found the prevalence of birth defects in children exposed to ATD in early pregnancy to be: PTU, 8.0%; MMI, 9.1%; MMI and PTU, 10.1%; no ATD, 5.4%; non-exposed, 5.7%; and P 0.001 [55]. Other studies, however, have not found an association between PTU and birth defects. In a Japanese cohort study by Yoshihara and colleagues, the incidence of birth defects was twice as high for women taking MMI than for those taking PTU or for untreated controls (4.1% vs 1.9% vs 2.1%, respectively) [56]. American Thyroid Association guidelines recommend PTU through 16 weeks' gestation and they cite insufficient evidence to recommend switching back to MMI vs continuing PTU after that time [17].

As previously stated, some studies have shown that PTU also has a recognized risk of birth defects with an incidence of about 1/40 pregnancies. However, the defects with PTU tend to be milder than those seen with methimazole/carbimazole and are primarily head, neck, or urinary anomalies. While milder, many of them still require surgery [57].

Both PTU and MMI are able to cross the placenta and are equally effective at controlling hyperthyroidism. The starting dose of PTI in pregnancy is typically 100–300 mg per day divided into every 8 h doses, while MMI is dosed at 5–30 mg once daily. The goal during pregnancy is to use the lowest dose possible [8]. Due to a decrease in autoimmunity, ATDs can typically be reduced or stopped in many patients in the third trimester.

Other drugs other than ATDs have been used in pregnancy. Prior to the advent of ATDs, iodine was used to treat hyperthyroidism. However, many patients suffered from breakthrough hyperthyroidism on this therapy. A retrospective study from Japan by Yoshihara and colleagues examined outcomes in patients treated with MMI in the first trimester compared to those among patients treated with potassium iodide. They demonstrated a birth defect rate of 4/260 (1.53%) in the iodine group and 47/1134 (4.14%) in the MMI group. The MMI group also had a higher rate of miscarriage [58]. Importantly, however, Japan is a high iodine intake country and results may not be reproducible in other parts of the world. For that reason, the ATA does not recommend this treatment outside of Japan [17].

Given the known risk of birth defects, discontinuation of ATDs is an option for select patients with Graves' disease. Potential candidates for ATD discontinuation are euthyroid on low doses of ATDs (5–10 mg/d of MMI or 100–200 mg/d of PTU) and do not have the following risk factors for relapse: palpable goiter at the time of diagnosis, current smoking, elevated TRAb levels at the time of ATD discontinuation, and duration of treatment <6 months [59]. When the decision is made to stop ATDs, the patient must be monitored closely with TSH and FT4 every 1–2 weeks, which can be extended to 2–4 weeks if thyroid labs are stable. In order to see the benefit, withdrawal of ATDs must occur before the major teratogenic period, which is weeks 6–10 of gestation [17].

Goals of Therapy

In a pregnant patient with hyperthyroidism from Graves' disease, toxic adenoma, or toxic multi-nodular goiter, the goals of treatment are to maintain the safety of the mother and the pregnancy while not inducing fetal hypothyroidism. TRAbs, maternal thyroid hormone, and ATDs are all able to cross the placental barrier and must be accounted for in monitoring the fetus. ATDs used to maintain maternal euthyroidism are often more potent in the fetus than in the mother. This can lead to fetal hypothyroidism in a mother whose hormone levels are rendered normal with ATDs. PTU and MMI have been found to impact the fetal thyroid gland equally [60]. Screening for fetal hypothyroidism found that 25% of cases were due to maternal ingestion of ATDs [60]. In order to avoid fetal hypothyroidism, the goal of therapy for ATDs in pregnancy is to maintain the TT4/FT4 values in the range of high normal or just above the nonpregnant normal range [17, 26, 36]. Overtreatment should be avoided because of risk of fetal hypothyroidism and fetal goiter. Due to decreases in thyroid autoimmunity as pregnancy progresses, discontinuation of ATDs is possible in 20–30% of patients [61]. TT4 or FT4 and TSH should be monitored every 2–4 weeks and 2 weeks after a dose of medication change.

Thyroidectomy is a treatment option for the management of Graves' disease during pregnancy, but it is typically the last resort due to the associated maternal and fetal risks. In a population-based study of pregnant patients undergoing thyroid and parathyroid surgery, the complication rates were higher than for the general population. The fetal and maternal complication rates were 5.5% and 4.5%, respectively, with fetal complications including induced, spontaneous, or missed abortion, early or threatened labor, fetal distress, intrauterine death, stillbirth, neonatal hypocalcemic tetany, and neonatal hypoparathyroidism [19].

Indications for surgery in a pregnant patient with Graves' disease include intolerance of or allergy to ATDs, requirement of large doses of ATDs to control hyperthyroidism (generally 40–60 mg of MMI per day or 800–1200 mg of PTU/day), poor adherence to ATDs [8, 17], or compressive goiter [8]. In a patient intolerant of ATDs, a short course of beta-blockers and potassium iodide (50–100 mg/day) should be given in preparation for surgery. Potassium iodide leads to a decrease in thyroidal iodine uptake, a decrease in iodide oxidation, and organification and blocks the release of thyroid hormone [62]. Surgical complications of thyroidectomy include both transient and permanent hypoparathyroidism, injury to the recurrent laryngeal nerve, and bleeding which can threaten the airway and the patient's life. Lugol's solution has been shown to reduce thyroidal blood flow and intraoperative blood loss prior to surgery [62]. With regard to the risk of pregnancy complications, the optimal time for surgery is during the second trimester.

Considerations in the Postpartum Period

As noted earlier, many women with Graves' disease will go into remission during the course of pregnancy due to a decrease in autoimmunity. These women still need close monitoring, as many have a rebound after pregnancy, during the postpartum period. In a study of 65 women whose ATDs were withdrawn during pregnancy, 71% had a relapse in the first postpartum year versus 29% of those who were continued on low-dose MMI. In another study of 41 pregnancies in 35 women with Graves' disease who had discontinued ATDs in pregnancy, 80% relapsed into hyperthyroidism after pregnancy [63]. For relapsed or newly diagnosed Graves' disease in the postpartum period, ATDs are the first-line therapy. Both PTU and MMI are excreted in the breast milk but in very small quantities. PTU excretion in breast milk is 0.025%, compared to 0.1–0.17% for MMI. Breastfeeding by mothers taking either MMI or PTU has not been shown to cause hypothyroidism or developmental problems in the infant. The goals of treatment in this population are similar to that of the nonpregnant population, with recommended maximum doses of 20 mg MMI and 450/d of PTU. These recommendations are based on trials demonstrating safety for breastfeeding infants [64]. In general, MMI is the preferred agent due to the risk of idiosyncratic hepatic damage with PTU [65].

Preconception Counseling of Women with Preexisting Hyperthyroidism

A large proportion of women with hyperthyroidism, especially Graves' disease, are of reproductive age. Women on methimazole for Graves' disease should be transitioned to PTU before attempting pregnancy and should not switch back to methimazole until at least 16 weeks gestation [17]. Patients undergoing radioactive iodine ablation should wait at least 6 months after treatment before attempting to conceive and should demonstrate stable euthyroidism off or on LT4 therapy. Finally, thyroidectomy can offer the benefit of faster time to definitive therapy and a decrease in maternal TRAbs. Pregnancy after surgery should be delayed at least 3 months to ensure stable euthyroidism before proceeding with surgery [17]. All women with Graves' disease must be followed during pregnancy for the presence of TRaB [17].

Special Therapy Considerations: Thyroid Storm

Thyroid storm is a rare, life-threatening condition that can occur in pregnancy, posing serious risk to the mother or fetus [66]. Moreover, parturition often precipitates thyroid storm. Patients require specific therapy directed against the thyroid but may require supportive therapy in an intensive care unit. Most importantly, prompt recognition is key since the mortality rate of thyroid storm may reach 30% [67]. Therapy options include beta-blockers to control the symptoms of increased adrenergic tone, thionamides to reduce thyroid hormone synthesis, iodine solution to block release of thyroid hormone, and glucocorticoids to reduce T4 to T3 conversion, promote vasomotor stability, and treat any associated relative adrenal insufficiency. Bile acid sequestrants may also be of benefit to decrease enterohepatic recycling of thyroid hormones [26]. The Burch and Wartofsky scoring system can be helpful to differentiate between impending storm versus probable storm. This encompasses heart rate, temperature, hepatic/gastrointestinal dysfunction, neuropsychiatric dysfunction, presence of arrhythmia, and precipitating factors. A score of 45 or greater is consistent with thyroid storm, while a score of less than 25 makes thyroid storm unlikely [68]. In patients with clinical features of thyroid storm or severe thyrotoxicosis who do not meet full criteria for thyroid storm, the recommendation is to begin immediate therapy with a beta-blocker. High-dose propranolol can provide additional T4 to T3 conversion reduction. Typically, 60–80 mg every 4–6 h is the dose required to achieve adequate control of heart rate. Additionally, PTU 200 mg every 4 h or methimazole 20 mg every 4 to 6 h is typically utilized. PTU is favored over MMI due to PTU's ability to decrease T4 to T3 conversion. One hour after the first dose of a thionamide, iodine solution can be administered. Options are the saturated solution of potassium iodide (SSKI), 5 drops orally every 6 h, or Lugol's solution, 10 drops every 8 h. Delaying administration of iodine by 1 h after thionamide prevents the iodine from being used as substrate for new hormone synthesis. If frank thyroid storm is present, hydrocortisone 100 mg every 8 h should be added. Lastly, cholestyramine 4 g orally four times a day may be of benefit as previously mentioned. Besides the above medications, supportive therapy and work-up of any precipitating factors are critical [26, 69].

Clinical Case and Discussion

A 25-year-old G2P1 female is referred to endocrinology for abnormal thyroid levels in pregnancy. She is currently 13 weeks gestational age. Upon review of records, her TSH (thyroid-stimulating hormone) was 0.1 mIU/L about 4 weeks prior with a free T4 within normal reference range at the upper range of normal. She denies a history of known thyroid disease and had no known thyroid problems in her first pregnancy. She denies recent iodine exposure, thyroid pain, or recent viral illness. She has had a confirmed viable singleton intrauterine pregnancy at her obstetrician's office via ultrasound. Upon interview, she denies weight loss, diarrhea, or tremor. She has noted some heat intolerance, racing heart, and insomnia. She is taking only a prenatal vitamin. She does not use tobacco products and does not drink alcohol. She reports her mother has Hashimoto's thyroiditis and takes levothyroxine supplementation. She has no other family history of thyroid disease.

Upon examination, her heart rate is 102 beats per minute. Her blood pressure is normal at 112/72 mmHG. She weighs 134 pounds and is five feet, three inches tall. Her temperature is normal. She has no obvious exophthalmos, lid lag, stare, scleral injection, or chemosis. Her skin is mildly warm and a bit smooth but dry. No tremor of the outstretched hands is noted and her reflexes are normal with a normal relaxation phase. Her hair has a normal distribution and there are no skin rashes. Her thyroid is about 20% above normal size, smooth, and without masses or bruit. What is your differential diagnosis? What tests will you order?

Your differential diagnosis includes GTT, Graves' disease, thyroiditis, toxic adenoma, and multinodular goiter, the latter two less likely given age and exam. Your evaluation should include a repeat TSH and total T4 and free T3 levels, in addition to thyroid peroxidase (TPO) and TSH receptor antibodies (TRAB). You counsel her that a thyroid uptake and scan is contraindicated in pregnancy. At this time, thyroid ultrasound is not warranted.

Her laboratory evaluation shows a TSH of 0.08 mIU/L (reference range 0.34–5.5 mIU/L), total T4 of 18 mcg/dL (reference range 5–12 mcg/dL), and free T3 of 5.75 pg/mL (reference range 2.0–3.80 pg/mL). TRAbs return as 150% of normal and TPO antibodies are negative. She had a normal white blood cell count and liver function tests with her primary care provider within the last month. You counsel her that you suspect Graves' disease as the etiology of her thyroid disorder.

You discuss medical therapy options. Radioactive iodine (RAI) is contraindicated in pregnancy and is therefore not an option. Surgery would not be first line if there are no compressive symptoms or concerning thyroid nodules. You discuss that propylthiouracil (PTU) is preferred in the first 16 weeks of pregnancy and that methimazole is preferred thereafter. You discuss goals in therapy, ideal thyroid levels in pregnancy, and monitoring strategies. She is started with PTU and will follow-up in 4 weeks.

References

1. Korelitz JJ, McNally DL, Masters MN, Li SX, Xu Y, Rivkees SA. Prevalence of thyrotoxicosis, antithyroid medication use, and complications among pregnant women in the United States. Thyroid. 2013;23(6):758–65.
2. Weetman AP. Graves' disease. N Engl J Med. 2000;343(17):1236–48.
3. Carle A, Pedersen IB, Knudsen N, Perrild H, Ovesen L, Rasmussen LB, Laurberg P. Epidemiology of subtypes of hyperthyroidism in Denmark: a population-based study. Eur J Endocrinol. 2011;164(5):801–9.
4. Abraham-Nordling M, Byström K, Törring O, Lantz M, Berg G, Calissendorff J, et al. Incidence of hyperthyroidism in Sweden. Eur J Endocrinol. 2011;165(6):899–905.
5. Laurberg P, Cerqueira C, Ovesen L, Rasmussen LB, Perrild H, Andersen S, et al. Iodine intake as a determinant of thyroid disorders in populations. Best Pract Res Clin Endocrinol Metab. 2010;24(1):13–27.
6. Andersen SL, Olsen J, Laurberg P. Maternal thyroid disease in the Danish National Birth Cohort: prevalence and risk factors. Eur J Endocrinol. 2016;174(2):203–12.
7. Andersen SL, Olsen J, Carlé A, Laurberg P. Hyperthyroidism incidence fluctuates widely in and around pregnancy and is at variance with some other autoimmune diseases: a Danish population-based study. J Clin Endocrinol Metab. 2015;100(3):1164–71.
8. Cooper DS, Laurberg P. Hyperthyroidism in pregnancy. Lancet Diabetes Endocrinol. 2013;1(3):238–49.
9. Forfar JC, Muir AL, Sawers SA, Toft AD. Abnormal left ventricular function in hyperthyroidism: evidence for a possible reversible cardiomyopathy. N Engl J Med. 1982;307(19):1165–70.
10. Klein I, Ojamaa K. Thyroid hormone and the cardiovascular system. N Engl J Med. 2001;344(7):501–9.

11. Kriplani A, Buckshee K, Bhargava VL, Takkar D, Ammini AC. Maternal and perinatal outcome in thyrotoxicosis complicating pregnancy. Eur J Obstet Gynecol Reprod Biol. 1994;54(3):159–63.
12. Sheffield JS, Cunningham FG. Thyrotoxicosis and heart failure that complicate pregnancy. Am J Obstet Gynecol. 2004;190(1):211–7.
13. Millar LK, Wing DA, Leung AS, Koonings PP, Montoro MN, Mestman JH. Low birth weight and preeclampsia in pregnancies complicated by hyperthyroidism. Obstet Gynecol. 1994;84(6):946–9.
14. Männistö T, Mendola P, Grewal J, Xie Y, Chen Z, Laughon SK. Thyroid diseases and adverse pregnancy outcomes in a contemporary US cohort. J Clin Endocrinol Metabol. 2013;98(7):2725–33.
15. van der Kaay DC, Wasserman JD, Palmert MR. Management of neonates born to mothers with Graves' disease. Pediatrics. 2016;137(4):1–14. https://doi.org/10.1542/peds.2015-1878 originally published online March 15, 2016.
16. Aggarawal N, Suri V, Singla R, Chopra S, Sikka P, Shah VN, Bhansali A. Pregnancy outcome in hyperthyroidism: a case control study. Gynecol Obstet Investig. 2014;77(2):94–9.
17. Alexander EK, Pearce EN, Brent GA, Brown RS, Chen H, Dosiou C, et al. 2017 guidelines of the American Thyroid Association for the diagnosis and management of thyroid disease during pregnancy and the postpartum. Thyroid. 2017;27(3):315–89.
18. Pakkila F, Männistö T, Hartikainen AL, Ruokonen A, Surcel HM, Bloigu A, et al. Maternal and child's thyroid function and child's intellect and scholastic performance. Thyroid. 2015;25(12):1363–74.
19. Bernal J. Thyroid hormones and brain development. Vitam Horm. 2005;71:95–122.
20. Korevaar TI, Muetzel R, Medici M, Chaker L, Jaddoe VW, de Rijke YB, et al. Association of maternal thyroid function during early pregnancy with offspring IQ and brain morphology in childhood: a population-based prospective cohort study. Lancet Diabetes Endocrinol. 2016;4(1):35–43.
21. Pitcher-Wilmott RW, Hindocha P, Wood CB. The placental transfer of IgG subclasses in human pregnancy. Clin Exp Immunol. 1980;41(2):303–8.
22. Polak M, Legac I, Vuillard E, Guibourdenche J, Castanet M, Luton D. Congenital hyperthyroidism: the fetus as a patient. Horm Res. 2006;65(5):235–42.
23. Zimmerman D. Fetal and neonatal hyperthyroidism. Thyroid. 1999;9(7):727–33.
24. Ogilvy-Stuart AL. Neonatal thyroid disorders. Arch Dis Child Fetal Neonatal Ed. 2002;87(3):F165–71.
25. De Groot L, Abalovich M, Alexander EK, Amino N, Barbour L, Cobin RH, et al. Management of thyroid dysfunction during pregnancy and postpartum: an Endocrine Society clinical practice guideline. J Clin Endocrinol Metab. 2012;97(8):2543–65.
26. Ross DS, Burch HB, Cooper DS, Greenlee MC, Laurberg P, Maia AL, et al. 2016 American Thyroid Association guidelines for diagnosis and management of hyperthyroidism and other causes of thyrotoxicosis. Thyroid. 2016;26(10):1343–421.
27. Haddow JE, Knight GJ, Palomaki GE, McClain MR, Pulkkinen AJ. The reference range and within-person variability of thyroid stimulating hormone during the first and second trimesters of pregnancy. J Med Screen. 2004;11(4):170–4.
28. Li C, Shan Z, Mao J, Wang W, Xie X, Zhou W, et al. Assessment of thyroid function during first-trimester pregnancy: what is the rational upper limit of serum TSH during the first trimester in Chinese pregnant women? J Clin Endocrinol Metab. 2014;99(1):73–9.
29. Lockwood CM, Grenache DG, Gronowski AM. Serum human chorionic gonadotropin concentrations greater than 400,000 IU/L are invariably associated with suppressed serum thyrotropin concentrations. Thyroid. 2009;19(8):863–8.
30. Glinoer D. The regulation of thyroid function in pregnancy: pathways of endocrine adaptation from physiology to pathology. Endocr Rev. 1997;18(3):404–33.
31. Moleti M, Trimarchi F, Vermiglio F. Thyroid physiology in pregnancy. Endocr Pract. 2014;20(6):589–96.

32. Lee RH, Spencer CA, Mestman JH, Miller EA, Petrovic I, Braverman LE, Goodwin TM. Free T4 immunoassays are flawed during pregnancy. Am J Obstet Gynecol. 2009;200(3): 260.e1–6.
33. Korevaar TI, Chaker L, Medici M, de Rijke YB, Jaddoe VW, Steegers EA, et al. Maternal total T4 during the first half of pregnancy: physiologic aspects and the risk of adverse outcomes in comparison with free T4. Clin Endocrinol. 2016;85(5):757–63.
34. Wilson KL, Casey BM, McIntire DD, Cunningham FG. Is total thyroxine better than free thyroxine during pregnancy? Am J Obstet Gynecol. 2014;211(2):132.e1–6.
35. Lazarus J, Brown RS, Daumerie C, Hubalewska-Dydejczyk A, Negro R, Vaidya B. 2014 European thyroid association guidelines for the management of subclinical hypothyroidism in pregnancy and in children. Eur Thyroid J. 2014;3(2):76–94.
36. Practice Bulletin No. 148: thyroid disease in pregnancy. Obstet Gynecol. 2015;125(4): 996–1005.
37. Yoshihara A, Noh JY, Mukasa K, Suzuki M, Ohye H, Matsumoto M, et al. Serum human chorionic gonadotropin levels and thyroid hormone levels in gestational transient thyrotoxicosis: is the serum hCG level useful for differentiating between active Graves' disease and GTT? Endocr J. 2015;62(6):557–60.
38. Tan JY, Loh KC, Yeo GS, Chee YC. Transient hyperthyroidism of hyperemesis gravidarum. BJOG. 2002;109(6):683–8.
39. Casey BM, Dashe JS, Wells CE, McIntire DD, Leveno KJ, Cunningham FG. Subclinical hyperthyroidism and pregnancy outcomes. Obstet Gynecol. 2006;107(2 Pt 1):337–41.
40. Bartalena L. Diagnosis and management of Graves disease: a global overview. Nat Rev Endocrinol. 2013;9(12):724–34.
41. Goldman AM, Mestman JH. Transient non-autoimmune hyperthyroidism of early pregnancy. J Thyroid Res. 2011;2011:142413.
42. Viard JP, Gilquin J. Graves' disease. N Engl J Med. 2017;376(2):184–5.
43. Bahn RS. Graves' ophthalmopathy. N Engl J Med. 2010;362(8):726–38.
44. Ross DS. Radioiodine therapy for hyperthyroidism. N Engl J Med. 2011;364(6):542–50.
45. Burch HB, Cooper DS. Management of Graves disease: a review. JAMA. 2015;314(23): 2544–54.
46. Watanabe N, Narimatsu H, Noh JY, Yamaguchi T, Kobayashi K, Kami M, et al. Antithyroid drug-induced hematopoietic damage: a retrospective cohort study of agranulocytosis and pancytopenia involving 50,385 patients with Graves' disease. J Clin Endocrinol Metab. 2012;97(1):E49–53.
47. Tajiri J, Noguchi S. Antithyroid drug-induced agranulocytosis: special reference to normal white blood cell count agranulocytosis. Thyroid. 2004;14(6):459–62.
48. Takata K, Kubota S, Fukata S, Kudo T, Nishihara E, Ito M, et al. Methimazole-induced agranulocytosis in patients with Graves' disease is more frequent with an initial dose of 30 mg daily than with 15 mg daily. Thyroid. 2009;19(6):559–63.
49. Cooper DS, Goldminz D, Levin AA, Ladenson PW, Daniels GH, Molitch ME, et al. Agranulocytosis associated with antithyroid drugs. Effects of patient age and drug dose. Ann Intern Med. 1983;98(1):26–9.
50. Andersen SL, Olsen J, Laurberg P. Antithyroid drug side effects in the population and in pregnancy. J Clin Endocrinol Metab. 2016;101(4):1606–14.
51. Wang MT, Lee WJ, Huang TY, Chu CL, Hsieh CH. Antithyroid drug-related hepatotoxicity in hyperthyroidism patients: a population-based cohort study. Br J Clin Pharmacol. 2014;78(3):619–29.
52. Noh JY, Yasuda S, Sato S, Matsumoto M, Kunii Y, Noguchi Y, et al. Clinical characteristics of myeloperoxidase antineutrophil cytoplasmic antibody-associated vasculitis caused by antithyroid drugs. J Clin Endocrinol Metab. 2009;94(8):2806–11.
53. Chen M, Gao Y, Guo XH, Zhao MH. Propylthiouracil-induced antineutrophil cytoplasmic antibody-associated vasculitis. Nat Rev Nephrol. 2012;8(8):476–83.
54. Cooper DS. Antithyroid drugs. N Engl J Med. 2005;352(9):905–17.

55. Andersen SL, Olsen J, Wu CS, Laurberg P. Birth defects after early pregnancy use of antithyroid drugs: a Danish nationwide study. J Clin Endocrinol Metab. 2013;98(11):4373–81.
56. Yoshihara A, Noh J, Yamaguchi T, Ohye H, Sato S, Sekiya K, et al. Treatment of Graves' disease with antithyroid drugs in the first trimester of pregnancy and the prevalence of congenital malformation. J Clin Endocrinol Metab. 2012;97(7):2396–403.
57. Andersen SL, Olsen J, Wu CS, Laurberg P. Severity of birth defects after propylthiouracil exposure in early pregnancy. Thyroid. 2014;24(10):1533–40.
58. Yoshihara A, Noh JY, Watanabe N, Mukasa K, Ohye H, Suzuki M, et al. Substituting potassium iodide for methimazole as the treatment for Graves' disease during the first trimester may reduce the incidence of congenital anomalies: a retrospective study at a single medical institution in Japan. Thyroid. 2015;25(10):1155–61.
59. Laurberg P, Krejbjerg A, Andersen SL. Relapse following antithyroid drug therapy for Graves' hyperthyroidism. Curr Opin Endocrinol Diabetes Obes. 2014;21(5):415–21.
60. Momotani N, Noh JY, Ishikawa N, Ito K. Effects of propylthiouracil and methimazole on fetal thyroid status in mothers with Graves' hyperthyroidism. J Clin Endocrinol Metab. 1997;82(11):3633–6.
61. Hamburger JI. Diagnosis and management of Graves' disease in pregnancy. Thyroid. 1992;2(3):219–24.
62. Erbil Y, Ozluk Y, Giriş M, Salmaslioglu A, Issever H, Barbaros U, et al. Effect of lugol solution on thyroid gland blood flow and microvessel density in the patients with Graves' disease. J Clin Endocrinol Metab. 2007;92(6):2182–9.
63. Amino N, Tanizawa O, Mori H, Iwatani Y, Yamada T, Kurachi K, et al. Aggravation of thyrotoxicosis in early pregnancy and after delivery in Graves' disease. J Clin Endocrinol Metab. 1982;55(1):108–12.
64. Mandel SJ, Cooper DS. The use of antithyroid drugs in pregnancy and lactation. J Clin Endocrinol Metab. 2001;86(6):2354–9.
65. Azizi F, Amouzegar A. Management of hyperthyroidism during pregnancy and lactation. Eur J Endocrinol. 2011;164(6):871–6.
66. Sarlis NJ, Gourgiotis L. Thyroid emergencies. Rev Endocr Metab Disord. 2003;4(2):129–36.
67. Angell TE, Lechner MG, Nguyen CT, Salvato VL, Nicoloff JT, LoPresti JS. Clinical features and hospital outcomes in thyroid storm: a retrospective cohort study. J Clin Endocrinol Metab. 2015;100(2):451–9.
68. Burch HB, Wartofsky L. Life-threatening thyrotoxicosis. Thyroid storm. Endocrinol Metab Clin N Am. 1993;22(2):263–77.
69. Chiha M, Samarasinghe S, Kabaker AS. Thyroid storm: an updated review. J Intensive Care Med. 2015;30(3):131–40.
70. Cooper DS, Laurberg P. Hyperthyroidism in pregnancy. Lancet Diabetes Endocrinol. 2013;1:239–49.
71. Glinoer D, de Nayer P. Regulation of maternal thyroid during pregnancy. J Clin Endocrinol Metab. 1990;71(2):276–87.

Chapter 8
Thyroid Nodules and Cancer in Pregnancy

Sarah E. Mayson and Linda A. Barbour

> **Clinical Case**
> An otherwise healthy 31-year-old G1P0 female patient is detected to have a firm 3 cm right thyroid nodule on clinical neck exam at 15 weeks gestation. She is completely asymptomatic, reports no history of head or neck radiation exposure, and has no family history of thyroid malignancy. What evaluation should be performed? What are her treatment options?

Thyroid Nodules

Definition

Thyroid nodules are discrete structural lesions that are distinct from the background thyroid parenchyma on ultrasound. They can represent multiple pathologic processes and may be caused by neoplastic and nonneoplastic conditions. Nonneoplastic causes of thyroid nodules include pure cysts, hyperplastic nodules, and pseudonodules occurring as a consequence of inflammation (Hashimoto's thyroiditis) or infection (bacterial or fungal abscess). Thyroid nodules can rarely also be due to non-thyroidal etiologies, such as parathyroid adenomas. Thyroid nodules may represent clonal lesions, including follicular and Hurthle cell adenomas, noninvasive follicular thyroid neoplasm with papillary-like nuclear features (NIFTP), and thyroid cancers of various types, the most common being papillary thyroid carcinoma (PTC) and follicular carcinoma (FC) [1]. Medullary thyroid carcinoma – which may occur in the context of multiple endocrine neoplasia (MEN) type 2 – thyroid lymphoma, and non-thyroid cancer metastasis to the thyroid gland are rare causes of thyroid nodules.

Epidemiology and Pathogenesis of Thyroid Nodules in Pregnant Women

Thyroid nodules are 3–5 times more common in women than men in the general population. The prevalence of thyroid nodules detected during pregnancy was 3–21% in three studies completed in populations with borderline iodine sufficiency to moderate deficiency and 30% in an area of severe deficiency [2–5]. Data from iodine-replete regions are not available. As in the nonpregnant population, thyroid nodules are more common with increasing age, but are also seen at a higher frequency with greater parity [2–4, 6]. A rise in the incidence of thyroid nodular disease has been observed from early to late pregnancy, increasing from 15% in the first trimester to 24% 3 months postpartum in a prospective study of Chinese women [2, 3]. A study from Belgium also found that 60% of nodules doubled in size during pregnancy, while the Chinese study and a more recent one from Italy that included 155 women detected no significant change in nodule size [2, 3, 7].

Both hormonal effects and relative iodine deficiency likely contribute to the development of thyroid enlargement and nodular development during pregnancy. Thyroid cancer is also more common in women than men with the incidence increasing in girls at puberty and declining after menopause. This suggests a possible role of estrogen and/or progesterone in thyroid tumorigenesis. Both the estrogen receptor (ER)-α and the progesterone receptor are commonly expressed in thyroid tumor tissue [8]. Estradiol has been shown to stimulate the growth of benign and malignant thyroid follicular cells in vitro. This is mediated through estrogen-dependent genomic and non-genomic signaling, including the mitogen-activated protein (MAP) kinase and phosphatidylinositol 3-kinase (PI_3K)-Akt pathways [9]. Progesterone may also play a role. In cultured thyroid follicular cells, progesterone has been shown to increase the mRNA expression of genes involved in thyroid cell function and proliferation, while these effects are blocked by mifepristone, a progesterone receptor antagonist [10]. Despite robust experimental evidence supporting a role of estrogen in thyroid tumorigenesis, ER-α and estrogen receptor (ER)-β expression patterns vary widely in thyroid cancer tissues, and epidemiologic studies do not show consistent associations between estrogen status and thyroid cancer risk [9].

Human chorionic gonadotropin (hCG) may also contribute to thyroid nodule formation during pregnancy. A fall in serum TSH occurs near the end of the first trimester of pregnancy in association with peak elevation in hCG. There is significant structural homology between the glycoprotein hormones TSH and hCG and between the TSH and LH/CG receptors with the alpha subunit being identical between these groups of hormones. High levels of serum hCG during pregnancy can lead to indiscriminant binding and activation of the TSH receptor on thyroid follicular cells by hCG, stimulating thyroid cell growth, likely nodular growth, and thyroid hormone synthesis and secretion [11].

Dietary iodine needs are higher in pregnant women owing to increased synthesis of maternal thyroid hormones, greater urinary losses, and fetal iodine requirements, and a deficiency can also stimulate thyroid and possibly nodular growth [12]. The 2005 to 2010 National Health and Nutrition Examination Surveys (NHANES) demonstrated lower median urine iodine concentrations consistent with mild iodine deficiency in US pregnant women [13]. Iodine stores remain stable in women with adequate intake before and during pregnancy, while a gradual decline in total-body iodine levels can be seen over the duration of pregnancy in women from geographic regions demonstrating mild to moderate deficiency. Relative iodine deficiency during pregnancy can lead to impaired maternal and fetal thyroid hormone synthesis, ensuing rises in TSH production, and subsequent maternal and fetal thyroid growth and goitrogenesis [12].

Initial Evaluation of Thyroid Nodules in Pregnant Women

The initial evaluation of a thyroid nodule detected during pregnancy is outlined in Fig. 8.1. This should begin with the history and physical exam. The patient should be questioned about risk factors for thyroid cancer. Patients who have had significant exposures to ionizing radiation should be identified, including childhood cancer survivors whose treatment included head or neck radiation therapy and patients who grew up in geographic areas directly affected by nuclear disasters (e.g., 1986 Chernobyl accident). A family history of thyroid cancer, multiple endocrine neoplasia type 2, and other predisposing genetic syndromes (Cowden syndrome, familial adenomatous polyposis, Carney complex, and Werner syndrome) should also be elicited. Patients should be questioned about compressive symptoms related to thyroid nodules, including dysphagia, hoarseness, difficulty breathing, and cough. Examination of the thyroid gland involves both visual examination and palpation of the gland while the patient swallows water. The thyroid gland can be palpated with the examiner behind the patient or with the examiner facing the patient. Bringing the chin down slightly decreases the tension on the skin and muscles and often makes palpation easier. The size, location, and consistency of any nodules should be noted. The patient's neck should also be examined for the presence or absence of adenopathy.

The next step in the evaluation of a thyroid nodule detected during pregnancy is measurement of serum TSH. The purpose of measuring serum TSH is to detect autonomously functioning or "hot" nodules, which account for 5–10% of palpable thyroid nodules in the general population. Autonomous nodules may cause hyperthyroidism and are associated with a very low risk (<1%) of malignancy. Conversely,

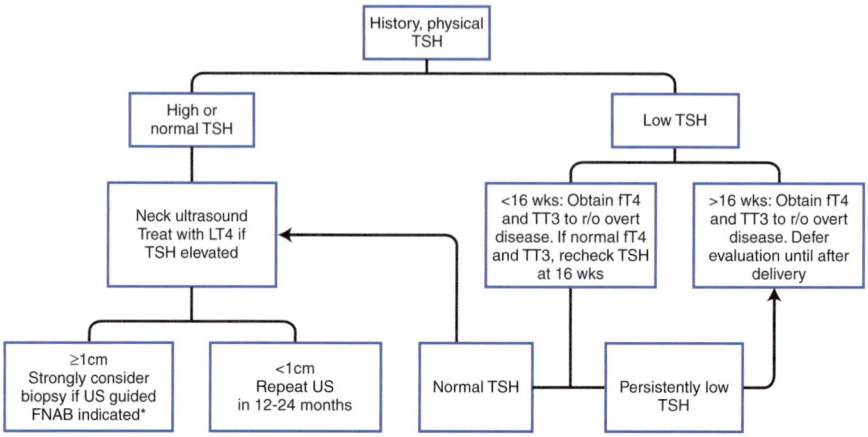

Fig. 8.1 Algorithm for the initial evaluation of thyroid nodules detected in pregnant women. Note: Need for FNAB should be determined based on a combination of patient-specific risk factors for thyroid cancer and the sonographic appearance of the thyroid nodule

most patients with thyroid cancer will have a normal or elevated serum TSH. An elevated TSH should be treated in pregnancy in the context of a nodule because a pseudo-nodule from Hashimoto's may resolve with treatment and a high TSH may stimulate growth of a true nodule. The interpretation of a low serum TSH level in early pregnancy is confounded by the fact that serum TSH may be suppressed as a result of high hCG levels and stay mildly suppressed in the second and third trimester. Serum TSH should be reassessed, and if serum TSH remains <0.5 beyond 16 weeks gestation, further evaluation of the thyroid nodule should be deferred until after delivery given the possibility of a warm or hot nodule [12]. Although recommended as the next step in the evaluation of the nonpregnant patient with a thyroid nodule and suppressed TSH, thyroid radionuclide scanning (I-123, I-131, technetium pertechnetate) and determination of radioiodine (RAI) uptake are contraindicated in pregnant women [12]. Concerns related to the administration of I-131 during pregnancy include whole-body radiation exposure of the fetus and, after 7–8 weeks gestation, damage to the fetal thyroid gland causing fetal/neonatal hypothyroidism [12]. I-123 is much less likely to cause destruction of the fetal thyroid than I-131.

Evaluation of a nodule suspected to be warm or hot (due to a TSH <0.5 in the second or third trimester) should be reassessed postpartum first with repeat measurement of serum TSH. If the TSH remains suppressed, an I-123 scan postpartum can be offered during lactation given the half-life of I-123 is only ~ 8 h as long as the mother agrees to pump and discard her milk for 48 h [14]. During the postpartum evaluation, a suppressed TSH in a patient with a nodule cannot be assumed to be due to a warm or hot nodule because it is also possible that the patient has Graves' disease with a cold nodule or has a multinodular goiter with both cold and warm nodules.

8 Thyroid Nodules and Cancer in Pregnancy

Image	Description	Image	Description
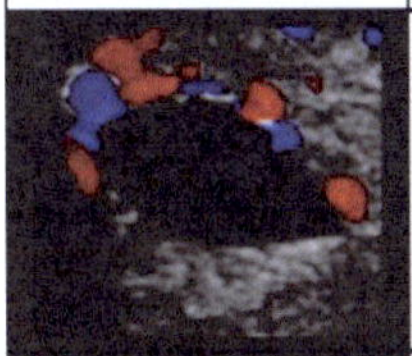	Pure cyst demonstrating no internal vascular flow	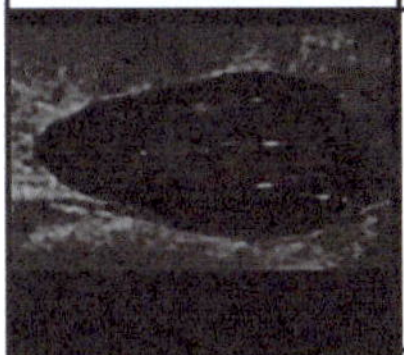	Spongiform nodule
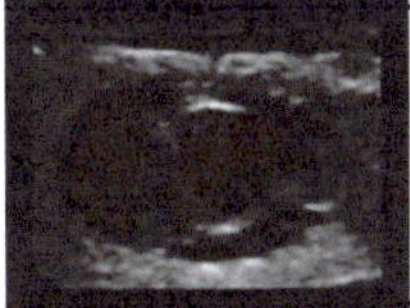	Mixed cystic and soild nodule	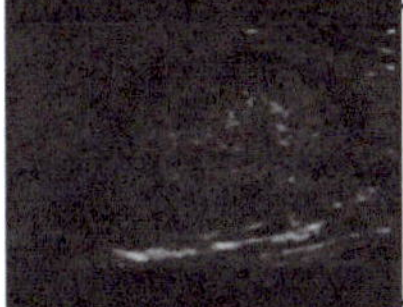	Isoechoic soild nodule
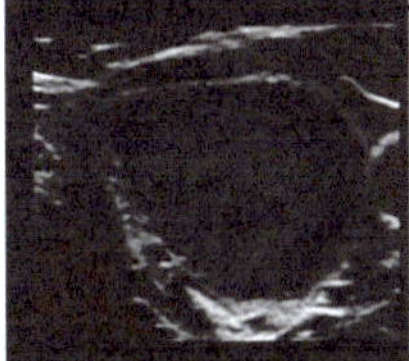	Hypoechoic soild nodule	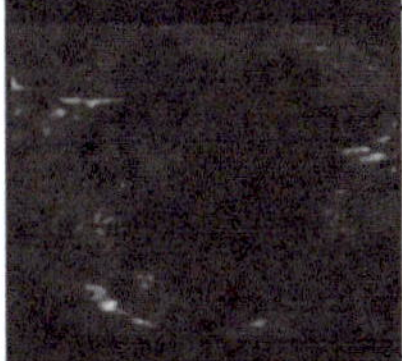	Nodule with irregular margins
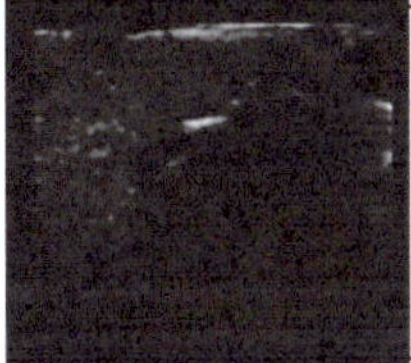	Nodule with interrupted rim calcification	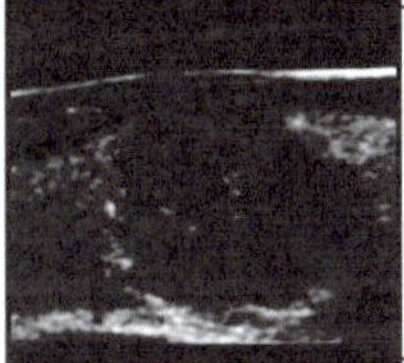	Nodule with microcalcifications
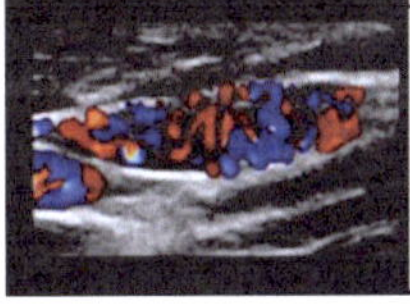	Abnormal lymph node with diffuse hypervascularity	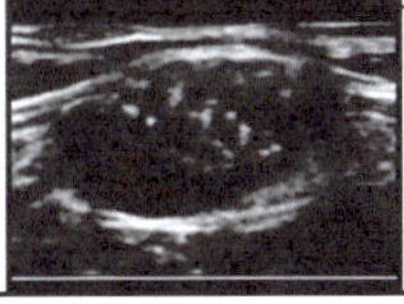	Abnormal lymph node with calcifications

Fig. 8.2 Sonographic features of thyroid nodules and images of abnormal lymph nodes

Ultrasound of the thyroid gland and lymph nodes in the central and lateral compartments of the neck should be performed in all pregnant women with thyroid nodules given that the presence of suspicious lymph nodes will usually mandate that a lymph node biopsy be done to evaluate for metastatic disease. Determination of which nodules require FNAB should take into account any patient-specific risk factors for thyroid cancer and both the sonographic appearance and size of the nodule, as well as the presence of any suspicious lymph nodes. Thyroid nodules can be described based on their composition, echogenicity, shape, margins, and the presence of additional features that are more likely to indicate benignity or malignancy. Representative images are shown in Fig. 8.2. The composition of a thyroid nodule is designated as solid, cystic, or mixed. Among 360 thyroid cancers evaluated at the Mayo Clinic, 88% had solid composition, 9.2% were <50% cystic, and only 2.5% were >50% cystic [15]. Mixed composition nodules with microcystic spaces occupying >50% of the nodule's volume are referred to as spongiform or honeycomb. Pure cysts and spongiform nodules are both very likely to be benign solely based on their sonographic appearance and are associated with a posttest probability of malignancy of 1% and 2%, respectively [16]. Echogenicity describes the brightness of a nodule compared to the background thyroid parenchyma on ultrasound. Hyperechoic nodules are brighter, isoechoic nodules are equally bright, and hypoechoic nodules are darker than the background thyroid parenchyma. The margins of isoechoic and hyperechoic nodules are defined by a hypoechoic halo surrounding the nodule, while hypoechoic nodules are demarcated from the background thyroid by their differing echogenicity. If well-defined, a nodule's margins can be described as regular or irregular.

Sonographic features of thyroid nodules that have been associated with malignancy include taller-than-wide shape, irregular margins, hypoechogenicity, microcalcifications, and intranodular vascularity. Among these, taller-than-wide shape and microcalcifications convey the highest specificity for cancer. Taller-than-wide shape is the ratio of a nodule's anterior-posterior (depth) to horizontal (width) diameter of >1 when measured in the transverse plane [17]. Microcalcifications are punctate echogenic foci without posterior acoustic shadowing that are the sonographic correlate of psammoma bodies seen in PTC. However, the presence of taller-than-wide shape or microcalcifications alone is not an accurate predictor that a thyroid nodule is malignant (posttest probability of malignancy: 60% and 50%, respectively) [16]. Moreover, the interobserver agreement for most sonographic features is only fair to moderate [18]. Because high- and low-risk features tend to associate with one another, several groups have recommended classifying thyroid nodules based on constellations of features (Table 8.1) [19, 20]. Sonographic

Table 8.1 Sonographic patterns and estimated risks of malignancy as proposed by the 2015 ATA guidelines and actual risks of malignancy determined in study populations

2015 ATA guidelines sonographic pattern	Description	Estimated ROM per 2015 ATA guidelines	Actual ROM (range)[a]
Benign	Pure cyst	<1%	ND
Very low suspicion	Spongiform and partially cystic nodules not meeting criteria for low, intermediate, or high suspicion patterns	<3%	3–5%
Low suspicion	Iso-/hyperechoic solid nodule or partially cystic nodule with eccentric solid areas and no suspicious feature[b]	5–10%	2–10%
Intermediate suspicion	Hypoechoic solid nodule with regular margins and no suspicious feature[b]	10–20%	10–22%
High suspicion	Hypoechoic solid nodule or partially cystic and solid nodule that is hypoechoic with ≥1 suspicious feature[b]	>70–90%	55–72%

Data from Haugen et al. [20], Rosario et al. [67], Yoon et al. [68], and Xu et al. [69]
Abbreviations: *ATA* American Thyroid Association, *ND* not determined, *ROM* risk of malignancy
[a]From Rosario et al. [67], Yoon et al. [68], and Xu et al. [69]
[b]Suspicious features: microcalcifications, taller-than-wide shape, irregular margins, extrathyroidal extension, interrupted rim calcification with soft tissue extrusion

patterns are associated with higher sensitivity and specificity and lower interobserver variability than individual features [21, 22].

Thyroid nodule FNAB can be safely performed in a pregnant woman. Indications for thyroid nodule FNAB are the same as in nonpregnant patients; however, patient preference with regard to timing (during or after pregnancy) should also be taken into account [12, 20, 23]. Most experts suggest that FNAB be performed during pregnancy according to nonpregnant criteria even if the patient would not elect surgery until postpartum so that a diagnosis can be determined and plans for postpartum management are not delayed. The 2015 American Thyroid Association (ATA) guidelines recommend classifying thyroid nodules into one of five sonographic patterns, each of which is associated with a different risk of malignancy. The ATA sonographic patterns are summarized in Table 8.1. Need for FNAB is determined accordingly, with higher-risk nodules prioritized for biopsy at smaller sizes. These guidelines recommend FNAB of nodules consistent with the ATA high and intermediate suspicion patterns if ≥ 1 cm in size, low suspicion pattern if ≥ 1.5 cm, and very low suspicion pattern if ≥ 2 cm in size or not at all with clinical observation being an acceptable alternative. FNAB of purely cystic nodules is not indicated for cytology determination. Abnormal-appearing cervical lymph nodes should also be targeted for biopsy. The ATA guidelines do not recommend FNAB for subcentimeter thyroid nodules unless associated with symptoms, pathologic lymphadenopathy, extrathyroidal extension, or a high-risk history (e.g., neck irradiation) [20].

Thyroid nodule FNAB should be performed under ultrasound guidance when possible due to improved diagnostic accuracy compared to palpation biopsy. For each nodule meeting FNAB criteria, 2–4 separate passes are made using 25 or 27 gauge needles and cytology smears are prepared. Thyroid cytopathology is interpreted according to criteria developed at the National Cancer Institute Thyroid Fine Needle Aspiration State of the Science Conference, also known as the Bethesda Conference. The Bethesda classification system was updated in 2017, as summarized in Table 8.2 [24]. The estimated risk of malignancy for each diagnostic category has not been specifically determined for pregnant patients; however, pregnancy does not appear to alter the cytology diagnosis of thyroid tissue obtained by FNAB based on retrospective data, and therefore the same criteria are used [25].

Subsequent Management of Benign and Indeterminate Thyroid Nodules

Thyroid nodules not meeting criteria for FNAB and nodules with benign cytology results should be managed as in nonpregnant patients [12]. This generally includes clinical follow-up and repeat ultrasound imaging in 12–24 months, although sonographic follow-up for very low suspicion nodules should be deferred for at least 24 months, if it is performed at all [20]. Conversely, nodules with suspicious ultrasound changes and those with benign cytology that demonstrate rapid growth should be targeted for repeat FNAB and may be considered for surgery [12].

Table 8.2 Cytology diagnoses obtained by fine-needle aspiration biopsy of thyroid nodules and management recommendations in pregnant women

FNAB cytology diagnosis	ROM (%) NIFTP not malignant[a]	ROM (%) NIFTP malignant[a]	Management
I. Nondiagnostic	5–10	5–10	Repeat FNAB, or defer until after delivery
II. Benign	0–3	0–3	Routine follow-up[b]
III. Atypia of uncertain significance or follicular lesion of uncertain significance	6–18	10–30	Repeat FNAB, or monitor and defer until after delivery[c]
IV. Follicular neoplasm or suspicious for follicular neoplasm	10–40	25–40	Monitor and defer until after delivery[c]
V. Suspicious for malignancy	45–60	50–75	Monitor and defer until after delivery[c]
VI. Malignant	94–96	97–99	Surgery in the second trimester, or defer until after delivery

Data from Alexander et al. [12], Cibas and Ali [24], and Haugen et al. [20]
[a]Risk of malignancy based on cytology diagnosis as determined for the general population. Noninvasive follicular thyroid neoplasm with papillary-like nuclear features (NIFTP) is considered a "precancerous" lesion. If counted as non-malignant, the risk of malignancy is reduced for all Bethesda categories except I and II
[b]Benign nodules should be followed as in nonpregnant patients with clinical follow-up and repeat ultrasound in 12–24 months. For nodules demonstrating the ATA high suspicion sonographic pattern, repeat ultrasound and FNAB should be performed within 12 months
[c]In nonpregnant patients, management strategies include surgery and/or molecular genetic testing of the nodule. Molecular testing should not be performed in pregnant women. Surgery may be considered during pregnancy if there is clinical suspicion of aggressive behavior

There are no prospective studies evaluating the outcome and prognosis of pregnant women with thyroid nodules of indeterminate cytology (Bethesda III–V) [12]. In nonpregnant patients, management strategies for Bethesda III (follicular lesion of uncertain significance, FLUS; atypia of uncertain significance, AUS) and Bethesda IV (suspicious for follicular neoplasm; follicular neoplasm) nodules may include clinical surveillance (Bethesda III only), repeat FNAB for cytology (Bethesda III only), molecular genetic testing, and surgery, usually thyroid lobectomy. Outside of pregnancy, nodules that are suspicious for malignancy (Bethesda V) are managed with lobectomy or near-total thyroidectomy similar to nodules with malignant cytology (Bethesda VI) [20]. However, during pregnancy, surgery is usually deferred until postpartum for thyroid nodules with indeterminate or suspicious cytology unless there is clinical suspicion of aggressive behavior (Table 8.2). Molecular genetic testing has not been validated in pregnant women due to the unknown influence of pregnancy on signaling biomarkers. It is not recommended in pregnancy, but may be useful postpartum to better stratify the risk of malignancy in an indeterminate nodule [12, 20].

Thyroid Cancer

Epidemiology

Thyroid cancer is second only to breast cancer in pregnancy, but the true prevalence is difficult to discern due to referral bias. The prevalence has significantly increased in all ages in the general population including women <45 years old, but mortality from thyroid cancer has only slightly increased. This reflects the indolent nature of the disease and increases in diagnosis due to more frequent imaging [26]. In addition to confirming an overall increase in the annual incidence of thyroid cancer from 1974 to 2013, a recent analysis of data from the Surveillance, Epidemiology, and End Results-9 cancer registry program demonstrated an increase in both the incidence (2.4% per year) and incidence-based mortality rate (2.9% per year) of advanced-stage PTC. This indicates that there has also been a true increase in the occurrence of thyroid cancer in the USA over the last several decades [27]. Epidemiologic studies such as the EPIC study, a prospective cohort of 345,157 women followed for a median of 11 years, did not find a strong association between reproductive factors and the risk of developing thyroid cancer [28]. However, a meta-analysis with 21 studies – including 406,329 cases and controls – suggested an association between ≥3 pregnancies and thyroid cancer and a transient increased risk within 5 years of recent pregnancy [29]. All of these studies are subject to surveillance bias given pregnant women are more likely to receive routine thyroid exams compared to nonpregnant women of the same reproductive age.

A number of studies have focused on determining the malignancy rate in thyroid nodules in pregnant women compared to nonpregnant women. In one of several retrospective series at the University of Toronto and Mount Sinai Hospital, 43% of 20 pregnant women referred for thyroid nodules between 1982 and 1985 had carcinoma [30]. In a follow-up study of 66 pregnant women, the malignancy rate was 50% [31]. In a Mayo Clinic series of 40 pregnant women, only 15% of nodules were malignant [32]. A cancer estimate of ~30% (21% PTC and 9% suspected PTC) was reported in 57 pregnant or postpartum women referred to George Washington University Medical Center [25]. Overall, these cohort studies suggest that the proportion of thyroid nodules that are malignant is increased during pregnancy, but these are likely overestimates due to the selection bias of women referred for diagnosis and treatment at major referral centers. In a small prospective study from China, in which all women with a nodule >5 mm underwent FNAB, the malignancy rate was 0/21; however, some nodules would not be biopsied by current guidelines [3].

Case-control studies have suggested a modestly increased risk of thyroid cancer in pregnancy. For example, in a study from Washington state that compared women with one or more pregnancies to a matched control group, the relative risk of thyroid cancer was 1.8 (95% CI 1.1–3.1) [33]. The overall prevalence of thyroid cancer in pregnancy in a California Cancer Registry was reported in 2003 at 14/100,000 live births, making it the second most common malignancy, but more recent estimates are not available [34]. Accurate unbiased prospective data estimating the prevalence of malignancy in nodules >1 cm during pregnancy are not available, but prevalence is unlikely to be less than for nonpregnant patients.

New Diagnosis of Thyroid Cancer in Pregnancy

Although the data are limited, there is no evidence that pregnancy worsens the survival from well-differentiated thyroid cancer (DTC) compared to the general population [35–38]. As a result, there is no rationale to recommend interruption of pregnancy for newly diagnosed DTC. However, there are limited but inconsistent retrospective data suggesting that thyroid cancers discovered during pregnancy may have a higher chance of recurrence using biochemical or ultrasound measures.

An earlier retrospective cohort by Moosa and Mazzaferri compared 61 patients with thyroid cancer diagnosed in pregnancy to 528 age-matched, nonpregnant women with similar tumor types (>80% PTC) and stage [36]. Thirteen percent of the tumors were stage 1, 69% stage 2, 16% stage 3, and 2% stage 4. Thirty percent of tumors were diagnosed in the first trimester, 43% in the second, and 28% in the third. Twenty percent of women were operated on in the second trimester and 77% of women underwent thyroidectomy after delivery. The recurrence rate was 15% in the pregnant women versus 23% in the nonpregnant women and cancer deaths were 0% and 1.2%, respectively. This study also looked at the difference in outcomes between the pregnant women who had early surgery versus those with delayed surgery, with a median follow-up of 22.4 years. The recurrence rate in the women who underwent surgery in pregnancy at a mean of 1.1 months after diagnosis was 14% versus 15% in women who delayed their surgery postpartum at a mean of 16 months after diagnosis. However, recurrence was based on positive whole-body scans and not thyroglobulin (TG) biomarkers or lymph node assessment.

A comparison of disease-related survival in 595 women diagnosed with thyroid cancer during pregnancy or within 1 year after delivery to an age-matched nonpregnant cohort also observed no significant difference in outcome during up to 11 years of follow-up [39]. Furthermore, no deleterious effect of surgery performed during pregnancy on pregnancy outcomes was found. Given the overall highly favorable long-term prognosis with thyroid cancer and the relatively early stage of cancers discovered in pregnancy, it is not surprising that survival would not appear to be affected by pregnancy.

However, using more sensitive measures of recurrence such as TG assays and ultrasound, there are data suggesting that recurrence may be higher when the diagnosis is made in pregnancy. In a small retrospective study of 123 women who were either nulliparous, currently pregnant, within 1 year of delivery, or more than 1 year since their last delivery, the definition of persistence or recurrence of thyroid cancer included a basal or stimulated TG >2 ug/l or progressively increasing TG antibodies [40]. This study suggested that a diagnosis of thyroid cancer during pregnancy or within 1 year after delivery carried a less favorable prognosis than cancers diagnosed outside of pregnancy; however, only 14 cases were diagnosed during or within 1 year of pregnancy. Although the pregnancy group was small, the data suggested that women who were diagnosed in or within 1 year of pregnancy had a higher risk of persistent or recurrent disease at a mean follow-up of ~5 years compared to nulliparas or those diagnosed more than 1 year after delivery. Persistence or recurrence was most often identified by positive lymph nodes, a TG >10 ug/l, or rising anti-TG antibodies. Of note, more women diagnosed in or within 1 year of pregnancy had lymph node involvement at diagnosis, which was an independent predictor of recurrence or persistence disease. Ten of the 11 pregnant women underwent surgery during pregnancy. Interestingly, although only 1/3 of the cases underwent testing for ERα, a higher percentage of pregnant women were ERα positive. The authors speculated that the high prevalence of ERα positivity in pregnancy may have contributed to proliferation and growth of thyroid cancer cells via MAP kinase cytoplasmic signaling based on previous data on the growth of thyroid tumor cells in culture [41]. Not surprisingly, there was no difference in survival in this shorter 5–6-year follow-up study.

A larger study compared recurrence rates among 152 women with DTC diagnosed at least 2 years after delivery, 150 nulliparous women, and 38 women diagnosed in pregnancy or up to 2 years postpartum. The recurrence rate was higher (10%) for patients diagnosed in or within 2 years of pregnancy compared to women diagnosed at least 2 years after delivery (1.3%) and nulliparous women (4.3%) [42]. Recurrence was defined using TG, stimulated TG, or increasing TG antibodies in addition to neck ultrasound. Staging and clinical risk factors appeared similar. Although expression of ERα positivity was explored in a subset (37 total), in addition to analyzing the presence of the NIS and BRAF mutations, there was no difference in these biomarkers in the pregnancy/postpartum group. However, another study of 24 women diagnosed in pregnancy or within 1 year postpartum compared to 30 nonpregnant age-matched controls showed no difference in recurrence by stimulated TG or ultrasound or in disease-free survival at ~44 months [43]. Despite tumors in the pregnancy group being larger with more regional lymph nodes, there were also no differences in specific microRNA profiles in a subset of samples. Although numbers are limited in all of the above studies, there are no data to suggest that deferring surgery until postpartum affects recurrence or survival.

Indications for Surgery in Pregnancy and Timing

Although deferring surgery until postpartum has not been shown to decrease disease specific survival or alter recurrence risk, there is evidence that surgery in the second trimester can be safely performed and likely poses no significant increased risk to the fetus. If surgery is performed in pregnancy, the preferred timing is in the second trimester after organogenesis has been completed and before viability (<23 weeks). Two studies have attempted to better define the risk of thyroid surgery in the second trimester. A retrospective cross-sectional analysis of hospital discharge data from the Healthcare Cost and Utilization Project-Nationwide Inpatient Sample (HCUP-NIS) database compared 201 pregnant women undergoing either thyroid ($n = 165$) or parathyroid surgery ($n = 36$) to ~31,155 age-matched nonpregnant controls [44]. Surgeries performed during pregnancy had a two- to threefold higher risk of endocrine or general surgical complications, a 0.3-day longer hospital course, and an additional $300 adjusted cost. However, the composite fetal complication rate (induced or spontaneous abortions, early or threatened labor, fetal distress, intrauterine death, stillbirth, neonatal hypocalcemia, tetany, or hypoparathyroidism) was documented to be only 5.5%. Further, there were no data to determine whether these complications were temporally related to the timing of the surgery or whether the surgery was performed for maternal hyperparathyroidism or thyroid disease. There were also no data on disease severity or stage of thyroid cancer in the women who received surgery during pregnancy versus those who underwent surgery in the nonpregnant state. Furthermore, the women who received surgery during the pregnancy were more likely to be black, of lower socioeconomic status, or have government insurance (Medicaid), all of which were associated with a higher risk of adverse surgical outcomes. Total composite maternal complications were listed as Cesarean section, dilation and curettage, and hysterectomy at 4.5%. However, these were unlikely to be related to the thyroid surgery, and the Cesarean section rate quoted is unusually low.

A more recent retrospective study from Japan reported a more homogeneous population of 45 patients with well-differentiated PTC, of whom 24 had a thyroidectomy in pregnancy (19/24 in the second) and 21 who had surgery within 1 year of delivery [45]. The groups were comparable for stage and risk factors. There were no surgical complications or pregnancy losses or differences in pregnancy outcomes and also no differences in recurrence of thyroid cancer. Lastly, in a series of 35 cases of DTC reported in the International Network on Cancer, Infertility and Pregnancy, in which all were stage 1 cancers and only 1 underwent lymph node resection, 29/35 (83%) had surgery in pregnancy (25 total thyroidectomies and 4 hemithyroidectomies) at a mean gestational age of 18–20 weeks gestation [46]. Maternal and neonatal outcomes were uncomplicated, and all were term live births.

Mothers can be reassured that there are no data that postponing surgery until after delivery within 1 year of diagnosis affects survival and there are no data that suggest that the recurrence risk is altered by the timing of surgery as long as the cancer is well differentiated. However, there are also no data suggesting an increased risk of adverse fetal outcomes if surgery is performed during the second trimester (Table 8.2). In the first trimester, there are some concerns over possible teratogenic effects on the fetus, and surgery of any type is associated with increased early fetal loss [47]. In the third trimester, although very unlikely, neck surgery might be associated with a higher incidence of preterm labor. For cancer found early in pregnancy, surgery during the second trimester (before 23 weeks) is an option, especially if the nodule is large and/or associated with suspicious lymphadenopathy or if patients are anxious and prefer that it be performed. However, most women with DTC can be reassured that waiting until postpartum does not appear to affect prognosis. Most importantly, any thyroid cancer surgery should be performed by a high-volume surgeon to minimize the risk of injury or complete removal of the parathyroid glands resulting in severe hypocalcemia.

Inadequate data are available for patients with advanced disease or thyroid cancers associated with a poorer prognosis including medullary, poorly differentiated, or anaplastic carcinomas. In these unusual cases, surgical treatment should be offered if the patient is <22 weeks, and consideration should be given regarding earlier timing of delivery, particularly closer to 37 weeks, if the patient is beyond 23 weeks [12, 20, 23, 48]. Patients with more advanced disease or tumor progression during pregnancy are also strong candidates for surgery in the second trimester and can also be reassured of fetal safety, although the risk of maternal and potentially fetal hypocalcemia from hypoparathyroidism may be higher with more extensive surgery or the need for lateral neck dissection. There are no specific guidelines for the management of pregnancy in women with DTC with distant metastases identified prior to pregnancy or at conception [49]. However, in seven patients with known pulmonary metastases reported in the Memorial Sloan Kettering Cancer Center cohort, only one of seven showed progression of distant metastases during pregnancy [50].

Structural imaging techniques such as CT or functional imaging using RAI or PET scanning should not be performed due to concerns about ionizing radiation to the fetus. The potential risk from the proliferative effects of estrogen, hCG, or other growth factors is not quantifiable in the mother with distant metastases. However, it is usually recommended that patients who have been properly treated for distant metastases be counseled that pregnancy is not contraindicated, even though some minor biochemical or structural disease progression is possible [50, 51]. For patients with inadequately treated metastatic disease, options include delaying treatment with RAI or the use of tyrosine kinase inhibitors, for which there are negligible human pregnancy data available but animal studies have demonstrated teratogenicity and embryo toxicity [12, 49]. A discussion about possibly deferring pregnancy until treatment is completed should occur.

Thyroid Hormone Suppression for Cancers or Suspicious Nodules

Among pregnant women with thyroid cancer or a suspicious nodule who delay surgery until postpartum, the risks and benefits of exogenously administered thyroid hormone at suppressive doses are unclear [12]. There are data that strongly support that subclinical hyperthyroidism does not appear to pose a risk during pregnancy [52]. If thyroid suppression is used, it is recommended to achieve a suppressed but detectable TSH level and not to increase the free T4 outside of the normal range [48, 52]. There are no studies in pregnancy examining the optimal degree of TSH suppression in women discovered to have thyroid cancers or who have highly suspicious nodules. The degree of TSH suppression should be dictated by an estimation of the likelihood that the tumor will behave aggressively and the TSH level. Because higher serum TSH levels may correlate with more advanced cancer and can stimulate cancer growth, if the patient's TSH is >2 mU/L, it is reasonable to initiate thyroid hormone therapy. The TSH should be maintained between 0.3 and 1.0 mU/L, ensuring the free T4 or the total T4 (TT4) is still within the normal range for pregnancy (i.e., TT4 to 1.5 times the normal nonpregnant range). Thyroid nodules that are benign and those for which cytology is indeterminate or not obtained should not be treated with suppressive therapy given there are no data demonstrating that levothyroxine decreases the size or arrests the growth of nodules during pregnancy.

In patients taking levothyroxine for previously diagnosed thyroid cancer, it must be remembered that the majority of patients will need close to a 30% increase in levothyroxine dose with pregnancy [12]. For patients on suppression for thyroid cancer prior to pregnancy, it is reasonable to maintain the same TSH level during pregnancy given the lack of any demonstrated maternal and neonatal complications with subclinical hyperthyroidism [52]. Although there are no outcome data in pregnancy, the same guidelines outside of pregnancy can be used to determine the degree of TSH suppression according to whether the woman has evidence of persistent disease (<0.1 mU/L) or appears clinically free of disease (0.1–0.5 mU/L) [20]. In patients with persistent structural disease or at high risk of recurrence in whom a TSH <0.1 is recommended, a free T4 within the upper limits of the normal range (or TT4 no more than 50% elevated from the nonpregnancy range) should be maintained and monitored to ensure that the mother does not become overtly hyperthyroid [12, 48].

Progression of Thyroid Cancer in Pregnancy and Monitoring

The 2015 ATA guidelines on thyroid nodules recommend that a nodule with PTC discovered early in pregnancy be monitored by ultrasound, and if it grows substantially by 24 weeks gestation (>50% in volume and >20% in diameter in two dimensions) or if suspicious cervical lymph nodes are present, surgery should be considered in the second trimester [20]. For nodules that remain stable by mid-gestation or are diagnosed after 24 weeks, surgery can be performed after delivery. TSH (and free T4 if the TSH is suppressed) should be monitored every 4 weeks until ~18 weeks, after every dose adjustment, and then can be monitored less often after 26 weeks. In a small series of 19 women who chose to delay surgery for thyroid cancer diagnosed just before conception or during early pregnancy, 13 of whom had PTC <1 cm, there were no clinically relevant changes in maximal tumor size after a median 9.5-month follow-up [53]. Furthermore, there were no newly developed lesions or cervical lymph nodes in this very low-risk group with small cancers, in whom suspicious lymph nodes were only present in 3/19 at baseline.

In patients with thyroid cancer diagnosed preconception, there are no data to suggest that subsequent pregnancy increases the risk for thyroid cancer recurrence. However, many studies were performed before contemporary monitoring surveillance tools were used [54, 55]. In a retrospective analysis of 36 women who became pregnant a median of 4.3 years after initial therapy for thyroid cancer, no evidence of recurrence was detected in the early postpartum period in women with a negative prepregnancy ultrasound and either undetectable or suppressed TG levels [56]. However, eight women who did not have suppressed TG, which is often a biomarker of residual disease, had TG values postpartum that were 20% higher than prepregnancy. This might suggest slight progression of disease, but the clinical significance of this is not known. In a study of 64 Brazilian women (48 PTC and 16 FC) with TG <2 ng/ml and negative neck ultrasound, there were no recurrences at 6 months postpartum, but surveillance was not reported after that period [57]. Similarly, in a study of 63 women who gave birth after being treated for PTC, none of the women categorized as disease-free by TG <0.9 ng/ml or normal neck ultrasounds had progression of disease when followed nearly 5 years later [58]. However, 6/13 women with persistent prepregnancy disease experienced progression with either an increase in metastatic cervical lymph nodes or new nodal metastases.

A recent retrospective review of 235 women followed at Memorial Sloan Kettering Cancer Center for DTC from 1997 to 2015 investigated the risk of progression or recurrence based on the response to therapy prior to pregnancy [50]. The authors determined that patients with an excellent, indeterminate, or biochemical incomplete response before pregnancy continued to show no evidence of structurally identifiable disease when evaluated 3–12 months after delivery. Furthermore, only a minority of patients demonstrated a postpartum TG that was higher than their prepregnancy level. In women with structural disease or incomplete response, evidence of structural progression (defined as at least 3 mm increase in size of known disease or new metastases) was identified in 29%. However, additional therapy was recommended during the first postpartum year in only 8% of those patients who had a structural incomplete response to therapy prior to pregnancy, while 92% continued to be followed with observation. These data confirm that the prepregnancy response to therapy status is an excellent predictor of progression in pregnancy and that those without structural disease predating the pregnancy should be reassured that pregnancy is safe and highly unlikely to be associated with new structural disease [12, 50].

The above studies suggest that pregnancy does not appear to increase the risk for recurrence in women without evidence of biochemical or structural disease prior to pregnancy. Therefore, more intensive monitoring with TG or ultrasound is not recommended during pregnancy or postpartum [12]. However, in women with structural or biochemical disease supporting an incomplete response, it is possible that pregnancy could stimulate growth and surveillance with TG, and ultrasound monitoring should be performed [12]. For women with known PTC prior to pregnancy who are undergoing active surveillance (usually due to a <1 cm nodule), ultrasound monitoring should be performed in pregnancy due to data which support an increased risk of tumor growth during pregnancy [59]. Furthermore, in women who have received RAI ablation, monitoring for evidence of recurrence using TG is recommended as in nonpregnant women. Increasing TG levels should raise concern for residual disease. Neck ultrasound and possible FNAB should be considered. It must be remembered when counseling women preconception, even those with persistent structural disease, that the long-term prognosis for most thyroid cancer patients <45 years is quite good with a 10-year disease-specific survival of >95% [51]. Thus the evidence to date suggests that in the vast majority of patients, pregnancy will not impact survival or overall thyroid cancer prognosis.

Effect of I-131 Ablative Therapy on Subsequent Pregnancy Outcome or in Breastfeeding Women

I-131 is contraindicated in pregnancy given the half-life of I-131 is ~8 days (~40 days to near-completely clear in circulation) and would be highly destructive to the fetal thyroid if it is given within 40 days (after 7–8 weeks from LMP) of when the fetus begins to concentrate and make thyroid hormone at ~10–12 weeks. However, prior ablative treatment with I-131 does not appear to affect subsequent neonatal outcomes. Several series have demonstrated that prior RAI administration did not adversely affect rates of congenital malformations, live birth, mode of delivery, or 1-year neonatal mortality [37, 54, 60–63]. There is also no evidence that previous I-131 affects rates of stillbirth, low birth weight, prematurity, or nonthyroidal malignancy in the children. In a retrospective study of 1044 women treated for thyroid cancer, the incidence of miscarriage was slightly increased in those treated with I-131 within 1 year of conception, thought to be due to inadequate control of thyroid hormone status following thyroidectomy and ablation [37]. However, in a follow-up study by the same authors 13 years later, with a larger cohort of 2673 pregnancies, there was no increased rate of miscarriage [62]. In a retrospective case-control study that evaluated the risk of miscarriage and congenital malformation in 126 pregnancies after I-131 treatment compared to 101 pregnancies before treatment, there was no difference in malformations or miscarriage [64]. A large systematic review including 16 studies and 3023 women who had received I-131 for thyroid cancer also concluded that there was not a significantly increased risk of long-term infertility, miscarriage, stillbirth, neonatal death, or congenital malformation but that RAI-treated women might experience a slightly earlier age of menopause [65]. Most recently, a retrospective cohort study using the California Cancer Registry and California Office of Statewide Health Planning and Development database evaluated 18,850 women with DTC [66]. This study reported that although the birthrate in the entire cohort was not affected by a history of RAI ablation, it was lower in women age 35–39 and there was a delay to the first live birth in women 20–39 by about 8 months (34.5 versus 26.1 months). Whether this is due to reproductive choice, a delay in obtaining an optimal TSH, decreasing fertility with advancing age, a perception of more severe chronic disease, or implications to reproductive health is not clear. Data on later childhood outcomes are sparse. One series of 78 live births to women with prior therapy showed no abnormal development at a mean of 8 years [61].

I-131 is contraindicated in breastfeeding because of concentration of the isotope in the lactating breast and transfer of the isotope to the infant. It has also been recommended that lactation be discontinued for 1–2 months prior to 131-I treatment in order to avoid excess breast exposure [26]. Conception should occur after remission of thyroid cancer has been documented and stability of thyroid function has been achieved at least 6 months after 131-I ablative treatment [12, 23, 48, 60, 61, 63].

> **Clinical Case and Discussion**
>
> An otherwise healthy 31-year-old G1P0 female patient is detected to have a firm 3 cm right thyroid nodule on clinical neck exam at 15 weeks gestation. She is completely asymptomatic, reports no history of head or neck radiation exposure, and no family history of thyroid malignancy. What evaluation should be performed? What are her treatment options?
>
> A neck ultrasound confirms a 3.5 × 1.8 × 2.4 cm hypoechoic nodule in the right thyroid lobe with microcalcifications and irregular borders. No abnormal lymph nodes are noted in the central or lateral compartments of the neck. Serum TSH is measured and is 1.5 mU/L. The patient undergoes an ultrasound-guided fine-needle aspiration biopsy (FNAB) of the nodule, which confirms a diagnosis of PTC.
>
> Given the lack of abnormal lymph nodes on neck ultrasound, the patient can be reassured that thyroidectomy can be postponed until after delivery without negatively impacting her survival or risk of recurrence. However, if preferred by the patient, there is also evidence that surgery can be safely performed in the second trimester after organogenesis has been completed and before viability (<23 weeks) without any significant increased risk to the fetus. TSH suppression therapy with levothyroxine can be deferred until after thyroidectomy is performed given the normal serum TSH level. The need for adjuvant 131-I therapy will be determined following surgery based on the final tumor pathology and postoperative TG level.

References

1. Nikiforov YE, Seethala RR, Tallini G, Baloch ZW, Basolo F, Thompson LD, et al. Nomenclature revision for encapsulated follicular variant of papillary thyroid carcinoma: a paradigm shift to reduce overtreatment of indolent tumors. JAMA Oncol. 2016;2(8):1023–9.
2. Glinoer D, Soto MF, Bourdoux P, Lejeune B, Delange F, Lemone M, et al. Pregnancy in patients with mild thyroid abnormalities: maternal and neonatal repercussions. J Clin Endocrinol Metab. 1991;73(2):421–7.
3. Kung AW, Chau MT, Lao TT, Tam SC, Low LC. The effect of pregnancy on thyroid nodule formation. J Clin Endocrinol Metab. 2002;87(3):1010–4.
4. Struve CW, Haupt S, Ohlen S. Influence of frequency of previous pregnancies on the prevalence of thyroid nodules in women without clinical evidence of thyroid disease. Thyroid. 1993;3(1):7–9.

5. Sahin SB, Ogullar S, Ural UM, Ilkkilic K, Metin Y, Ayaz T. Alterations of thyroid volume and nodular size during and after pregnancy in a severe iodine-deficient area. Clin Endocrinol. 2014;81(5):762–8.
6. Zhu J, Zhu X, Tu C, Li YY, Qian KQ, Jiang C, et al. Parity and thyroid cancer risk: a meta-analysis of epidemiological studies. Cancer Med. 2016;5(4):739–52.
7. Vannucchi G, Covelli D, Vigo B, Perrino M, Mondina L, Fugazzola L. Thyroid volume and serum calcitonin changes during pregnancy. J Endocrinol Investig. 2017;40(7):727–32.
8. Sturniolo G, Zafon C, Moleti M, Castellvi J, Vermiglio F, Mesa J. Immunohistochemical expression of estrogen receptor-alpha and progesterone receptor in patients with papillary thyroid Cancer. Eur Thyroid J. 2016;5(4):224–30.
9. Derwahl M, Nicula D. Estrogen and its role in thyroid cancer. Endocr Relat Cancer. 2014;21(5):T273–83.
10. Bertoni AP, Brum IS, Hillebrand AC, Furlanetto TW. Progesterone upregulates gene expression in normal human thyroid follicular cells. Int J Endocrinol. 2015;2015:864852.
11. Glinoer D. The regulation of thyroid function in pregnancy: pathways of endocrine adaptation from physiology to pathology. Endocr Rev. 1997;18(3):404–33.
12. Alexander EK, Pearce EN, Brent GA, Brown RS, Chen H, Dosiou C, et al. 2017 guidelines of the American Thyroid Association for the diagnosis and Management of Thyroid Disease during Pregnancy and the postpartum. Thyroid. 2017;27(3):315–89.
13. Caldwell KL, Pan Y, Mortensen ME, Makhmudov A, Merrill L, Moye J. Iodine status in pregnant women in the National Children's study and in U.S. women (15-44 years), National Health and nutrition examination survey 2005-2010. Thyroid. 2013;23(8):927–37.
14. King JR, Lachica R, Lee RH, Montoro M, Mestman J. Diagnosis and Management of Hyperthyroidism in pregnancy: a review. Obstet Gynecol Surv. 2016;71(11):675–85.
15. Henrichsen TL, Reading CC, Charboneau JW, Donovan DJ, Sebo TJ, Hay ID. Cystic change in thyroid carcinoma: prevalence and estimated volume in 360 carcinomas. J Clin Ultrasound. 2010;38(7):361–6.
16. Brito JP, Gionfriddo MR, Al Nofal A, Boehmer KR, Leppin AL, Reading C, et al. The accuracy of thyroid nodule ultrasound to predict thyroid cancer: systematic review and meta-analysis. J Clin Endocrinol Metab. 2014;99(4):1253–63.
17. Grant EG, Tessler FN, Hoang JK, Langer JE, Beland MD, Berland LL, et al. Thyroid ultrasound reporting lexicon: white paper of the ACR thyroid imaging, reporting and data system (TIRADS) committee. J Am Coll Radiol. 2015;12(12 Pt A):1272–9.
18. Choi SH, Kim EK, Kwak JY, Kim MJ, Son EJ. Interobserver and intraobserver variations in ultrasound assessment of thyroid nodules. Thyroid. 2010;20(2):167–72.
19. Horvath E, Majlis S, Rossi R, Franco C, Niedmann JP, Castro A, et al. An ultrasonogram reporting system for thyroid nodules stratifying cancer risk for clinical management. J Clin Endocrinol Metab. 2009;94(5):1748–51.
20. Haugen BR, Alexander EK, Bible KC, Doherty GM, Mandel SJ, Nikiforov YE, et al. 2015 American Thyroid Association management guidelines for adult patients with thyroid nodules and differentiated thyroid Cancer: The American Thyroid Association guidelines task force on thyroid nodules and differentiated thyroid Cancer. Thyroid. 2016;26(1):1–133.
21. Russ G, Royer B, Bigorgne C, Rouxel A, Bienvenu-Perrard M, Leenhardt L. Prospective evaluation of thyroid imaging reporting and data system on 4550 nodules with and without elastography. Eur J Endocrinol. 2013;168(5):649–55.
22. Haugen BR. 2015 American Thyroid Association management guidelines for adult patients with thyroid nodules and differentiated thyroid Cancer: what is new and what has changed? Cancer. 2017;123(3):372–81.
23. Gharib H, Papini E, Garber JR, Duick DS, Harrell RM, Hegedus L, et al. American Association of Clinical Endocrinologists, American College of Endocrinology, and Associazioni Medici Endocrinologi medical guidelines for clinical practice for the diagnosis and Management of Thyroid Nodules--2016 update. Endocr Pract. 2016;22(5):622–39.
24. Cibas ES, Ali SZ. The 2017 Bethesda system for reporting thyroid cytopathology. Thyroid. 2017;27(11):1341–6.

25. Marley EF, Oertel YC. Fine-needle aspiration of thyroid lesions in 57 pregnant and postpartum women. Diagn Cytopathol. 1997;16(2):122–5.
26. Khaled H, Al Lahloubi N, Rashad N. A review on thyroid cancer during pregnancy: multitasking is required. J Adv Res. 2016;7(4):565–70.
27. Lim H, Devesa SS, Sosa JA, Check D, Kitahara CM. Trends in thyroid Cancer incidence and mortality in the United States, 1974-2013. JAMA. 2017;317(13):1338–48.
28. Zamora-Ros R, Rinaldi S, Biessy C, Tjonneland A, Halkjaer J, Fournier A, et al. Reproductive and menstrual factors and risk of differentiated thyroid carcinoma: the EPIC study. Int J Cancer. 2015;136(5):1218–27.
29. Zhou YQ, Zhou Z, Qian MF, Gong T, Wang JD. Association of thyroid carcinoma with pregnancy: a meta-analysis. Mol Clin Oncol. 2015;3(2):341–6.
30. Rosen IB, Walfish PG, Nikore V. Pregnancy and surgical thyroid disease. Surgery. 1985;98(6):1135–40.
31. Rosen IB, Korman M, Walfish PG. Thyroid nodular disease in pregnancy: current diagnosis and management. Clin Obstet Gynecol. 1997;40(1):81–9.
32. Tan GH, Gharib H, Goellner JR, van Heerden JA, Bahn RS. Management of thyroid nodules in pregnancy. Arch Intern Med. 1996;156(20):2317–20.
33. McTiernan AM, Weiss NS, Daling JR. Incidence of thyroid cancer in women in relation to reproductive and hormonal factors. Am J Epidemiol. 1984;120(3):423–35.
34. Smith LH, Danielsen B, Allen ME, Cress R. Cancer associated with obstetric delivery: results of linkage with the California cancer registry. Am J Obstet Gynecol. 2003;189(4):1128–35.
35. Choe W, McDougall IR. Thyroid cancer in pregnant women: diagnostic and therapeutic management. Thyroid. 1994;4(4):433–5.
36. Moosa M, Mazzaferri EL. Outcome of differentiated thyroid cancer diagnosed in pregnant women. J Clin Endocrinol Metab. 1997;82(9):2862–6.
37. Schlumberger M, De Vathaire F, Ceccarelli C, Francese C, Pinchera A, Parmentier C. Outcome of pregnancy in women with thyroid carcinoma. J Endocrinol Investig. 1995;18(2):150–1.
38. Vini L, Hyer S, Pratt B, Harmer C. Management of differentiated thyroid cancer diagnosed during pregnancy. Eur J Endocrinol. 1999;140(5):404–6.
39. Yasmeen S, Cress R, Romano PS, Xing G, Berger-Chen S, Danielsen B, et al. Thyroid cancer in pregnancy. Int J Gynaecol Obstet. 2005;91(1):15–20.
40. Vannucchi G, Perrino M, Rossi S, Colombo C, Vicentini L, Dazzi D, et al. Clinical and molecular features of differentiated thyroid cancer diagnosed during pregnancy. Eur J Endocrinol. 2010;162(1):145–51.
41. Zeng Q, Chen GG, Vlantis AC, van Hasselt CA. Oestrogen mediates the growth of human thyroid carcinoma cells via an oestrogen receptor-ERK pathway. Cell Prolif. 2007;40(6):921–35.
42. Messuti I, Corvisieri S, Bardesono F, Rapa I, Giorcelli J, Pellerito R, et al. Impact of pregnancy on prognosis of differentiated thyroid cancer: clinical and molecular features. Eur J Endocrinol. 2014;170(5):659–66.
43. Lee JC, Zhao JT, Clifton-Bligh RJ, Gill AJ, Gundara JS, Ip J, et al. Papillary thyroid carcinoma in pregnancy: a variant of the disease? Ann Surg Oncol. 2012;19(13):4210–6.
44. Kuy S, Roman SA, Desai R, Sosa JA. Outcomes following thyroid and parathyroid surgery in pregnant women. Arch Surg. 2009;144(5):399–406; discussion.
45. Uruno T, Shibuya H, Kitagawa W, Nagahama M, Sugino K, Ito K. Optimal timing of surgery for differentiated thyroid cancer in pregnant women. World J Surg. 2014;38(3):704–8.
46. Boucek J, de Haan J, Halaska MJ, Plzak J, Van Calsteren K, de Groot CJM, et al. Maternal and obstetrical outcome in 35 cases of well-differentiated thyroid carcinoma during pregnancy. Laryngoscope. 2018;128(6):1493–500.
47. Sam S, Molitch ME. Timing and special concerns regarding endocrine surgery during pregnancy. Endocrinol Metab Clin N Am. 2003;32(2):337–54.
48. De Groot L, Abalovich M, Alexander EK, Amino N, Barbour L, Cobin RH, et al. Management of thyroid dysfunction during pregnancy and postpartum: an Endocrine Society clinical practice guideline. J Clin Endocrinol Metab. 2012;97(8):2543–65.

49. Rowe CW, Murray K, Woods A, Gupta S, Smith R, Wynne K. Management of metastatic thyroid cancer in pregnancy: risk and uncertainty. Endocrinol Diabetes Metab Case Rep. 2016;2016 pii: 16-0071. Epub 2016 Dec 2.
50. Rakhlin L, Fish S, Tuttle RM. Response to therapy status is an excellent predictor of pregnancy-associated structural disease progression in patients previously treated for differentiated thyroid Cancer. Thyroid. 2017;27(3):396–401.
51. Haymart MR, Pearce EN. How much should thyroid Cancer impact plans for pregnancy? Thyroid. 2017;27(3):312–4.
52. Casey BM, Dashe JS, Wells CE, McIntire DD, Leveno KJ, Cunningham FG. Subclinical hyperthyroidism and pregnancy outcomes. Obstet Gynecol. 2006;107(2 Pt 1):337–41.
53. Oh HS, Kim WG, Park S, Kim M, Kwon H, Jeon MJ, et al. Serial neck Ultrasonographic evaluation of changes in papillary thyroid carcinoma during pregnancy. Thyroid. 2017;27(6):773–7.
54. Hill CS Jr, Clark RL, Wolf M. The effect of subsequent pregnancy on patients with thyroid carcinoma. Surg Gynecol Obstet. 1966;122(6):1219–22.
55. Rosvoll RV, Winship T. Thyroid carcinoma and pregnancy. Surg Gynecol Obstet. 1965;121(5):1039–42.
56. Leboeuf R, Emerick LE, Martorella AJ, Tuttle RM. Impact of pregnancy on serum thyroglobulin and detection of recurrent disease shortly after delivery in thyroid cancer survivors. Thyroid. 2007;17(6):543–7.
57. Rosario PW, Barroso AL, Purisch S. The effect of subsequent pregnancy on patients with thyroid carcinoma apparently free of the disease. Thyroid. 2007;17(11):1175–6.
58. Hirsch D, Levy S, Tsvetov G, Weinstein R, Lifshitz A, Singer J, et al. Impact of pregnancy on outcome and prognosis of survivors of papillary thyroid cancer. Thyroid. 2010;20(10):1179–85.
59. Shindo H, Amino N, Ito Y, Kihara M, Kobayashi K, Miya A, et al. Papillary thyroid microcarcinoma might progress during pregnancy. Thyroid. 2014;24(5):840–4.
60. Casara D, Rubello D, Saladini G, Piotto A, Pelizzo MR, Girelli ME, et al. Pregnancy after high therapeutic doses of iodine-131 in differentiated thyroid cancer: potential risks and recommendations. Eur J Nucl Med. 1993;20(3):192–4.
61. Chow SM, Yau S, Lee SH, Leung WM, Law SC. Pregnancy outcome after diagnosis of differentiated thyroid carcinoma: no deleterious effect after radioactive iodine treatment. Int J Radiat Oncol Biol Phys. 2004;59(4):992–1000.
62. Garsi JP, Schlumberger M, Rubino C, Ricard M, Labbe M, Ceccarelli C, et al. Therapeutic administration of 131I for differentiated thyroid cancer: radiation dose to ovaries and outcome of pregnancies. J Nucl Med. 2008;49(5):845–52.
63. Lin JD, Wang HS, Weng HF, Kao PF. Outcome of pregnancy after radioactive iodine treatment for well differentiated thyroid carcinomas. J Endocrinol Investig. 1998;21(10):662–7.
64. Fard-Esfahani A, Hadifar M, Fallahi B, Beiki D, Eftekhari M, Saghari M, et al. Radioiodine treatment complications to the mother and child in patients with differentiated thyroid carcinoma. Hell J Nucl Med. 2009;12(1):37–40.
65. Sawka AM, Lakra DC, Lea J, Alshehri B, Tsang RW, Brierley JD, et al. A systematic review examining the effects of therapeutic radioactive iodine on ovarian function and future pregnancy in female thyroid cancer survivors. Clin Endocrinol. 2008;69(3):479–90.
66. Wu JX, Young S, Ro K, Li N, Leung AM, Chiu HK, et al. Reproductive outcomes and nononcologic complications after radioactive iodine ablation for well-differentiated thyroid cancer. Thyroid. 2015;25(1):133–8.
67. Rosario PW, da Silva AL, Nunes MS, Ribeiro Borges MA, Mourao GF, Calsolari MR. Risk of malignancy in 1502 solid thyroid nodules >1 cm using the new ultrasonographic classification of the American Thyroid Association. Endocrine. 2017;56(2):442–5.
68. Yoon JH, Lee HS, Kim EK, Moon HJ, Kwak JY. Malignancy risk stratification of thyroid nodules: comparison between the thyroid imaging reporting and data system and the 2014 American Thyroid Association management guidelines. Radiology. 2016;278(3):917–24.
69. Xu T, Gu JY, Ye XH, Xu SH, Wu Y, Shao XY, et al. Thyroid nodule sizes influence the diagnostic performance of TIRADS and ultrasound patterns of 2015 ATA guidelines: a multicenter retrospective study. Sci Rep. 2017;7:43183.

Chapter 9
Thyroid Dysfunction and Infertility

Shweta J. Bhatt, Emily C. Holden, and Aimee Seungdamrong

> **Clinical Case**
> A 37-year-old G0 female presents with 2 years of infertility despite regular menses. Her workup reveals bilaterally patent fallopian tubes, a normal semen analysis for her partner, and ovarian reserve testing showing an anti-Mullerian hormone (AMH) of 1.8 ng/ml, day 3 follicle-stimulating hormone (FSH) of 8.4 mIU/ml, and day 3 estradiol of 48 pg/ml. Her thyroid-stimulating hormone (TSH) is 3.87 mIU/L. How would you counsel her?

Introduction

Female fertility is a cumulative process of ovarian function, oocyte development, endometrial receptivity, and male factors. Infertility is defined as 12 months or more of regular unprotected intercourse without conception and occurs in about 15% of couples. After this timeframe, an evaluation of infertility is recommended. In women over age 35 years old, an evaluation is recommended after 6 months [1].

S. J. Bhatt · E. C. Holden
Rutgers New Jersey Medical School, Department of Obstetrics, Gynecology, and Women's Health, Newark, NJ, USA

A. Seungdamrong (✉)
Rutgers New Jersey Medical School, Department of Obstetrics, Gynecology, and Women's Health, Newark, NJ, USA

Damien Fertility Partners, Shrewsbury, NJ, USA

The infertility evaluation frequently involves testing of thyroid function. As described in Chap. 1 of this book, thyroid hormone is produced in the thyroid gland, transported through cell membranes, and deiodinated within the cytoplasm. Its effects are mediated through nuclear transport and interaction with thyroid hormone receptors. In this chapter, we will examine the relationship between dysfunction and female reproductive potential. Table 9.1 summarizes the Society Practice Guidelines for Screening and Treatment of Thyroid Dysfunction in Women with Infertility.

Table 9.1 Summary of the Society Practice Guidelines for Screening and Treatment of Thyroid Dysfunction in Women with Infertility

Society	Indications for screening	Indications for treatment
Endocrine Society 2012 (Pubmed ID 22869843)	Some members of the committee recommend universal screening for thyroid disease; others reserve testing for "high-risk" patients, includes infertility. Universal screening for TPO antibodies **not** routinely recommended; if +TPO antibody testing, recommended TSH screening	Recommended for TSH ≥ 2.5 mIU/L if attempting pregnancy; may discontinue if not pregnant or postpartum. Monitor TSH in euthyroid women with +TPO antibody before and during pregnancy
American College of Obstetrics and Gynecology (ACOG) 2015 (Pubmed ID 25798985)	Universal screening of thyroid disease **not** recommended. Testing recommended only for personal history of thyroid disease or presence of symptoms. No specific recommendations for infertility patients	Recommended for overt hypothyroidism
American Society for Reproductive Medicine (ASRM) [12] 2015	TSH testing recommended for infertility patients. TPO antibody testing **not** routinely recommended, may consider for TSH ≥ 2.5 mIU/L or risk factors for thyroid disease	Recommended for overt hypothyroidism (TSH ≥ 4.0 mIU/L). Consider monitoring with repeat testing or treatment for SCH (TSH 2.5–4 mIU/L). Consider treatment for SCH with +TPO antibodies
American Thyroid Association (ATA) [13] 2017	TSH testing recommended for infertility patients	Recommended for overt hypothyroidism. Natural conception: Consider treatment for SCH and -ATA. No recommendation for euthyroid with +ATA. ART: Recommend treatment for SCH. Consider treatment for euthyroid with +ATA

TSH thyroid-stimulating hormone, *TPO* thyroid peroxidase, *SCH* subclinical hypothyroidism, *ATA* antithyroid antibody, *ART* assisted reproductive technology

Thyroid Function and the Menstrual Cycle

The occurrence of regular cyclic menses is the end result of a series of signaling pathways within the hypothalamic-pituitary-ovarian axis. Changes in the axis result in irregularities of ovulation and menstruation.

Hypothyroidism is associated with changes in menstrual patterns including decreased menstrual cycle frequency and increased volume of menses [2]. Primary hypofunction of the thyroid gland results in increased secretion of thyroid-releasing hormone (TRH) which in turn increases pituitary TSH and prolactin secretion. These changes then affect pituitary gonadotropin secretion. Irregularities in the hypothalamic-pituitary axis can result in oligo- or anovulation and subsequent subfertility or infertility [2]. These alterations are mediated through a decrease in sex hormone-binding globulin (SHBG), an increase in prolactin (PRL), and changes in the frequency of gonadotropin-releasing hormone (GnRH) secretion [3].

Hyperthyroidism can also lead to changes in the hypothalamic-pituitary-ovarian axis and the menstrual cycle [2]. Increased SHBG and estradiol levels have been observed in women with hyperthyroidism as well as a variety of menstrual irregularities including oligomenorrhea and amenorrhea [2]. However, compared to hypothyroidism, hyperthyroidism less frequently results in anovulation and infertility [2].

Thyroid Function and the Ovary

The cellular processes regulated by thyroid hormones within the ovarian follicle and in the oocyte itself have been a subject of active investigation. Existing literature has demonstrated the presence of thyroid hormone receptors in the ovary. An early study by Zhang and colleagues examined the expression of thyroid hormone receptors in follicular fluid specimens from fourteen patients undergoing in vitro fertilization [4]. Human oocytes, granulosa cells, and cumulus cells were examined for the presence of mRNA of thyroid hormone receptors α1, β1, and β2. Thyroid hormone receptor mRNA was found in all three cell types [4]. Another group studied both primary human ovarian tissue from human surgical specimens and follicular fluid from patients undergoing IVF [5]. Thyroid hormone receptor proteins were localized to the ovarian surface epithelium, ovarian follicles, and oocytes at various stages of development. Evaluation for deiodinases 2 and 3 showed localization to luteinized granulosa cells. Additionally, granulosa cells stimulated in vitro with TSH showed a significant increase in cAMP concentrations indicating activation through TSHR [5].

Other studies have examined the potential role of thyroid hormone in ovarian follicular function. For example, T3 has been shown to amplify FSH-induced granulosa cell proliferation in vitro [1]. This interaction is mediated through the PI3/Akt pathway [1]. Liu and colleagues demonstrated that the combination of T3 and FSH increased CYP51 expression in mouse granulosa cells, thereby inducing steroidogenesis [6]. Another study showed that T3 can prevent apoptosis in a human granulosa cell line [7]. Glucose transporters GLUT-1 and GLUT-4 may also play a role in preantral follicle development [8]. After 48 h co-treatment of rat granulosa cells with FSH and T3, expression of GLUT-1 and GLUT-4 was significantly enhanced, and glucose uptake was significantly elevated [8]. Furthermore, the PI3K/Akt pathway as well as NOS/NO were found to be involved in this regulatory system [8]. While the precise changes that occur within the human ovarian granulosa cell and oocyte in the setting of thyroid dysfunction are still unclear, this body of evidence suggests that thyroid hormone and thyroid hormone receptors play an active role in ovarian physiology.

Thyroid Function and the Endometrium

Thyroid hormone receptors are found at the surface of the endometrium and are thought to be involved in the interaction between the endometrium and the blastocyst. At the time of implantation, TSH increases leukemia inhibitory factor (LIF) and leukemia inhibitory factor receptor (LIFR) while increasing GLUT-1 expression and glucose uptake [9]. Thyroid hormone transporters in syncytiotrophoblast cells are involved in actively mediating uptake of thyroid hormone from maternal blood after implantation [9].

Aghajanova and colleagues characterized the expression and cellular distribution of thyroid hormone pathway components in human endometrial biopsy samples from fertile women throughout the menstrual cycle [10]. Thyroid hormone receptors $\alpha 1$ and $\beta 1$ were present throughout the menstrual cycle and were significantly more abundant during the mid-secretory phase. Deiodinases were also expressed in the endometrium throughout the menstrual cycle but were less present during the mid-secretory phase of the menstrual cycle. These mid-secretory changes were associated with the electron microscopic finding of the presence of pinopodes, which are expressed during the window of implantation. The authors also found changes in the expression of leukemia inhibitory factor (LIF) and its receptor (LIFR) and an increased concentration of thyroid hormone in conditioned media from cultured endometrial epithelial cells after TSH stimulation. While the downstream effects of these changes are unclear, they suggest a potential impact of thyroid hormone on endometrial function [10].

Ovarian hyperstimulation for the treatment of infertility may alter the signaling pathways for thyroid hormones in the endometrium. In an elegant study of endometrial biopsy samples obtained day 3 after ovulation, samples from oocyte donors undergoing ovarian hyperstimulation were compared with normal fertile controls [11]. The mRNA expression levels of thyroid stimulating hormone receptor, thyroid hormone receptor $\beta 1$, and deiodinase 2 were decreased in oocyte donors compared to controls. There were no differences in the mRNA levels of thyroid hormone receptors $\alpha 1$ and $\alpha 2$ [11].

The presence of thyroid hormone receptors and deiodinases in the endometrium and the cyclic variation in expression point to a role of thyroid hormone in endometrial function. However, the ovarian and endometrial specific effects of thyroid dysfunction on overall female fertility remain to be elucidated.

Subclinical Hypothyroidism and Infertility

As discussed in Chaps. 2 and 6, subclinical hypothyroidism is usually defined by thyroid-stimulating hormone (TSH) levels exceeding the upper limit of normal despite a normal free T4 level [12–14]. While overt hypothyroidism and hyperthyroidism carry clear detrimental effects on fertility, the effect of subclinical hypothyroidism has been a subject of great debate. This is secondary to a lack of controls and varying definitions of subclinical hypothyroidism present in the literature including the use of a thyrotropin-releasing hormone (TRH) test or different values for the upper limit of normal with the TSH assay. The prevalence of subclinical hypothyroidism in the general population is estimated to be between 4.5% and 9%, based on a large cross-sectional study from Colorado [12] and the National Health and Nutrition Examination Survey (NHANES III) [13]. In the infertile population, the prevalence of subclinical hypothyroidism has been reported to be as high as 13.9% [15], although other studies have reported rates similar to those of the general population [16, 17].

In the largest study to date, authors used the Danish General Suburban Population Study (GESUS) to perform a retrospective cross-sectional analysis of 11,254 women. Subclinical hypothyroidism was defined as a TSH >3.7 mIU/L. After adjusting for covariates, they found that subclinical hypothyroidism was significantly associated with childlessness and lack of conception [18]. Similarly, in a retrospective, case control study comparing 244 infertile women and 155 healthy women, the prevalence of subclinical hypothyroidism was higher in the infertile population (13.9%) than in female controls (3.9%) [15]. In that study, subclinical hypothyroidism was defined by a TSH >4.22 mIU/mL with a normal free T4 or a positive TRH stimulation test when TSH levels were between 2 and 4.22 mIU/mL [17]. In contrast, a prospective study of 884 women with a TSH <2.5 mIU/L and 303 women with a TSH ≥2.5 mIU/L showed no difference in the time to conception, pregnancy loss, or live birth [19]. Other studies have found similar outcomes [16, 17]. Due to conflicting data, the American Society for Reproductive Medicine concludes there are insufficient data to conclude that SCH is associated with infertility [12].

In infertile women with subclinical hypothyroidism who are not undergoing assisted reproductive technologies, there are little high-quality data regarding treatment with levothyroxine and pregnancy outcomes. Yoshioka and colleagues conducted a prospective observational study of 69 infertile women treated with levothyroxine for subclinical hypothyroidism. The pregnancy rate was 84% during the study period [20]. In another study of 394 infertile women, Verma and colleagues demonstrated benefit of treating women with TSH >4.2 mIU/L but did not distinguish those with subclinical hypothyroidism from those with overt hypothyroidism [21]. Due to the paucity of data, the American Thyroid Association concludes that "insufficient data exist for recommending for or against routine LT4 therapy in subclinically hypothyroid, thyroid autoantibody–negative infertile women who are attempting conception but not undergoing ART" [13]. The American Society for Reproductive Medicine states that there is insufficient evidence for treating TSH between 2.5 and 4 mIU/L; however, it does advocate for treatment when TSH levels are greater than 4 mIU/L [12]. However, both groups concede that the overall risk of treatment is low. Given the potential benefit of treating certain subgroups, it may still be reasonable to treat these patients [12, 13].

There are even fewer data available regarding the association between subclinical hypothyroidism and male subfertility. For a long time, the testes were not thought to be responsive to thyroid hormone [22]. However, it has since been determined that spermatogenesis is affected by thyroid hormone [22, 23]. Most of the data comes from studies of overt hypothyroidism in men and not subclinical hypothyroidism. In a cross-sectional study by Lotti and colleagues, there was no significant difference in seminal or hormonal parameters of men with subclinical hypothyroidism when compared to euthyroid and hyperthyroid patients [24]. However, given the paucity of data on this subject, further studies are needed.

Subclinical Hypothyroidism and Miscarriage

There is much stronger evidence linking SCH to miscarriage than to infertility. Overall, the evidence suggests that the risk of miscarriage is positively correlated with the level of TSH. For example, in a large prospective cohort study of 3315 Chinese women with spontaneous pregnancies, Liu and colleagues demonstrated a higher miscarriage rate in women with TSH greater than 5.2 mIU/L than those with TSH less than 2.5 mIU/L. However, TSH between 2.5 mIU/L and upper limit of the prepregnancy assay may not increase the chance of miscarriage [19, 25–27]. This is influenced by the presence or absence of thyroid peroxidase (TPO) antibodies, as discussed in more detail in Chap. 10.

Multiple studies have shown that treating SCH with TSH >4.5 mIU/L, or the upper limit of normal in the assay, may decrease miscarriage rates [27–29]. Two randomized controlled trials have shown a benefit of levothyroxine treatment in women with subclinical hypothyroidism based on a TSH greater than 4.5 mIU/L. Both studies demonstrated reduced miscarriage rates after treatment [28, 29]. In a prospective study, miscarriage rates were increased in patients with subclinical hypothyroidism as defined by TSH >2.5 mIU/L [30]. However, in that same study, the miscarriage rate did not significantly decrease after levothyroxine treatment [30].

Controlled Ovarian Hyperstimulation and Thyroid Function

Controlled ovarian hyperstimulation (COH), the first step in both intrauterine insemination (IUI) and in vitro fertilization (IVF) cycles, is the process by which medications are given to stimulate growth and maturity of multiple ovarian follicles. Existing literature suggests that COH may impact thyroid function. An elevation in the serum estradiol level leads to an increase in thyroid binding globulin (TBG), thus decreasing free thyroid hormone and increasing TSH levels [31]. Additionally, use of human chorionic gonadotropin (hCG) to trigger oocyte maturation may act on the TSH receptor to increase free thyroxine and decrease TSH [32]. A prospective cohort study demonstrated increased serum TSH, free T4, and thyroid-binding globulin with controlled ovarian hyperstimulation, with a peak noted at 1 week after hCG trigger administration. This peak in TSH was significantly higher in women with hypothyroidism compared to euthyroid women [33]. A prospective cohort study of women taking levothyroxine for overt hypothyroidism demonstrated an increase in TSH from 1.7 mIU/L prior to COH to 2.9 mIU/mL at the time of hCG trigger administration and up to 3.2 mIU/L 2 weeks later [34]. These elevations in TSH normalize in women who do not conceive, though persistent elevations in pregnancy may warrant treatment with levothyroxine. Given the likely transient nature of elevations in TSH with COH, the American Thyroid Association (ATA) recommends repeat serum TSH measurement 2–4 weeks after controlled ovarian hyperstimulation in nonpregnant women with mild TSH elevations [13].

Thyroid Dysfunction and Intrauterine Insemination

There are sparse data on the impact of thyroid function on outcomes of intrauterine insemination. One retrospective study examined IUI outcomes in euthyroid women and those with a "high normal" TSH (2.5–4.8 mIU/L) [35]. The clinical pregnancy rate, miscarriage rate, and live birth rate were similar between groups. Another retrospective study demonstrated comparable pregnancy, miscarriage, and live birth rates in women with or without subclinical hypothyroidism; furthermore, the presence of TPO antibodies had no effect on outcomes [36]. A secondary analysis of two large RCTs examined the association between pregnancy outcomes and preconception TPO antibody status among euthyroid women undergoing ovulation induction with intrauterine insemination. TSH elevation above 2.5 mIU/L was not associated with adverse pregnancy outcomes; however, TPO antibodies were associated with an increased miscarriage rate (25.3% vs 43.9%) and decreased live birth rate (25.4% vs 17.1) [37]. Based on these studies, there are insufficient data to support an association between subclinical hypothyroidism and outcomes of IUI. Thyroid antibodies, however, may negatively impact outcomes. There is currently insufficient evidence to recommend levothyroxine supplementation in patients with subclinical hypothyroidism and/or presence of thyroid antibodies undergoing intrauterine insemination without well-designed, prospective studies.

Thyroid Dysfunction and Assisted Reproductive Technology

Assisted reproductive technology (ART) is defined as fertility treatment in which the eggs and sperm are handled outside the body. In vitro fertilization (IVF) is the most common form of ART. Patients undergoing IVF undergo controlled ovarian hyperstimulation with gonadotropins, followed by oocyte retrieval. The oocytes are fertilized with sperm, and one or more embryos are transferred back into the uterus. Embryo transfers may be performed with either fresh or frozen embryos. Given the negative impact of hypothyroidism on pregnancy, preconception assessment and management of thyroid disease prior to the use of ART treatments has become a topic of both great interest and debate. Evidence suggests that subclinical hypothyroidism and thyroid autoimmunity, in addition to overt hypothyroidism, may be associated with negative outcomes in women undergoing infertility treatment using advanced reproductive technology.

While treatment of overt hypothyroidism is recommended to reduce the rate of pregnancy complications after in vitro fertilization, management of women with subclinical hypothyroidism is less straightforward. Retrospective studies have demonstrated mixed results, with some supporting an association between subclinical hypothyroidism and negative IVF outcomes [38, 39] and others demonstrating no effect [25, 26, 40]. These retrospective studies have prompted further study with prospective randomized controlled trials. In one study, 70 subclinically hypothyroid women with IVF were randomized to either levothyroxine treatment or placebo. Subclinical hypothyroidism was defined as normal free thyroxine and TSH greater than 4.2 mIU/L. The women who received levothyroxine treatment had a lower miscarriage rate, higher clinical pregnancy rate, and higher live birth rate than the placebo-treated group [29]. A second, similar RCT included 64 women with subclinical hypothyroidism, defined as normal free thyroxine and TSH greater than 4.5mIU/L. Patients were randomized to levothyroxine supplementation initiated on day 1 of ovarian stimulation or control. The mean number of oocytes retrieved was similar between groups, but the levothyroxine group had significantly higher rates of clinical pregnancy and live birth with a decreased miscarriage rate [28].

The current evidence suggests that levothyroxine treatment improves IVF outcomes among women with TSH levels greater than 4.0 mIU/L, as recommended by ASRM [17]. However, there is insufficient evidence to recommend levothyroxine treatment in women with TSH 2.5–4 mIU/L undergoing IVF. For women with TSH values in the 2.5 and 4 mIU/L range, clinicians may either monitor TSH values or treat to maintain TSH less than 2.5 mIU/L.

The relevance of thyroid autoantibodies in women undergoing in vitro fertilization, and the potential role of levothyroxine treatment for antibody-positive women, is controversial. One retrospective cohort study demonstrated that women with antithyroid antibodies had significantly lower fertilization rates, implantation rates, and pregnancy rates in addition to higher miscarriage rates than antibody-negative controls [41]. Another retrospective study found a clinical pregnancy rate of 23.9% with

IVF in women without thyroid antibodies compared to no pregnancies in the group of women positive for TPO antibodies [39]. In contrast, however, a prospective study comparing euthyroid women with and without thyroid antibodies demonstrated no difference in peak estradiol, number of oocytes retrieved, fertilization rate, implantation rate, miscarriage rate, and ongoing pregnancy rate [42]. A meta-analysis pooling data from six retrospective studies and six prospective studies demonstrated no difference in the number of oocytes retrieved or rates of fertilization, implantation, and clinical pregnancy in euthyroid women undergoing IVF who had positive thyroid antibodies compared to women without antibodies. However, the live birth rate was lower in women with thyroid antibodies, suggesting a negative association between thyroid antibodies and ongoing pregnancy. Finally, a recent RCT assessed the potential role of levothyroxine supplementation compared to control in euthyroid women with positive antithyroid peroxidase antibodies. The study demonstrated no difference in miscarriage rate or live birth rate with or without treatment with levothyroxine, suggesting no benefit to thyroid supplementation in euthyroid women with positive thyroid peroxidase antibody undergoing in vitro fertilization [43]. Despite limitations in existing data, given the minimal risk and potential benefit of levothyroxine treatment, the ATA recommends consideration of levothyroxine supplementation (25–50 micrograms per day) in euthyroid women undergoing ART who are thyroid peroxidase antibody positive [13].

In summary, while a transient change in thyroid function may occur with controlled ovarian hyperstimulation, levothyroxine supplementation is not currently indicated for euthyroid women. However, it may improve reproductive outcomes in women with subclinical hypothyroidism undergoing treatment with ART. Although pregnancy outcomes after ART may be affected by the presence of thyroid antibodies, current evidence does not support routine supplementation of levothyroxine in euthyroid women (TSH <2.5 mIU/ml) with positive thyroid antibodies. Treatment with levothyroxine can be considered on an individual basis, given that there is potential benefit and minimal risk.

Clinical Case and Discussion

A 37-year-old G0 female presents with 2 years of infertility despite regular menses. Her workup reveals bilaterally patent fallopian tubes, a normal semen analysis for her partner, and ovarian reserve testing showing an AMH of 1.8 ng/ml, day 3 FSH of 8.4 mIU/ml, and day 3 estradiol of 48 pg/ml. Her TSH is 3.87 mIU/L. How would you counsel her?

Our next step based on multiple society guidelines would be to consider repeat TSH testing and thyroid peroxidase antibody testing. If her thyroid peroxidase antibodies are negative, we would counsel her to proceed with recommended fertility treatment after completing her workup. If her thyroid peroxidase antibodies are positive, we would consider thyroid supplementation.

References

1. Vissenberg R, Manders VD, Mastenbroek S, Fliers E, Afink GB, Ris-Stalpers C, et al. Pathophysiological aspects of thyroid hormone disorders/thyroid peroxidase autoantibodies and reproduction. Hum Reprod Update. 2015;21(3):378–87.
2. Krassas GE, Poppe K, Glinoer D. Thyroid function and human reproductive health. Endocr Rev. 2010;31(5):702–55.
3. Dittrich R, Beckmann MW, Oppelt PG, Hoffmann I, Lotz L, Kuwert T, et al. Thyroid hormone receptors and reproduction. J Reprod Immunol. 2011;90:58–66.
4. Zhang SS, Carrillo AJ, Darling DS. Expression of multiple thyroid hormone receptor mRNAs in human oocytes, cumulus cells, and granulosa cells. Mol Hum Reprod. 1997;3(7):555–62.
5. Aghajanova L, Lindeberg M, Carlsson IB, Stavreus-Evers A, Zhang P, Scott JE, et al. Receptors for thyroid-stimulating hormone and thyroid hormones in human ovarian tissue. Reprod Biomed Online. 2009;18(3):337–47.
6. Liu J, Tian Y, Ding Y, Heng D, Xu K, Liu W, et al. Role of CYP51 in the regulation of T3 and FSH-induced steroidogenesis in female mice. Endocrinology. 2017;158(11):3974–87.
7. Verga Falzacappa C, Mangialardo C, Patriarca V, Bucci B, Amendola D, Raffa S, et al. Thyroid hormones induce cell proliferation and survival in ovarian granulosa cells COV434. J Cell Physiol. 2009;221(1):242–53.
8. Tian Y, Ding Y, Liu J, Heng D, Xu K, Liu W, et al. Nitric oxide-mediated regulation of GLUT by T3 and follicle-stimulating hormone in rat granulosa cells. Endocrinology. 2017;158(6):1898–915.
9. Colicchia M, Campagnolo L, Baldini E, Ulisse S, Valensise H, Moretti C. Molecular basis of thyrotropin and thyroid hormone action during implantation and early development. Hum Reprod Update. 2014;20(6):884–904.
10. Aghajanova L, Stavreus-Evers A, Lindeberg M, Landgren B-M, Sparre LS, Hovatta O. Thyroid-stimulating hormone receptor and thyroid hormone receptors are involved in human endometrial physiology. Fertil Steril. 2011;95(1):237.e1–2.
11. Detti L, Uhlmann RA, Fletcher NM, Diamond MP, Saed GM. Endometrial signaling pathways during ovarian stimulation for assisted reproduction technology. Fertil Steril. 2013;100(3):889–94.
12. Practice Committee of the American Society for Reproductive Medicine. Subclinical hypothyroidism in the infertile female population: a guideline. Fertil Steril. 2015;104(3):545–53.
13. Alexander EK, Pearce EN, Brent GA, Brown RS, Chen H, Dosiou C, et al. 2017 guidelines of the American Thyroid Association for the diagnosis and Management of Thyroid Disease during Pregnancy and the postpartum. Thyroid. 2017;27(3):315–89.
14. Surks MI, Ortiz E, Daniels GH, Sawin CT, Col NF, Cobin RH, et al. Subclinical thyroid disease: scientific review and guidelines for diagnosis and management. JAMA. 2004;291(2):228–38.
15. Abalovich M, Mitelberg L, Allami C, Gutierrez S, Alcaraz G, Otero P, et al. Subclinical hypothyroidism and thyroid autoimmunity in women with infertility. Gynecol Endocrinol. 2007;23(5):279–83.
16. Poppe K, Glinoer D, Van Steirteghem A, Tournaye H, Devroey P, Schiettecatte J, et al. Thyroid dysfunction and autoimmunity in infertile women. Thyroid. 2002;12(11):997–1001.
17. Lincoln SR, Ke RW, Kutteh WH. Screening for hypothyroidism in infertile women. J Reprod Med. 1999;44(5):455–7.
18. Feldthusen A-D, Pedersen PL, Larsen J, Toft Kristensen T, Ellervik C, Kvetny J. Impaired fertility associated with subclinical hypothyroidism and thyroid autoimmunity: the Danish general suburban population study. J Pregnancy. 2015;2015:132718.
19. Plowden TC, Schisterman EF, Sjaarda LA, Zarek SM, Perkins NJ, Silver R, et al. Subclinical hypothyroidism and thyroid autoimmunity are not associated with fecundity, pregnancy loss, or live birth. J Clin Endocrinol Metab. 2016;101(6):2358–65.

20. Yoshioka Y, Amino N, Ide A, Kang S, Kudo T, Nishihara E, et al. Thyroxine treatment may be useful for subclinical hypothyroidism in patients with female infertility. Endocr J. 2015;62(1):87–92.
21. Verma I, Sood R, Juneja S, Kaur S. Prevalence of hypothyroidism in infertile women and evaluation of response of treatment for hypothyroidism on infertility. Int J Appl Basic Med Res. 2012;2(1):17–9.
22. La Vignera S, Vita R, Condorelli RA, Mongioì LM, Presti S, Benvenga S, et al. Impact of thyroid disease on testicular function. Endocrine. 2017;58(3):397–407.
23. Rajender S, Monica MG, Walter L, Agarwal A. Thyroid, spermatogenesis, and male infertility. Front Biosci (Elite Ed). 2011;3:843–55.
24. Lotti F, Maseroli E, Fralassi N, Degl'Innocenti S, Boni L, Baldi E, et al. Is thyroid hormones evaluation of clinical value in the work-up of males of infertile couples? Hum Reprod. 2016;31(3):518–29.
25. Cai Y, Zhong L, Guan J, Guo R, Niu B, Ma Y, et al. Outcome of in vitro fertilization in women with subclinical hypothyroidism. Reprod Biol Endocrinol. 2017;15(1):39.
26. Chai J, Yeung W-YT, Lee C-YV, Li H-WR, Ho PC, Ng H-YE. Live birth rates following in vitro fertilization in women with thyroid autoimmunity and/or subclinical hypothyroidism. Clin Endocrinol. 2014;80(1):122–7.
27. Liu H, Shan Z, Li C, Mao J, Xie X, Wang W, et al. Maternal subclinical hypothyroidism, thyroid autoimmunity, and the risk of miscarriage: a prospective cohort study. Thyroid. 2014;24(11):1642–9.
28. Kim CH, Ahn J-W, Kang SP, Kim SH, Chae H-D, Kang B-M. Effect of levothyroxine treatment on in vitro fertilization and pregnancy outcome in infertile women with subclinical hypothyroidism undergoing in vitro fertilization/intracytoplasmic sperm injection. Fertil Steril. 2011;95(5):1650–4.
29. Abdel Rahman AH, Aly Abbassy H, Abbassy AAE. Improved in vitro fertilization outcomes after treatment of subclinical hypothyroidism in infertile women. Endocr Pract. 2010;16(5):792–7.
30. Wang S, Teng WP, Li JX, Wang WW, Shan ZY. Effects of maternal subclinical hypothyroidism on obstetrical outcomes during early pregnancy. J Endocrinol Investig. 2012;35(3):322–5.
31. Ain KB, Mori Y, Refetoff S. Reduced clearance rate of thyroxine-binding globulin (TBG) with increased sialylation: a mechanism for estrogen-induced elevation of serum TBG concentration. J Clin Endocrinol Metab. 1987;65(4):689–96.
32. Yoshimura M, Hershman JM. Thyrotropic action of human chorionic gonadotropin. Thyroid. 1995;5(5):425–34.
33. Gracia CR, Morse CB, Chan G, Schilling S, Prewitt M, Sammel MD, et al. Thyroid function during controlled ovarian hyperstimulation as part of in vitro fertilization. Fertil Steril. 2012;97(3):585–91.
34. Busnelli A, Somigliana E, Benaglia L, Sarais V, Ragni G, Fedele L. Thyroid axis dysregulation during in vitro fertilization in hypothyroid-treated patients. Thyroid. 2014;24(11):1650–5.
35. Karmon AE, Batsis M, Chavarro JE, Souter I. Preconceptional thyroid-stimulating hormone levels and outcomes of intrauterine insemination among euthyroid infertile women. Fertil Steril. 2015;103(1):258–63.
36. Unuane D, Velkeniers B, Bravenboer B, Drakopoulos P, Tournaye H, Parra J, et al. Impact of thyroid autoimmunity in euthyroid women on live birth rate after IUI. Hum Reprod. 2017;32(4):915–22.
37. Seungdamrong A, Steiner AZ, Gracia CR, Legro RS, Diamond MP, Coutifaris C, et al. Preconceptional antithyroid peroxidase antibodies, but not thyroid-stimulating hormone, are associated with decreased live birth rates in infertile women. Fertil Steril. 2017.; pii: S0015–0282(17)31748-X.
38. Baker VL, Rone HM, Pasta DJ, Nelson HP, Gvakharia M, Adamson GD. Correlation of thyroid stimulating hormone (TSH) level with pregnancy outcome in women undergoing in vitro fertilization. Am J Obstet Gynecol. 2006;194(6):1668–74. discussion 1674–5

39. Fumarola A, Grani G, Romanzi D, Del Sordo M, Bianchini M, Aragona A, et al. Thyroid function in infertile patients undergoing assisted reproduction. Am J Reprod Immunol. 2013;70(4):336–41.
40. Reh A, Grifo J, Danoff A. What is a normal thyroid-stimulating hormone (TSH) level? Effects of stricter TSH thresholds on pregnancy outcomes after in vitro fertilization. Fertil Steril. 2010;94(7):2920–2.
41. Zhong Y, Ying Y, Wu HT, Zhou CQ, Xu YW, Wang Q, et al. Relationship between antithyroid antibody and pregnancy outcome following in vitro fertilization and embryo transfer. Int J Med Sci. 2012;9(2):121–5.
42. Karacan M, Alwaeely F, Cebi Z, Berberoglugil M, Batukan M, Ulug M, et al. Effect of antithyroid antibodies on ICSI outcome in antiphospholipid antibody-negative euthyroid women. Reprod Biomed Online. 2013;27(4):376–80.
43. Wang H, Gao H, Chi H, Zeng L, Xiao W, Wang Y, et al. Effect of levothyroxine on miscarriage among women with normal thyroid function and thyroid autoimmunity undergoing in vitro fertilization and embryo transfer: a randomized clinical trial. JAMA. 2017;318(22):2190–8.

Chapter 10
Thyroid Autoimmunity and Miscarriage

Kelly S. Acharya and Jennifer L. Eaton

Abbreviations

ASRM	American Society for Reproductive Medicine
ATA	American Thyroid Association
hCG	human chorionic gonadotropin; SAB, spontaneous abortion
RPL	recurrent pregnancy loss
T3	triiodothyronine
T4	thyroxine
TBG	thyroid-binding globulin
Tg	thyroglobulin
TgAb	thyroglobulin antibodies
TPO	thyroid peroxidase
TPOAb	thyroid peroxidase antibodies
TRAb	thyroid receptor antibodies
TSH	thyroid-stimulating hormone
TSI	thyroid-stimulating immunoglobulin

Prevalence and Natural History of Thyroid Autoimmunity in Fertility, Infertility, and Pregnancy

Thyroid peroxidase (TPO) is an enzyme present on the cell membrane of thyroid cells; it catalyzes a critical step in the conversion of thyroglobulin (Tg) to triiodothyronine (T3) and thyroxine (T4) (Fig. 10.1). Thyroglobulin is a precursor protein

K. S. Acharya · J. L. Eaton (✉)
Duke University Medical Center, Division of Reproductive Endocrinology and Infertility, Department of Obstetrics and Gynecology, Durham, NC, USA
e-mail: jennifer.eaton@duke.edu

© Springer Nature Switzerland AG 2019
J. L. Eaton (ed.), *Thyroid Disease and Reproduction*,
https://doi.org/10.1007/978-3-319-99079-8_10

Clinical Case
A 31-year-old woman presents for consultation for recurrent pregnancy loss. She has had two first-trimester spontaneous abortions, each at approximately 6 weeks gestation. Her history is unremarkable except for the two miscarriages, and her partner is healthy and had a normal semen analysis. Parental karyotypes are normal, and a saline-infusion sonogram revealed a normal uterine cavity. Her thyroid stimulation hormone (TSH) level is normal at 1.7 mIU/L, but thyroid peroxidase (TPO) antibody testing returns positive. How should she be counseled, and what is the recommended course of action?

to the active forms of thyroid hormone. In the case of thyroid autoimmunity, either TPO or Tg (or both) can have antibodies directed against them. The TPO antibodies, produced largely by infiltrating lymphocytes in the thyroid gland, have been found to activate complement and may cause damage to the thyroid gland itself [1]. Interestingly, the Tg antibodies have not been found to activate complement and are believed to exert their effect through a different, complement-independent mechanism. Initial studies suggest that this may be caused by direct hydrolytic cleavage of thyroglobulin when exposed to anti-Tg antibodies, causing Tg depletion and eventual depletion of the thyroid hormones T3 and T4 [2, 3].

In iodine-replete populations, the most common cause of thyroid dysfunction is chronic autoimmune thyroiditis. The prevalence of thyroid peroxidase antibodies (TPOAb) and thyroglobulin antibodies (TgAb) varies by ethnicity, with the highest prevalence in Caucasian and Asian women and the lowest prevalence in African American women [4, 5]. Some evidence also suggests that thyroid autoimmunity can vary based on iodine intake [6] and has been found to be associated with altered vitamin D levels as well [7]. It is common to have concomitantly positive TPOAb and TgAb; these are found together in approximately 8% of women, while isolated TPOAb or TgAb are each found in approximately 4–5% of women, respectively [8]. In the same study, women with either antibody present had a higher average thyroid stimulating hormone (TSH) value than those without the antibodies present [8]. The American Thyroid Association (ATA) recommends testing for TPOAb but not for TgAb, as testing for TPOAb alone will identify the majority of women with thyroid autoimmunity [9].

Antithyroid peroxidase antibodies (TPOAb) or anti-thyroglobulin antibodies (TgAb) are found in pregnant women at a prevalence of approximately 2–18% [5, 10–15]. In patients with infertility, defined as the inability to conceive after 1 year of unprotected intercourse or appropriately timed inseminations, the prevalence of thyroid autoimmunity is estimated to be as high as 10–27% [16–20]. The prevalence of thyroid autoimmunity appears to be even higher among women with recurrent pregnancy loss, with studies showing thyroid autoimmunity rates between 14 and 36% [19, 21–23].

During pregnancy, normal physiologic changes in the thyroid hormones include a stimulation of the TSH receptor by hCG in the first trimester, thereby decreasing

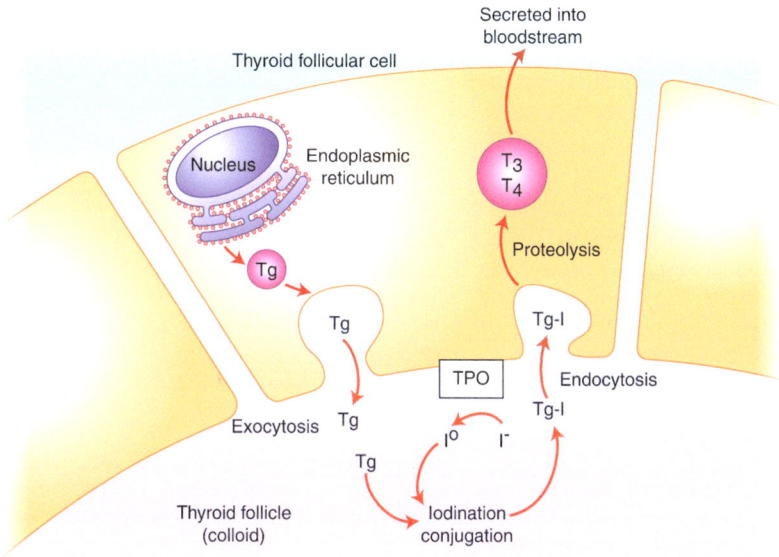

Fig. 10.1 Thyroglobulin (Tg) is synthesized and then packaged by the endoplasmic reticulum in the thyroid follicular cell, and it is secreted into the colloid of the thyroid follicle by exocytosis. Meanwhile, thyroid peroxidase (TPO) on the follicular cell membrane catalyzes the conversion of iodide (I^-) to iodine (I^0). The iodine then combines with the thyroglobulin, which undergoes iodination and conjugation. The iodinated and conjugated thyroglobulin (Tg-I) then reenters the follicular cell by endocytosis and undergoes proteolysis to create triiodothyronine (T3) and thyroxine (T4), which are secreted into the bloodstream

the circulating TSH level and increasing the circulating thyroid-binding globulin (TBG) and total T4. Thyroid peroxidase antibodies and TgAb can cross the placenta and may be detected in infant cord blood after delivery; however, the antibodies themselves are not thought to provoke neonatal thyroid dysfunction. Women positive for TPOAb and TgAb are at risk for progression from euthyroidism to hypothyroidism throughout the course of pregnancy; in a study of 87 euthyroid, TPOAb-positive women before and during pregnancy, 20% developed hypothyroidism with TSH >4.0 mU/L during pregnancy [24]. In another study of euthyroid, antibody-positive women during pregnancy, the mean TSH increased throughout pregnancy and averaged 3.5 mU/L by term, with 19% having overt hypothyroidism by the time of delivery [25].

The American Thyroid Association (ATA) recommends that serum TSH concentration should be measured in euthyroid but TPO or Tg antibody-positive pregnant women when pregnancy is confirmed and then every 4 weeks through midpregnancy (*strong recommendation, high-quality evidence*) [9]. A summary of the ATA recommendations regarding thyroid autoimmunity can be found in Table 10.1.

Thyroid Autoantibodies and Risk of Miscarriage

In the general population, between 27% and 31% of pregnancies end in spontaneous abortion [26, 27]. As was discussed in previous chapters of this textbook, thyroid dysfunction as a whole has been associated with increased rates of spontaneous

Table 10.1 American Thyroid Association guidelines: thyroid autoimmunity and miscarriage

Strong recommendation, high-quality evidence	Strong recommendation, moderate-quality evidence	Weak recommendation, moderate-quality evidence	Weak recommendation, low-quality evidence	Recommendation level: None
Euthyroid but TPO or Tg antibody-positive pregnant women: serum TSH concentration should be measured at pregnancy confirmation and then every 4 weeks through midpregnancy	Approach to subclinical hypothyroidism in pregnancy: for TPO antibody-positive women with a TSH greater than the pregnancy-specific reference range, levothyroxine therapy recommended	TPOAb-positive women during pregnancy: selenium supplementation is not recommended	Euthyroid women with history of recurrent pregnancy loss: intravenous immunoglobulin treatment is not recommended	Evaluate pregnant women with TSH concentrations >2.5 mIU/L for TPO antibody status
Monitor women at risk for hypothyroidism (e.g., patients who are euthyroid but TPO or TgAb-positive, post-hemithyroidectomy, or treated with radioactive iodine) with serum TSH measurement approximately every 4 weeks until mid-gestation and then once in the third trimester (at approximately 30 weeks)		Approach to subclinical hypothyroidism in pregnancy: TPO antibody-positive women with TSH concentrations >2.5 mIU/L and below the upper limit of the pregnancy-specific reference range, levothyroxine therapy can be considered	TPOAb-positive, euthyroid women who are newly pregnant: insufficient evidence to conclusively determine if levothyroxine therapy decreases pregnancy loss risk. TPOAb-positive, euthyroid pregnant women with a prior history of loss: Levothyroxine may be considered given its potential benefits compared to its minimal risk. Typical starting dose in these cases: 25–50 mcg	

Data from Alexander et al. [9]

abortion (SAB) compared with euthyroid controls [28, 29]. To what extent, if any, does thyroid autoimmunity impact the risk of miscarriage?

Multiple studies have demonstrated an association between the presence of thyroid autoantibodies and miscarriage; the risk of miscarriage in women with autoantibodies has been shown to be two to six times that of the antibody-negative population, depending on the characteristics of the patients studied [25, 29–32]. These studies are all complicated by the fact that it is difficult to parse out the relative effects of antibody positivity and elevated TSH, especially with the knowledge that positive thyroid antibodies are associated with increased TSH levels in general [14]. One large prospective study divided women into those with isolated thyroid autoimmunity, thyroid autoimmunity and subclinical hypothyroidism with TSH <5.22 mIU/L, and thyroid autoimmunity and TSH ≥5.22; they found the adjusted odds of miscarriage increased with increasing TSH level. With antibody positivity but normal TSH, the adjusted odds of miscarriage were 2.7 compared with controls; this increased to an odds ratio of 5–9.5 in the presence of thyroid autoimmunity *and* subclinical hypothyroidism [29]. A recent large study compared miscarriage rates among TPOAb-positive and TPOAb-negative infertile women undergoing ovulation induction with and without elevated TSH (≥2.5 mIU/L). The study found that elevated TSH did not confer an elevated risk of miscarriage, but patients with TPOAb had significantly higher risk of miscarriage when compared with TPOAb-negative women (OR 2.17, 95% CI 1.12–4.22) [33].

Other studies have examined the miscarriage risk in thyroid antibody-positive women undergoing treatment with assisted reproductive technology (ART). A prospective study of infertile TPOAb-positive women (without overt hypothyroidism) and TPOAb-negative women demonstrated 3.7 times higher odds of miscarriage in the antibody-positive women [32]. Another study examined patients undergoing intrauterine insemination (IUI) and found no difference in miscarriage rates between TPOAb-positive and TPOAb-negative patients after correction for TSH level; however, that analysis was underpowered. Additionally, it included women that were TPOAb negative but with subclinical hypothyroidism in the "euthyroid" control group [34]. Other studies have similarly shown mixed results [20, 35, 36]. Most recently, a meta-analysis compared miscarriage rates in women with and without thyroid autoimmunity undergoing treatment with ART. After adjustment for TSH level, thyroid antibodies were not associated with an increased risk of miscarriage [37]. Thus, in studies correcting for TSH and including women undergoing ART without a history of recurrent pregnancy loss, thyroid autoantibodies alone do not appear to increase the risk of miscarriage.

Still more studies have examined thyroid antibody prevalence in patients with recurrent pregnancy loss (RPL), inconsistently defined in the literature as two or three miscarriages. These studies found a two- to threefold increased prevalence of thyroid antibodies in women with RPL compared with controls [19, 38, 39]. Two meta-analyses of cohort and case-control studies examined the risk of miscarriage in the recurrent pregnancy loss (RPL) population with the presence or absence of thyroid antibodies and found the odds of miscarriage to be 1.8–3.9 times higher in the presence of thyroid antibodies compared with antibody-negative patients [40,

41]; however, these findings may have been confounded by older age and higher serum TSH among the women with thyroid antibodies present. Due to this finding, the American Thyroid Association considers women with recurrent pregnancy loss and thyroid autoimmunity to be at risk for further pregnancy loss and recommends consideration of treatment for this patient population [9]; see below for further details regarding treatment recommendations.

In terms of perinatal outcomes in TPO and Tg antibody-positive euthyroid women, existing data are limited. Cohort studies and case-control studies have shown mixed results, with some studies showing increased risk of preterm delivery [42–44] and others showing no significant association [45, 46]. The three meta-analyses of the subject do show an increased risk for preterm delivery among TPOAb+ euthyroid women [41, 47, 48]. There are little data, however, as to whether treatment helps to prevent preterm birth. One prospective interventional trial showed a lower rate of preterm delivery in the levothyroxine-treated group [25].

It is unknown whether thyroid antibodies impact other perinatal outcomes. Possible associations have been noted between the presence of thyroid autoantibodies and respiratory distress syndrome [42], placental abruption [13], and postpartum depression [49, 50]. In terms of long-term childhood outcomes, small studies have demonstrated associations between thyroid autoantibodies and neurocognitive outcomes, including perceptual performance, sensorineural hearing loss, IQ, ADHD, and autism [15, 51–55].

Thyroid Autoimmunity and Miscarriage: Possible Mechanisms of Action

Although an association has been noted between the presence of thyroid autoimmunity and the risk of miscarriage, causality has not been proven [56–58]. Hypotheses for the potential mechanism of action abound. One hypothesis is that the presence of thyroid autoimmunity places increased stress on the thyroid gland and that activation of complement may play a role. In turn, this damage may render the thyroid gland less able to accommodate the increased demands of pregnancy. TSH levels have repeatedly been shown to be higher in antibody-positive women as compared with antibody-negative controls [14, 25]. As mentioned in section "Prevalence and Natural History of Thyroid Autoimmunity in Fertility, Infertility, and Pregnancy", in euthyroid women with thyroid autoimmunity, the TSH level typically increases throughout pregnancy. Approximately 20% of these women develop a TSH level greater than 4.0 mU/L by the end of pregnancy [24]. The hypothesis that a general insult to the thyroid gland causes the increased pregnancy risk is supported by the fact that similar patterns of thyroid dysfunction are found in pregnant women with other types of thyroid injury, such as history of thyroid ablation or hemithyroidectomy [9]. These findings have prompted some groups to propose that the presence of TSH autoantibodies may be considered when determining trimester-specific cutoffs for "normal" TSH during pregnancy [7, 14].

Others have questioned whether there may be an association between thyroid autoantibodies and antiphospholipid antibody syndrome, as these are the two most commonly recognized autoimmune contributors to pregnancy loss. A retrospective case series of 156 women with recurrent miscarriages showed a significant association between TPOAb and TgAb positivity and antiphospholipid antibodies, including anti-β2-glycoprotein and anticardiolipin antibodies [59]. This is supported by previous work showing both reduced fecundity and increased pregnancy loss in women with recurrent pregnancy loss, antiphospholipid antibody syndrome, and thyroid autoantibodies, when compared with women with recurrent pregnancy loss and antiphospholipid antibody syndrome alone [60].

Other proposed mechanisms of action include cross-reactivity of thyroid antibodies with human chorionic gonadotropin (HCG) receptors on the zona pellucida, increased levels of endometrial cytokines causing increased stress and damage to the endometrium, and the potential presence of concurrent non-organ-specific autoimmunity [7]. Furthermore, the TPOAb are known to cross the placenta, and there is some evidence that the presence of the antibodies in utero may cause increased fetal resorption and pregnancy loss [56, 58]. Finally, multiple studies have proposed vitamin D deficiency as a "dual contributor" affecting both fertility and thyroid autoimmunity. This proposed mechanism of action entails vitamin D deficiency leading to altered expression of homeobox genes and altered innate and adaptive immune response; this may affect both the thyroid gland and the pregnancy itself [7, 61–63]. However, no studies have compared pregnancy outcomes in women with thyroid autoimmunity with and without vitamin D supplementation.

Treatment Strategies for Pregnant Patients with Thyroid Autoimmunity

Given the association between thyroid autoimmunity and miscarriage, the natural next step is to ask whether levothyroxine treatment may improve pregnancy outcomes. Several studies have examined levothyroxine treatment in prospectively screened antibody-positive, euthyroid women without a history of recurrent pregnancy loss. Some prospective trials have shown that levothyroxine treatment decreases miscarriage rates by 1.5- to 4-fold [25, 64]. Other studies, however, failed to detect a statistically significant difference [35]. There are two ongoing trials of euthyroid, antibody-positive women attempting pregnancy: the Thyroid Antibodies and Levothyroxine (TABLET) trial in the United Kingdom is enrolling women with infertility or with at least one previous miscarriage [65], and the T4Life Trial in the Netherlands is enrolling women with two or more previous miscarriages [66]. Both studies are randomizing women to treatment with levothyroxine versus placebo. Given the available data, the American Thyroid Association (ATA) has stated that, for TPOAb-positive, euthyroid women without a history of pregnancy loss, there is no sufficient evidence to determine conclusively if levothyroxine administration decreases pregnancy loss risk. But, in cases of TPOAb-positive, euthyroid pregnant women with a prior history of loss, levothyroxine administration can be considered due to its potential benefits when compared to its minimal risk; the typical starting dose in such cases would be 25–50 mcg of levothyroxine (weak recommendation, low-quality evidence) [9]. Note that these recommendations differentiate between newly pregnant antibody-positive euthyroid women without a history of pregnancy loss (for which there is insufficient evidence and no recommendation is made) and those with a history of pregnancy loss (for which consideration of low-dose levothyroxine treatment is recommended).

The recommendation for patients with positive thyroid autoantibodies and subclinical hypothyroidism is to consider treatment with levothyroxine; these recommendations are addressed as well in Chap. 6 on hypothyroidism in pregnancy. The rationale for treatment of women with both thyroid antibodies and subclinical hypothyroidism is apparent in a 2017 meta-analysis of 3 studies, including 1500 women; this showed that women with both thyroid antibodies and subclinical hypothyroidism had a higher miscarriage risk than those with isolated subclinical hypothyroidism or thyroid antibody positivity (RR 2.47, 95% CI 1.77–3.45) [67]. A randomized controlled trial examined pregnancy outcomes in treated versus untreated women with thyroid dysfunction (including "hypothyroid" women with TPOAb and TSH >2.5 mIU/L) and found fewer composite adverse outcomes in the treated patients [68]. The ATA recommends that subclinically hypothyroid, infertile women undergoing ART should be treated with levothyroxine with the goal of treatment to achieve a TSH <2.5 [9]. They further recommend that pregnant women with TSH >2.5 mU/L should be evaluated for TPO antibody status. If antibody positive and TSH is greater than the pregnancy-specific reference range, treatment with levothyroxine is recommended. Furthermore, treatment with levothyroxine should be considered if the patient is antibody positive and has a TSH concentration >2.5 mIU/L and below the upper limit of the pregnancy-specific reference range [9]. The American Society for Reproductive Medicine (ASRM) recommends consideration of TPOAb testing for repeated TSH >2.5 mIU/L or other risk factors (68). For women with known TPOAb positivity, TSH should be evaluated and treatment with levothyroxine considered for those with TSH >2.5 mIU/L [69].

There are limited data on the use of levothyroxine for the prevention of preterm labor in antibody-positive women. Small studies have shown mixed results, with some indicating a decrease in preterm deliveries [70], while others failed to detect a difference [71]. The ATA maintains that, regarding levothyroxine treatment recommendations for the prevention of preterm delivery in cases of euthyroid, thyroid autoantibody-positive pregnant women, there is insufficient evidence (no recommendation, insufficient evidence) [9].

Still fewer studies have examined treatment of antibody-positive women with agents other than levothyroxine. The ATA specifically addresses intravenous immunoglobulin, maintaining that, in the cases of euthyroid women with a history of recurrent pregnancy loss, intravenous immunoglobulin treatment is not recommended (weak recommendation, low-quality evidence) [9]. Similarly, studies regarding selenium supplementation have shown mixed results; one study found that selenium supplementation was associated with lower risk of postpartum thyroid dysfunction in antibody-positive euthyroid women [72], but other studies failed to show an effect [73, 74]. The ATA does not recommend selenium supplementation in TPOAb-positive women during pregnancy [9].

Graves' Disease and Miscarriage

Graves' disease is discussed in detail in Chaps. 3 and 7 but will also be discussed in this chapter, given the autoimmune nature of the disorder. Graves' disease is typically characterized by the presence of TSH receptor *antibodies* (TRAb, also known as thyroid-stimulating immunoglobulin or TSI). Obtaining TRAb in a pregnant patient who appears clinically hyperthyroid can help to distinguish between gestational transient thyrotoxicosis and Graves' disease [75, 76]. Approximately 95% of patients with Graves' disease will have detectable TRAb [77]. The prevalence of Graves' disease in pregnancy is 0.2–0.5% [78, 79] and thus is less common than subclinical hypothyroidism or thyroid autoimmunity by TPOAb or TgAb.

There are limited studies regarding the risk of miscarriage in Graves' disease. A small study examining pregnant women with Graves' disease found no difference in the TRAb levels between pregnancies ending in SAB versus those progressing to live birth [80]. A Danish study reviewed all pregnant and postpartum women with the diagnosis of hyperthyroidism. When maternal hyperthyroidism was diagnosed before or during pregnancy, the risk of SAB (delivery <22 wks) was 16% vs 13% in patients without thyroid dysfunction; there were also higher rates of stillbirth in patients diagnosed postpartum with hyperthyroidism. They concluded that SABs and stillbirths were more common in women with hyperthyroidism, although stillbirths remained a rare occurrence [79]. Of note, data on pregnancy outcomes and Graves' disease are confounded by the fact that the antithyroid drugs (ATDs) methimazole and PTU can also have adverse pregnancy effects [78]. More studies are needed on this subject.

Clinical Case and Discussion

A 31-year-old gravida 2, para 0 presents for consultation for recurrent pregnancy loss. She has had two first-trimester spontaneous abortions, each at approximately 6 weeks gestation. Her history is unremarkable except for the two miscarriages, and her partner is healthy and had a normal semen analysis. Parental karyotypes are normal, and a saline-infusion sonogram revealed a normal uterine cavity. Her thyroid stimulation hormone (TSH) level is normal at 1.7 mIU/L, but thyroid peroxidase (TPO) antibody testing returns positive. How should she be counseled, and what is the recommended course of action?

The patient should be counseled that, given her history of two prior miscarriages, she is already at slightly increased risk for miscarriage in future pregnancies. While her TSH was in the normal range, her TPOAb testing was positive. She should be counseled that this is a relatively common finding in women of reproductive age, but it may further increase her risk of miscarriage. She and her provider should discuss the possibility of initiation of levothyroxine treatment; while the benefit of levothyroxine in TPOAb women with recurrent pregnancy loss has not been clearly shown in large randomized trials, some observational studies have shown a possible benefit. Furthermore, the risk of this treatment is very low. If she and her provider decide upon initiation of levothyroxine treatment, a low dose such as 25 to 50 mcg daily should be used, with plans to increase this dose by 30% or two doses per week if she conceives. She should have her TSH checked at the time of confirmation of pregnancy as well as every 4 weeks thereafter, until about midpregnancy; this recommendation is due to increased risk of thyroid dysfunction and overt hypothyroidism in the presence of thyroid autoantibodies.

References

1. Chardès T, Chapal N, Bresson D, Bès C, Giudicelli V, Lefranc M-P, Péraldi-Roux S. The human anti-thyroid peroxidase autoantibody repertoire in graves' and Hashimoto's autoimmune thyroid diseases. Immunogenetics. 2002;54:141–57.
2. Li L, Paul S, Tyutyulkova S, Kazatchkine MD, Kaveri S. Catalytic activity of anti-thyroglobulin antibodies. J Immunol. 1995;154(7):3328–32.
3. Wootla B, Lacroix-Desmazes S, Warrington AE, Bieber AJ, Kaveri SV, Rodriguez M. Autoantibodies with enzymatic properties in human autoimmune diseases. J Autoimmun. 2011;37:144–50.
4. Hollowell JG, Staehling NW, Flanders WD, Hannon WH, Gunter EW, Spencer CA, Braverman LE. Serum TSH, T(4), and thyroid antibodies in the United States population (1988 to 1994): National Health and nutrition examination survey (NHANES III). J Clin Endocrinol Metab. 2002;87:489–99.
5. La'ulu SL, Roberts WL. Second-trimester reference intervals for thyroid tests: the role of ethnicity. Clin Chem. 2007;53:1658–64.

6. Shi X, Han C, Li C, et al. Optimal and safe upper limits of iodine intake for early pregnancy in iodine-sufficient regions: a cross-sectional study of 7190 pregnant women in China. J Clin Endocrinol Metab. 2015;100:1630–8.
7. Twig G, Shina A, Amital H, Shoenfeld Y. Pathogenesis of infertility and recurrent pregnancy loss in thyroid autoimmunity. J Autoimmun. 2012;38:J275–81.
8. Unuane D, Velkeniers B, Anckaert E, Schiettecatte J, Tournaye H, Haentjens P, Poppe K. Thyroglobulin autoantibodies: is there any added value in the detection of thyroid autoimmunity in women consulting for fertility treatment? Thyroid. 2013;23:1022–8.
9. Alexander EK, Pearce EN, Brent GA, et al. 2017 guidelines of the American Thyroid Association for the diagnosis and Management of Thyroid Disease during Pregnancy and the postpartum. Thyroid. 2017;27:315–89.
10. Moreno-Reyes R, Glinoer D, Van Oyen H, Vandevijvere S. High prevalence of thyroid disorders in pregnant women in a mildly iodine-deficient country: a population-based study. J Clin Endocrinol Metab. 2013;98:3694–701.
11. Ashoor G, Maiz N, Rotas M, Jawdat F, Nicolaides KH. Maternal thyroid function at 11 to 13 weeks of gestation and subsequent fetal death. Thyroid. 2010;20:989–93.
12. Benhadi N, Wiersinga WM, Reitsma JB, Vrijkotte TGM, van der Wal MF, Bonsel GJ. Ethnic differences in TSH but not in free T4 concentrations or TPO antibodies during pregnancy. Clin Endocrinol. 2007;66:765–70.
13. Abbassi-Ghanavati M, Casey BM, Spong CY, McIntire DD, Halvorson LM, Cunningham FG. Pregnancy outcomes in women with thyroid peroxidase antibodies. Obstet Gynecol. 2010;116:381–6.
14. Pearce EN, Oken E, Gillman MW, Lee SL, Magnani B, Platek D, Braverman LE. Association of first-trimester thyroid function test values with thyroperoxidase antibody status, smoking, and multivitamin use. Endocr Pract. 2008;14:33–9.
15. Wasserman EE, Nelson K, Rose NR, Eaton W, Pillion JP, Seaberg E, Talor MV, Burek L, Duggan A, Yolken RH. Maternal thyroid autoantibodies during the third trimester and hearing deficits in children: an epidemiologic assessment. Am J Epidemiol. 2008;167:701–10.
16. Geva E, Vardinon N, Lessing JB, Lerner-Geva L, Azem F, Yovel I, Burke M, Yust I, Grunfeld R, Amit A. Organ-specific autoantibodies are possible markers for reproductive failure: a prospective study in an in-vitro fertilization-embryo transfer programme. Hum Reprod. 1996;11:1627–31.
17. Kaider AS, Kaider BD, Janowicz PB, Roussev RG. Immunodiagnostic evaluation in women with reproductive failure. Am J Reprod Immunol. 1999;42:335–46.
18. Janssen OE, Mehlmauer N, Hahn S, Offner AH, Gärtner R. High prevalence of autoimmune thyroiditis in patients with polycystic ovary syndrome. Eur J Endocrinol. 2004;150:363–9.
19. Kutteh WH, Yetman DL, Carr AC, Beck LA, Scott RT. Increased prevalence of antithyroid antibodies identified in women with recurrent pregnancy loss but not in women undergoing assisted reproduction. Fertil Steril. 1999;71:843–8.
20. Negro R, Formoso G, Coppola L, Presicce G, Mangieri T, Pezzarossa A, Dazzi D. Euthyroid women with autoimmune disease undergoing assisted reproduction technologies: the role of autoimmunity and thyroid function. J Endocrinol Investig. 2007;30:3–8.
21. Bussen S, Steck T. Thyroid autoantibodies in euthyroid non-pregnant women with recurrent spontaneous abortions. Hum Reprod. 1995;10:2938–40.
22. Pratt D, Novotny M, Kaberlein G, Dudkiewicz A, Gleicher N. Antithyroid antibodies and the association with non-organ-specific antibodies in recurrent pregnancy loss. Am J Obstet Gynecol. 1993;168:837–41.
23. Muller AF, Verhoeff A, Mantel MJ, Berghout A. Thyroid autoimmunity and abortion: a prospective study in women undergoing in vitro fertilization. Fertil Steril. 1999;71:30–4.
24. Glinoer D, Riahi M, Grün JP, Kinthaert J. Risk of subclinical hypothyroidism in pregnant women with asymptomatic autoimmune thyroid disorders. J Clin Endocrinol Metab. 1994;79:197–204.

25. Negro R, Formoso G, Mangieri T, Pezzarossa A, Dazzi D, Hassan H. Levothyroxine treatment in euthyroid pregnant women with autoimmune thyroid disease: effects on obstetrical complications. J Clin Endocrinol Metab. 2006;91:2587–91.
26. Ellish NJ, Saboda K, O'Connor J, Nasca PC, Stanek EJ, Boyle C. A prospective study of early pregnancy loss. Hum Reprod. 1996;11:406–12.
27. Wilcox AJ, Weinberg CR, O'Connor JF, Baird DD, Schlatterer JP, Canfield RE, Armstrong EG, Nisula BC. Incidence of early loss of pregnancy. N Engl J Med. 1988;319:189–94.
28. De Vivo A, Mancuso A, Giacobbe A, Moleti M, Maggio Savasta L, De Dominici R, Priolo AM, Vermiglio F. Thyroid function in women found to have early pregnancy loss. Thyroid. 2010;20:633–7.
29. Liu H, Shan Z, Li C, et al. Maternal subclinical hypothyroidism, thyroid autoimmunity, and the risk of miscarriage: a prospective cohort study. Thyroid. 2014;24:1642–9.
30. Stagnaro-Green A, Roman SH, Cobin RH, el-Harazy E, Alvarez-Marfany M, Davies TF. Detection of at-risk pregnancy by means of highly sensitive assays for thyroid autoantibodies. JAMA. 1990;264:1422–5.
31. Sieiro Netto L, Medina Coeli C, Micmacher E, Mamede Da Costa S, Nazar L, Galvão D, Buescu A, Vaisman M. Influence of thyroid autoimmunity and maternal age on the risk of miscarriage. Am J Reprod Immunol. 2004;52:312–6.
32. Poppe K, Glinoer D, Tournaye H, Devroey P, van Steirteghem A, Kaufman L, Velkeniers B. Assisted reproduction and thyroid autoimmunity: an unfortunate combination? J Clin Endocrinol Metab. 2003;88:4149–52.
33. Seungdamrong A, Steiner AZ, Gracia CR, et al. Preconceptional antithyroid peroxidase antibodies, but not thyroid-stimulating hormone, are associated with decreased live birth rates in infertile women. Fertil Steril. 2017. pii: S0015-0282(17)31748-X; https://doi.org/10.1016/j.fertnstert.2017.08.026.
34. Unuane D, Velkeniers B, Bravenboer B, Drakopoulos P, Tournaye H, Parra J, De Brucker M. Impact of thyroid autoimmunity in euthyroid women on live birth rate after IUI. Hum Reprod. 2017;32:915–22.
35. Negro R, Mangieri T, Coppola L, et al. Levothyroxine treatment in thyroid peroxidase antibody-positive women undergoing assisted reproduction technologies: a prospective study. Hum Reprod. 2005;20:1529–33.
36. Singh A, Dantas ZN, Stone SC, Asch RH. Presence of thyroid antibodies in early reproductive failure: biochemical versus clinical pregnancies. Fertil Steril. 1995;63:277–81.
37. Leiva P, Schwarze JE, Vasquez P, Ortega C, Villa S, Crosby J, Balmaceda J, Pommer R. There is no association between the presence of anti-thyroid antibodies and increased reproductive loss in pregnant women after ART: a systematic review and meta-analysis. JBRA Assist Reprod. 2017;21(4):361–5.
38. Iravani AT, Saeedi MM, Pakravesh J, Hamidi S, Abbasi M. Thyroid autoimmunity and recurrent spontaneous abortion in Iran: a case-control study. Endocr Pract. 2008;14:458–64.
39. Dendrinos S, Papasteriades C, Tarassi K, Christodoulakos G, Prasinos G, Creatsas G. Thyroid autoimmunity in patients with recurrent spontaneous miscarriages. Gynecol Endocrinol. 2000;14:270–4.
40. Chen L, Hu R. Thyroid autoimmunity and miscarriage: a meta-analysis. Clin Endocrinol. 2011;74:513–9.
41. Thangaratinam S, Tan A, Knox E, Kilby MD, Franklyn J, Coomarasamy A. Association between thyroid autoantibodies and miscarriage and preterm birth: meta-analysis of evidence. BMJ. 2011;342:d2616.
42. Negro R, Schwartz A, Gismondi R, Tinelli A, Mangieri T, Stagnaro-Green A. Thyroid antibody positivity in the first trimester of pregnancy is associated with negative pregnancy outcomes. J Clin Endocrinol Metab. 2011;96:E920–4.
43. Haddow JE, Cleary-Goldman J, McClain MR, et al. Thyroperoxidase and thyroglobulin antibodies in early pregnancy and preterm delivery. Obstet Gynecol. 2010;116:58–62.

44. Korevaar TIM, Schalekamp-Timmermans S, de Rijke YB, et al. Hypothyroxinemia and TPO-antibody positivity are risk factors for premature delivery: the generation R study. J Clin Endocrinol Metab. 2013;98:4382–90.
45. Glinoer D, Soto MF, Bourdoux P, Lejeune B, Delange F, Lemone M, Kinthaert J, Robijn C, Grun JP, de Nayer P. Pregnancy in patients with mild thyroid abnormalities: maternal and neonatal repercussions. J Clin Endocrinol Metab. 1991;73:421–7.
46. Männistö T, Vääräsmäki M, Pouta A, Hartikainen A-L, Ruokonen A, Surcel H-M, Bloigu A, Järvelin M-R, Suvanto-Luukkonen E. Perinatal outcome of children born to mothers with thyroid dysfunction or antibodies: a prospective population-based cohort study. J Clin Endocrinol Metab. 2009;94:772–9.
47. Negro R. Thyroid autoimmunity and pre-term delivery: brief review and meta-analysis. J Endocrinol Investig. 2011;34:155–8.
48. He X, Wang P, Wang Z, He X, Xu D, Wang B. Thyroid antibodies and risk of preterm delivery: a meta-analysis of prospective cohort studies. Eur J Endocrinol. 2012;167:455–64.
49. Groer MW, Vaughan JH. Positive thyroid peroxidase antibody titer is associated with dysphoric moods during pregnancy and postpartum. J Obstet Gynecol Neonatal Nurs. 2013;42:E26–32.
50. Kuijpens JL, Vader HL, Drexhage HA, Wiersinga WM, van Son MJ, Pop VJ. Thyroid peroxidase antibodies during gestation are a marker for subsequent depression postpartum. Eur J Endocrinol. 2001;145:579–84.
51. Li Y, Shan Z, Teng W, et al. Abnormalities of maternal thyroid function during pregnancy affect neuropsychological development of their children at 25-30 months. Clin Endocrinol. 2010;72:825–9.
52. Williams FLR, Watson J, Ogston SA, Visser TJ, Hume R, Willatts P. Maternal and umbilical cord levels of T4, FT4, TSH, TPOAb, and TgAb in term infants and neurodevelopmental outcome at 5.5 years. J Clin Endocrinol Metab. 2013;98:829–38.
53. Wasserman EE, Pillion JP, Duggan A, Nelson K, Rohde C, Seaberg EC, Talor MV, Yolken RH, Rose NR. Childhood IQ, hearing loss, and maternal thyroid autoimmunity in the Baltimore collaborative perinatal project. Pediatr Res. 2012;72:525–30.
54. Ghassabian A, Bongers-Schokking JJ, de Rijke YB, et al. Maternal thyroid autoimmunity during pregnancy and the risk of attention deficit/hyperactivity problems in children: the generation R study. Thyroid. 2012;22:178–86.
55. Brown AS, Surcel H-M, Hinkka-Yli-Salomäki S, Cheslack-Postava K, Bao Y, Sourander A. Maternal thyroid autoantibody and elevated risk of autism in a national birth cohort. Prog Neuro-Psychopharmacol Biol Psychiatry. 2015;57:86–92.
56. Lee YL, Ng HP, Lau KS, Liu WM, O WS, Yeung WSB, Kung AWC. Increased fetal abortion rate in autoimmune thyroid disease is related to circulating TPO autoantibodies in an autoimmune thyroiditis animal model. Fertil Steril. 2009;91:2104–9.
57. Imaizumi M, Pritsker A, Kita M, Ahmad L, Unger P, Davies T. Pregnancy and murine thyroiditis: thyroglobulin immunization leads to fetal loss in specific allogeneic pregnancies. Endocrinology. 2001;142:823–9.
58. Matalon ST, Blank M, Levy Y, et al. The pathogenic role of anti-thyroglobulin antibody on pregnancy: evidence from an active immunization model in mice. Hum Reprod. 2003;18:1094–9.
59. Promberger R, Walch K, Seemann R, Pils S, Ott J. A retrospective study on the association between thyroid autoantibodies with β2-glycoprotein and Cardiolipin antibodies in recurrent miscarriage. Iran J Allergy Asthma Immunol. 2017;16:72–6.
60. De Carolis C, Greco E, Guarino MD, Perricone C, Dal Lago A, Giacomelli R, Fontana L, Perricone R. Anti-thyroid antibodies and antiphospholipid syndrome: evidence of reduced fecundity and of poor pregnancy outcome in recurrent spontaneous aborters. Am J Reprod Immunol. 2004;52:263–6.
61. Penna G, Adorini L. 1 Alpha,25-dihydroxyvitamin D3 inhibits differentiation, maturation, activation, and survival of dendritic cells leading to impaired alloreactive T cell activation. J Immunol. 2000;164:2405–11.

62. Boonstra A, Barrat FJ, Crain C, Heath VL, Savelkoul HF, O'Garra A. 1alpha,25-Dihydroxyvitamin d3 has a direct effect on naive CD4(+) T cells to enhance the development of Th2 cells. J Immunol. 2001;167:4974–80.
63. Stefanić M, Papić S, Suver M, Glavas-Obrovac L, Karner I. Association of vitamin D receptor gene 3'-variants with Hashimoto's thyroiditis in the Croatian population. Int J Immunogenet. 2008;35:125–31.
64. Lepoutre T, Debiève F, Gruson D, Daumerie C. Reduction of miscarriages through universal screening and treatment of thyroid autoimmune diseases. Gynecol Obstet Investig. 2012;74:265–73.
65. TABLET trial. www.birmingham.ac.uk/research/activity/mds/trials/bctu/trials/womens/tablet/index.aspx.
66. T4Life trial. http://www.studies-obsgyn.nl/T4-LIFE/page.asp?page_id=1326.
67. Zhang Y, Wang H, Pan X, Teng W, Shan Z. Patients with subclinical hypothyroidism before 20 weeks of pregnancy have a higher risk of miscarriage: a systematic review and meta-analysis. PLoS One. 2017;12:e0175708.
68. Negro R, Schwartz A, Gismondi R, Tinelli A, Mangieri T, Stagnaro-Green A. Universal screening versus case finding for detection and treatment of thyroid hormonal dysfunction during pregnancy. J Clin Endocrinol Metab. 2010;95:1699–707.
69. Practice Committee of the American Society for Reproductive Medicine. Subclinical hypothyroidism in the infertile female population: a guideline. Fertil Steril. 2015;104:545–53.
70. Nazarpour S, Ramezani Tehrani F, Simbar M, Tohidi M, Alavi Majd H, Azizi F. Effects of levothyroxine treatment on pregnancy outcomes in pregnant women with autoimmune thyroid disease. Eur J Endocrinol. 2017;176:253–65.
71. Negro R, Schwartz A, Stagnaro-Green A. Impact of levothyroxine in miscarriage and preterm delivery rates in first trimester thyroid antibody-positive women with TSH less than 2.5 mIU/L. J Clin Endocrinol Metab. 2016;101:3685–90.
72. Negro R, Greco G, Mangieri T, Pezzarossa A, Dazzi D, Hassan H. The influence of selenium supplementation on postpartum thyroid status in pregnant women with thyroid peroxidase autoantibodies. J Clin Endocrinol Metab. 2007;92:1263–8.
73. Karanikas G, Schuetz M, Kontur S, Duan H, Kommata S, Schoen R, Antoni A, Kletter K, Dudczak R, Willheim M. No immunological benefit of selenium in consecutive patients with autoimmune thyroiditis. Thyroid. 2008;18:7–12.
74. Mao J, Pop VJ, Bath SC, Vader HL, Redman CWG, Rayman MP. Effect of low-dose selenium on thyroid autoimmunity and thyroid function in UK pregnant women with mild-to-moderate iodine deficiency. Eur J Nutr. 2016;55:55–61.
75. Goodwin TM, Montoro M, Mestman JH. Transient hyperthyroidism and hyperemesis gravidarum: clinical aspects. Am J Obstet Gynecol. 1992;167:648–52.
76. Tan JYL, Loh KC, Yeo GSH, Chee YC. Transient hyperthyroidism of hyperemesis gravidarum. BJOG. 2002;109:683–8.
77. Laurberg P, Wallin G, Tallstedt L, Abraham-Nordling M, Lundell G, Tørring O. TSH-receptor autoimmunity in graves' disease after therapy with anti-thyroid drugs, surgery, or radioiodine: a 5-year prospective randomized study. Eur J Endocrinol. 2008;158:69–75.
78. Cooper DS, Laurberg P. Hyperthyroidism in pregnancy. Lancet Diabetes Endocrinol. 2013;1:238–49.
79. Andersen SL, Olsen J, Wu CS, Laurberg P. Spontaneous abortion, stillbirth and hyperthyroidism: a danish population-based study. Eur Thyroid J. 2014;3:164–72.
80. Uenaka M, Tanimura K, Tairaku S, Morioka I, Ebina Y, Yamada H. Risk factors for neonatal thyroid dysfunction in pregnancies complicated by graves' disease. Eur J Obstet Gynecol Reprod Biol. 2014;177:89–93.

Chapter 11
Postpartum Thyroiditis

Benjamin S. Harris and Jennifer L. Eaton

> **Clinical Case**
> A 25-year-old gravida 1, para 1, with Type 1 diabetes presents to her primary care physician for a follow-up visit 5 months postpartum. Her pregnancy and delivery were uncomplicated. She is exclusively breastfeeding without any issues, and she had an IUD placed at her 6-week postpartum visit. She reports having palpitations, irritability, and fatigue from about 6 to 12 weeks postpartum, which she attributed to the stress of taking care of the new baby. Her palpitations have improved, but more recently she has noticed weight gain and continued fatigue despite exercising 3 days a week.

Introduction

Postpartum thyroiditis (PPT) is defined as a transient autoimmune thyroid disorder, in the absence of Graves' disease, occurring within 1 year postpartum in patients who were euthyroid prior to pregnancy [1]. The clinical presentation of postpartum thyroiditis is highly variable. Approximately 22% of cases have a classical presentation of an initial transient thyrotoxic phase, followed by transient hypothyroidism with subsequent return to euthyroid state by 1 year postpartum [1].

B. S. Harris · J. L. Eaton (✉)
Duke University Medical Center, Division of Reproductive Endocrinology and Infertility, Department of Obstetrics and Gynecology, Durham, NC, USA
e-mail: jennifer.eaton@duke.edu

The remainder of case presentations varies between isolated thyrotoxicosis (25%) and isolated hypothyroidism (48%), respectively [1]. The transient thyrotoxic phase commonly presents between 2 and 6 months postpartum, with rare cases presenting up to 1 year postpartum [1, 2]. The hypothyroid phase typically presents between 3 and 12 months postpartum and can become permanent in up to 50% of affected individuals [1, 3].

Epidemiology and Natural History

The prevalence of postpartum thyroiditis ranges from 1.1% to 16.7% and is subject to geographic variation [1, 2, 4]. In a systematic review of prospective studies, the prevalence of postpartum thyroiditis in the general population was estimated to be 8.1% [4].

Postpartum thyroiditis is more common in individuals with a history of autoimmune disease. Among women with a history of Graves' disease, the incidence of PPT is as high as 44% [5]. Individuals with a history of Type 1 diabetes mellitus have three to four times the rate of postpartum thyroiditis compared to the general population, with an incidence that approaches 25% [1, 2]. The prevalence of PPT in women with a history of chronic viral hepatitis or systemic lupus erythematosus is 25% and 14%, respectively [1, 6, 7]. Individuals that fully recover from postpartum thyroiditis have up to a 70% chance of recurrence in subsequent pregnancy [8].

Etiology

Postpartum thyroiditis is an autoimmune disorder characterized by increased natural killer cell activity, complement activation, and lymphocyte abnormalities [9–11]. Development of PPT is strongly associated with the presence of underlying thyroid autoimmunity during pregnancy. The presence of thyroid peroxidase (TPO) or thyroglobulin antibodies during the first trimester of pregnancy is associated with a 33–50% risk of developing subsequent PPT [12]. Given that pregnancy is considered an immune suppressed state, onset of postpartum thyroiditis may be attributed to the postpartum rebound of the immune system [12]. Specifically, the gradual return of cellular and humoral immunity at 1–4 and 7–10 months, after delivery, respectively, plays an essential role in the development of PPT in susceptible women [12].

Postpartum thyroiditis is considered a variant form of chronic autoimmune (Hashimoto's) thyroiditis. The two conditions share association with human leukocyte antigen HLA-B and HLA-D, suggesting an inherited aspect of the disease pathogenesis [13]. In postpartum thyroiditis, autoimmune thyroid inflammation causes damage to thyroid follicles and induces proteolysis of thyroglobulin stores leading to increased serum levels of triiodothyronine (T3) and thyroxine (T4) and subsequent hyperthyroidism. The transient of nature of postpartum thyrotoxicosis is due to exhaustion of thyroglobulin stores and feedback inhibition of thyroid-stimulating hormone (TSH) secretion by increased T3 and T4 levels. The subsequent hypothyroid phase is characterized by thyroid regeneration after the thyrotoxic phase of inflammation; the thyroid undergoes a period of regeneration and the eventual return of normal thyroid hormone synthesis in most patients.

Clinical Presentation

Postpartum thyroiditis is typically a painless condition. Although the majority of women are asymptomatic, the clinical course may vary. Symptoms during the hyperthyroid phase, when present, are typically mild and consist of fatigue, weight loss, palpitations, heat intolerance, irritability, tachycardia, and tremor [1, 14–16]. Symptoms during the hypothyroid phase are more frequent, tend to be mild, and include cold intolerance, fatigue, dry skin, paresthesias, constipation, and concentration difficulties [15, 16]. Diagnosis of postpartum thyroiditis can prove to be difficult due to overlapping symptoms with normal stresses of sleep deprivation, breastfeeding, and adapting to a newborn. There are inconsistent data surrounding the association between postpartum thyroiditis and postpartum depression [15, 17–19]. As a result, the ATA recommends screening for thyroid dysfunction in all patients with depression, including postpartum depression [2]. See Table 11.1.

Table 11.1 American Thyroid Association Guidelines: postpartum thyroiditis

Strong recommendation, high-quality evidence	Strong recommendation, moderate-quality evidence	Strong recommendation, low-quality evidence	Weak recommendation, moderate-quality evidence	Weak recommendation, low-quality evidence
After resolution of the thyrotoxic phase of PPT: to screen for hypothyroid phase, measure TSH in approximately 4–8 weeks (or if new symptoms develop)	Thyrotoxic phase of PPT: treat symptomatic women with a β-blocker safe for lactating women (such as propranolol or metoprolol) at the lowest possible dose to alleviate symptoms Therapy duration: typically a few weeks	Thyroid dysfunction screening for all patients with depression (including postpartum depression)	Consider LT4 therapy for women with symptomatic hypothyroidism due to PPT; check TSH levels every 4–8 weeks if treatment is not started until thyroid function normalizes. LT4 should also be started in hypothyroid women attempting pregnancy or are breastfeeding; LT4 therapy should be initiated	Attempt discontinuation of LT4 therapy for PPT after 12 months. Avoid tapering of LT4 if a woman is actively attempting pregnancy or is pregnant

Data from Alexander et al. [2]

Thyrotoxic Phase

Thyroid inflammation may lead to the thyrotoxic phase of PPT, which is characterized by a destructive thyroiditis in which preformed thyroid hormone is released [20]. Symptoms occur 2–4 months postpartum and are generally transient, lasting approximately 6–9 weeks [20].

Given that the thyrotoxic phase is due to the release of preformed thyroid hormone rather than an increase in thyroid hormone production, propylthiouracil and methimazole are not effective treatments. Symptoms are usually mild, but if they are clinically significant, beta-blockers (propranolol or metoprolol) can be used at the lowest effective dose. The thyrotoxic phase typically resolves spontaneously, and treatment is usually required for only a few weeks. A TSH should be repeated 4–8 weeks after symptom resolution in order to screen for the hypothyroid phase [2].

The thyrotoxic phase of PPT can be difficult to distinguish from Graves' disease. Clinically, goiter with bruits or ophthalmopathy is diagnostic of Graves' disease. Ide and colleagues retrospectively evaluated 42 patients with new-onset postpartum thyrotoxicosis and demonstrated that most (86%) patients with PPT with thyrotoxicosis present within 3 months postpartum, whereas patients with Graves' disease in this cohort all had an onset of 6 months or more [21]. Laboratory testing can also be used to differentiate between the two diagnoses. Antibodies to the TSH receptor are found in almost all cases of Graves' disease but rarely in women with PPT. Additionally, an elevated T4 to T3 ratio is also suggestive of PPT [2]. Lastly, radioiodine uptake during the thyrotoxic phase of postpartum thyroiditis is typically less than 1% compared to high uptake in patients with Graves' disease.

Hypothyroid Phase

The hypothyroid phase of PPT begins once the thyroid hormone stores have been depleted [20]. This occurs around 3–12 months postpartum. If patients are symptomatic with a TSH between 4 and 10 mU/l, or when TSH is greater than 10 mU/l regardless of symptoms, treatment with levothyroxine should be initiated [22]. Patients who have significant symptoms, are currently breastfeeding, or are actively trying to conceive should also be treated in order to maintain a euthyroid state. For many patients, thyroid function will return to normal in 12 months, and it is reasonable to consider weaning off treatment. Though duration of treatment has not been systematically evaluated, gradual discontinuation of LT4 treatment at 12 months will help to differentiate between transient and permanent hypothyroidism. For surveillance, TSH levels should be checked every 6–8 weeks during medication taper. In those patients not requiring treatment, a TSH level should be obtained every 4–8 weeks until euthyroid [2].

In contrast to the thyrotoxic phase, 10–20% of cases do not resolve and result in permanent hypothyroidism [2]. Multiparity, greater maternal age, a history of pregnancy loss, higher thyroid peroxidase antibody titers, and thyroid hypoechogenicity on ultrasound are associated with a higher risk of developing hypothyroidism [2, 22].

Clinical Case and Discussion

A 25-year-old gravida 1, para 1, with Type 1 diabetes presents to her primary care physician for a follow-up visit 5 months postpartum. Her pregnancy was uncomplicated, and she had a successful vaginal delivery at term. She is exclusively breastfeeding without any issues, and she had an IUD placed at her 6-week postpartum visit. She reports having palpitations, irritability, and fatigue from about 6 to 12 weeks postpartum, which she attributed to the stress of taking care of the new baby. Her palpitations have improved, but more recently she has noticed weight gain and continued fatigue despite exercising 3 days a week.

The patient's clinical history is suggestive of postpartum thyroiditis with the classical presentation of a transient period of hyperthyroidism followed by hypothyroidism. She developed palpitations, irritability, and fatigue within 2 months, lasting 6 weeks with spontaneous resolution. This was followed by continued fatigue and weight gain suspicious for hypothyroidism. If she had presented during the thyrotoxic phase, Graves' disease would have been on the differential diagnosis, and thyroid antibody testing may have helped distinguish the two conditions if ophthalmopathy or goiter were not present. Given her current clinical picture, measurement of TSH is indicated, with the initiation of treatment with levothyroxine titrated up until TSH is within normal range. She should be maintained on levothyroxine for as long as she is breastfeeding. After 12 months, if she is not breastfeeding and not considering another pregnancy, she can begin to wean off levothyroxine with TSH measurements every 6–8 weeks until reaching a euthyroid state. She should be counseled that she is at high risk of recurrence of PPT in future pregnancies and that she is also at risk of developing permanent hypothyroidism, especially given her preexisting autoimmune disorder, Type 1 diabetes.

References

1. Stagnaro-Green A. Approach to the patient with postpartum thyroiditis. J Clin Endocrinol Metab. 2012;97(2):334–42.
2. Alexander EK, Pearce EN, Brent GA, Brown RS, Chen H, Dosiou C, et al. 2017 guidelines of the American Thyroid Association for the diagnosis and Management of Thyroid Disease during pregnancy and the postpartum. Thyroid. 2017;27(3):315–89.

3. Stagnaro-Green A, Schwartz A, Gismondi R, Tinelli A, Mangieri T, Negro R. High rate of persistent hypothyroidism in a large-scale prospective study of postpartum thyroiditis in southern Italy. J Clin Endocrinol Metab. 2011;96(3):652–7.
4. Nicholson WK, Robinson KA, Smallridge RC, Ladenson PW, Powe NR. Prevalence of postpartum thyroid dysfunction: a quantitative review. Thyroid. 2006;16(6):573–82.
5. Tagami T, Hagiwara H, Kimura T, Usui T, Shimatsu A, Naruse M. The incidence of gestational hyperthyroidism and postpartum thyroiditis in treated patients with Graves' disease. Thyroid. 2007;17(8):767–72.
6. Elefsiniotis IS, Vezali E, Pantazis KD, Saroglou G. Post-partum thyroiditis in women with chronic viral hepatitis. J Clin Virol. 2008;41(4):318–9.
7. Stagnaro-Green A, Akhter E, Yim C, Davies TF, Magder L, Petri M. Thyroid disease in pregnant women with systemic lupus erythematosus: increased preterm delivery. Lupus. 2011;20(7):690–9.
8. Lazarus JH, Ammari F, Oretti R, Parkes AB, Richards CJ, Harris B. Clinical aspects of recurrent postpartum thyroiditis. Br J Gen Pract. 1997;47(418):305–8.
9. Muller AF, Drexhage HA, Berghout A. Postpartum thyroiditis and autoimmune thyroiditis in women of childbearing age: recent insights and consequences for antenatal and postnatal care. Endocr Rev. 2001;22(5):605–30.
10. Kuijpens JL, De Hann-Meulman M, Vader HL, Pop VJ, Wiersinga WM, Drexhage HA. Cell-mediated immunity and postpartum thyroid dysfunction: a possibility for the prediction of disease? J Clin Endocrinol Metab. 1998;83(6):1959–66.
11. Stagnaro-Green A, Roman SH, Cobin RH, el-Harazy E, Wallenstein S, Davies TF. A prospective study of lymphocyte-initiated immunosuppression in normal pregnancy: evidence of a T-cell etiology for postpartum thyroid dysfunction. J Clin Endocrinol Metab. 1992;74(3):645–53.
12. Smallridge RC. Postpartum thyroid disease a model of immunologic dysfunction. Clin Appl Immunol Rev. 2000;1(2):89–103.
13. Kologlu M, Fung H, Darke C, Richards CJ, Hall R, McGregor AM. Postpartum thyroid dysfunction and HLA status. Eur J Clin Investig. 1990;20(1):56–60.
14. Walfish PG, Meyerson J, Provias JP, Vargas MT, Papsin FR. Prevalence and characteristics of post-partum thyroid dysfunction: results of a survey from Toronto, Canada. J Endocrinol Investig. 1992;15(4):265–72.
15. Hayslip CC, Fein HG, O'Donnell VM, Friedman DS, Klein TA, Smallridge RC. The value of serum antimicrosomal antibody testing in screening for symptomatic postpartum thyroid dysfunction. Am J Obstet Gynecol. 1988;159(1):203–9.
16. Lazarus JH. Clinical manifestations of postpartum thyroid disease. Thyroid. 1999;9(7):685–9.
17. Pop VJ, de Rooy HA, Vader HL, van der Heide D, van Son M, Komproe IH, et al. Postpartum thyroid dysfunction and depression in an unselected population. N Engl J Med. 1991;324(25):1815–6.
18. Lazarus JH, Hall R, Othman S, Parkes AB, Richards CJ, McCulloch B, et al. The clinical spectrum of postpartum thyroid disease. QJM. 1996;89(6):429–35.
19. Le Donne M, Settineri S, Benvenga S. Early postpartum alexithymia and risk for depression: relationship with serum thyrotropin, free thyroid hormones and thyroid autoantibodies. Psychoneuroendocrinology. 2012;37(4):519–33.
20. Pearce EN. Thyroid disorders during pregnancy and postpartum. Best Pract Res Clin Obstet Gynaecol. 2015;29(5):700–6.
21. Ide A, Amino N, Kang S, Yoshioka W, Kudo T, Nishihara E, et al. Differentiation of postpartum Graves' thyrotoxicosis from postpartum destructive thyrotoxicosis using antithyrotropin receptor antibodies and thyroid blood flow. Thyroid. 2014;24(6):1027–31.
22. Stagnaro-Green A. Postpartum thyroiditis. Best Pract Res Clin Endocrinol Metab. 2004;18(2):303–16.

Index

A
Allan-Herndon-Dudley syndrome, 9
Amiodarone-induced thyrotoxicosis (AIT), 48
　treatment of, 63–64
Anoctamin 1, 7
Anti-neutrophil cytoplasmic antibody
　　medicated vasculitis (ANCA), 128
Anti-thyroglobulin antibodies, 21
Antithyroid drugs (ATDs)
　adverse effects, for Graves' disease
　　agranulocytosis, 57
　　hepatotoxicity, 57
　　minor, 57
　　vasculitis, 58
　agranulocytosis, 127, 128
　anti-neutrophil cytoplasmic antibody
　　medicated vasculitis, 128
　cessation of therapy, 58–59
　complete blood count and liver function
　　tests, 128
　hepatotoxicity, 127, 128
　methimazole, 56
　monitoring, 57–58
　in nonpregnant patient, 127
　pregnant patients, considerations for,
　　128–129
　propylthiouracil, 56, 57
　side effects, 127
Armour thyroid, 33
Assisted reproductive technology (ART), 164
Autoimmune hypothyroidism, 21, 25

B
Beta blockers, 55, 125, 131
Burch-Wartofsky Point Scale, 50, 51

C
Calcitonin, 5
Cardiovascular system, hypothyroidism in, 25
Central hypothyroidism, 19
　See also Secondary hypothyroidism
Chronic autoimmune hypothyroidism, 21
Congenital hypothyroidism (CH), 80
　central, 94
　classification and epidemiology, 86
　clinical presentation, 87
　definition, 86
　diagnosis, 94–95
　Iodine-123, 94
　levothyroxine tablets, 95
　permanent, 89
　　iodide organification defects, 92
　　iodide recycling defects, 93
　　iodide transport defects, 92
　　Pendred syndrome, 93
　　thyroglobulin deficiency, 93
　　thyroid dysgenesis, 89–92
　　thyroid dyshormonogenesis, 92
　scintigraphy, 94
　thyroid US, 94
　transient, 87
　　DUOX2 and DUOXA2 mutations, 89
　　hepatic hemangiomas, 89
　　iodine deficiency, 87
　　iodine excess, 88
　　maternal hyperthyroidism, 88–89
Controlled ovarian hyperstimulation (COH),
　　162–163

D
DEHAL1 mutations, 93

Deiodinases, in endometrium, 160, 161
Desiccated thyroid, 33
Diffuse autoimmune hyperthyroidism, *see* Graves' disease
Dual oxidase 2 (DUOX2), 4

E
Estradiol, 138
Euthyroid hyperthyroxinemia, 54

F
Familial gestational hyperthyroidism, 124
Fetal development, maternal thyroid function and, 74
Fetal hyperthyroidism, 120
Fetal thyroid physiology
    fetal thyroid function, development of, 82–84
    maternal-fetal interaction, 81–82
    thyroid hormones role, 82–85
Fine needle aspiration biopsy (FNAB), 143, 144

G
Gastrointestinal system, hypothyroidism in, 24
Gestational transient thyrotoxicosis (GTT), 70, 71, 118
    clinical features, 124
    vs. Graves' disease, 126
    incidence, 124
    supportive care, 125
Glucocorticoids, for Graves' orbitopathy, 61
Goiters, 46
Goitrous congenital hypothyroidism, 92
Graves' acropachy, 126
Graves' disease, 47
    anti-thyroidal agents during pregnancy, 120
    antithyroid drugs
        adverse effects, 57–58
        cessation of therapy, 59
        methimazole, 56
        monitoring, 58
        propylthiouracil, 56, 57
    characterization, 177
    clinical features, 126
    vs. gestational transient thyrotoxicosis, 126
    incidence, 118
    maternal TRAb levels, 120–121
    and miscarriage, 177
    in postpartum period, 130–131
    in pregnancy, 133
        antithyroidal drugs, 127–129
        categories, 125
        indications for surgery, 130
        thyroidectomy, 130
    radioactive iodine ablation, 59
    thyroidectomy, 59–60
    thyroid-stimulating immunoglobulins, 2
    treatment options, 56
Graves' orbitopathy (GO)/Graves' ophthalmopathy, 52, 126
    treatment of, 60–61

H
Hashimoto's encephalopathy, 27
Hashimoto's thyroiditis, 38
Hematological system, hypothyroidism in, 26
Hoffman syndrome, 28
Hypercholesterolemia, 26
Hyperthyroidism, 159
    clinical case presentation, 46
    defined, 74
    epidemiology, 46–47
    methimazole, 65
    preconception counseling, 131
    in pregnancy
        causes, 118
        differential diagnosis, 121
        intrauterine growth restriction, 119
        neurocognitive development, 120
        prevalence, 118
        risk factors, 118
        treatment goals, 129
    prevalence, 2
    subclinical, treatment of, 63
    symptomatic management, 55
    thyroidectomy, (*see also* Thyrotoxicosis), 65
Hyponatremia, 25
Hypothalamic-pituitary-thyroid (HPT) axis, Hypothyroidism, 2–4, 19, 159
    causes, 20
    chronic autoimmune, 21
    clinical features, 20
    clinical manifestations, 23
    cognitive disturbances, 27
    diagnosis, 28–30
    etiology, 20
    incidence, 20
    levothyroxine, 31, 110
        coronary artery disease, 32
        in elderly patients, 32
        pregnant patients, 32

Index 191

   thyroid cancer patients, 32
   timing of administration, 31
   treatment, 20
   L-triiodothyronine role, (*see also*
      Myxedema coma), 32–33
   overt (*see* Overt hypothyroidism, in
      pregnancy)
   pathophysiology and clinical features, 22
      cardiovascular system, 25–26
      gastrointestinal system, 23–25
      hematological system, 26
      integumentary system, 22
      musculoskeletal system, 27–28
      neurological system, 26–27
      pulmonary system, 22–24
      renal system, 24–25
      reproductive system, 26–27
   preconception counselling, 110
   prevalence, 2
   screening, 30
   subclinical, (*see also* Subclinical
      hypothyroidism), 36
Hypothyroid phase, of PPT, 186

I
I-131 ablative therapy, 150–153
Infertility
   clinical case presentation, 157
   defined, 157
   ovarian hyperstimulation, 160
   thyroid autoimmunity, prevalence of, 170
   thyroid peroxidase antibody testing, 165
Integumentary system, hypothyroidism, 22
Intrauterine insemination (IUI), 163
In vitro fertilization (IVF), 164, 165
Isolated maternal hypothyroxinemia, in
      pregnancy
   adverse obstetric outcomes, 108
   child neurobehavioral disorders, 109
   child neurocognition, 108
   defined, 102
   treatment benefits, 110

J
Jod-Basedow phenomenon, 48

L
Levothyroxine, 95, 110, 175, 176, 178, 187
   hypothyroidism, 20
      coronary artery disease, 32
      dosing, adjustment and timing, 31
      pregnant patients, 32

   thyroid cancer patients, 32
   subclinical hypothyroidism, 37
L-triiodothyronine role, 32
Lymphocyte infiltration, 21

M
Maternal thyroid dysfunction, screening for,
   74–76
Methimazole (MMI), 56, 127, 129
Miscarriage
   and Graves' disease, 177
   recurrent pregnancy loss (RPL), 173
   subclinical hypothyroidism, 162
   thyroid autoantibodies, 172–174
   and thyroid autoimmunity, 174
Monocarboxylate transporter 8 (MCT8), 9
Musculoskeletal system, hypothyroidism in,
   28
Myxedema, 22
Myxedema coma, 33
   clinical features, 34
   diagnosis, 34
   glucocorticoids, 35–36
   hyponatremia, 35
   hypothermia, 35
   laboratory evaluation, 34
   physical exam, 34
   respiratory depression, 35
   thyroid hormone replacement therapy,
      35–36
Myxedematous madness, 27

N
Neonatal Graves' disease, 120
Neonatal hyperthyroidism, 95–96
Neonatal thyroid disorders, 85
   congenital hypothyroidism, 86–94
   hypothyroidism in premature infants, 86
Neonatal thyroid physiology, 85
Neuropathies, in hypothyroid patients, 27
Newborn screening (NBS), 86
Nongoitrous congenital hypothyroidism, 91
Non-thyroidal illness, 53

O
Obstructive sleep apnea (OSA), in
   hypothyroidism, 24
Ovarian follicular function, thyroid hormone
   role in, 159
Ovarian hyperstimulation, (*see also*
      Controlled ovarian hyperstimulation
      (COH)), 160

Overt hypothyroidism, in pregnancy
adverse obstetric outcomes, 103
defined, 102, 122
levothyroxine, 111
maternal, adverse effects of, 103
treatment benefits, 104

P
Pendred syndrome, 7, 93
Pendrin, 7
Pericardial effusions, in hypothyroidism, 26
Postablative hypothyroidism, 22
Postpartum thyroiditis (PPT)
American Thyroid Association guidelines, 185
autoimmune thyroid inflammation, 184
clinical presentation, 185
definition, 183
etiology, 184–185
hypothyroid phase, 186–187
natural history, 184
prevalence, 184
thyroid stimulating hormone secretion (TSH) level, 186
thyrotoxic phase, 186
Postsurgical hypothyroidism, 22
PPT, *see* Postpartum thyroiditis (PPT)
Pregnancy
abnormal thyroid levels, 117, 132
clinical case presentation, 69, 101, 117, 132
hyperemesis gravidarum, 76
iodine deficiency, 139
isolated maternal hypothyroxinemia, 108–110
levothyroxine during, 111
overt hypothyroidism, 102, 103
physiological changes in hypothalamic-thyroid axis, 12
physiologic changes of thyroid gland
free T4 (FT4) thyroxine level, 73
human chorionic gonadotropin (hCG) level, 70, 71
human chorionic thyrotropin (HCT), 71
hypothalamic-pituitary-thyroid (HPT) axis, down-regulation of, 71
iodine requirement, 70
thyroxine-binding globulin (TBG), 72–73
total T4 (TT4) levels, 73
TSH levels, 71
PPT and, 184

propylthiuracil and methimazole, 133
subclinical hypothyroidism, 102, 104–108
thyroid cancer (*see* Thyroid cancer, in pregnant women)
thyroid dysfunction, universal screening for, 75
thyroid nodules (*see* Thyroid nodules, in pregnant women)
TSH reference ranges, 102
Primary hypothyroidism, 19, 20
diagnosis, 28–30
levothyroxine dose, 31
Progesterone, 138
Propylthiouracil (PTU), 56, 57, 127–129

R
Radioactive iodine ablation (RAI), for Graves' disease, 59–60
Recurrent pregnancy loss (RPL)
clinical case presentation, 170
counseling, 178
levothyroxine treatment, 178
miscarriage risk, 173
thyroid antibody prevalence, 173
thyroid autoimmunity, prevalence of, 170
Renal system, hypothyroidism in, 25
Reproductive system, hypothyroidism in, 27
Resistance to thyroid hormone β (RTHβ), 10
Resistance to TSH (RTSH), 90
Riedel's thyroiditis, 51

S
Secondary hypothyroidism, 21
diagnosis, 28–30
levothyroxine dose, 31
Sick euthyroid syndrome, 53
Struma ovarii, 48
Subclinical hypothyroidism, 36–37
definition, 161
and infertility, 161–162
levothyroxine treatment in women, 162
and male subfertility, 162
miscarriage, 162
in pregnancy
adverse child neurodevelopmental outcomes, 105–106
on adverse obstetric and neonatal outcomes, 104–105
defined, 102, 122
treatment benefits, 106–108
prevalence, 161

Index 193

thyrotropin releasing hormone (TRH)
    test, 161
    treatment, 62–63

T
Thyroid autoimmunity
    ATA recommendations, 171, 172
    infertility, 170
    levothyroxine treatment, 175
    and miscarriage, 174–175
    pregnant patients, treatment strategies
        for, 175–177
    prevalence and natural history, 169–172
    selenium supplementation, 177
    thyroid peroxidase and thyroglobulin, 170
    vitamin D deficiency, 175
Thyroid binding index (TBI), 73
Thyroid cancer
    disease-related survival, 146
    epidemiology, 145–146
    in pregnant women
        diagnosis, 145–147
        ERα positivity, 147
        I-131 ablative therapy, 152
        indications for surgery and timing,
            146–149
        progression and monitoring,
            150–152
        thyroid hormone suppression,
            149–150
Thyroid dysfunction
    and assisted reproductive technology,
        164–165
    chronic autoimmune thyroiditis, 170
    in infertile women, screening and
        treatment, 158
    intrauterine insemination, 163
Thyroid dysgenesis (TD), 90
Thyroidectomy, 130, 131
    for Graves' disease, 60
Thyroid embryology, 80–81
Thyroid function
    controlled ovarian hyperstimulation, 163
    endometrium, 160–161
    medications interfering with, 29
    and menstrual cycle, 159
    and ovary, 159–160
    and pregnancy (see Pregnancy)
Thyroid gland morphogenesis, 80
Thyroid hormone receptor (TRab), 21
Thyroid hormone replacement therapy
    myxedema coma, 36

overt hypothyroidism in pregnancy, 104
Thyroid hormones
    action, 10–12
    gonadal axis, impact on, 12
    mechanism of action, 11
    modification by deiodinases, 6
    physiology, 1–2
    structure, 6
    synthesis, 5
        apical iodide efflux, 7
        dehalogenation of MIT and DIT, 9
        hydrogen peroxide generating
            system, 8
        iodide uptake by sodium-iodide
            symporter, 6–7
        processing and secretion, 9
        sodium-iodide symporter, 4
        spherical thyroid follicles, 4
        thyroglobulin, 7–8
        thyroperoxidase, 7–8
    transport, 9
    uptake into target cells, 10
Thyroiditis, 47
    Riedel's, 51
    suppurative/infectious, 51
    treatment, 64
Thyroid nodules
    ATA sonographic patterns, 143
    benign and indeterminate, management
        strategies, 139–144
    clonal lesions, 137
    composition, 141
    definition, 137
    echogenicity, 142
    isoechoic and hyperechoic nodules, 142
    non-neoplastic causes, 137
    in pregnant women
        clinical case presentation, 137
        epidemiology and pathogenesis,
            138–139
        fine needle aspiration biopsy,
            143, 144
        human chorionic gonadotropin, 138
        initial evaluation, 139–143
        neck ultrasound, 153
        prevalence, 138
        thyroidectomy, 153
    sonographic features, 141–143
Thyroid peroxidase (TPO) antibodies, 21
Thyroid storm
    mortality rates, 50, 131
    therapy options, 131, 132
    treatment, 61–62

Thyrotoxicosis
    amiodarone-induced thyrotoxicosis, 48
    causes, 48
    clinical manifestation, 49
    etiology, 46–48
    eye examination, 52
    laboratory evaluation
        amiodarone-related thyrotoxicosis, etiology, 54
        high uptake etiologies, 53
        low uptake etiologies, 53–54
        thyroid function studies, 52–53
        thyroid labs, considerations for, 54–55
        thyroid uptake and scan, 53
        TSH level, 52
    in pregnancy
        causes, 121
        diagnosis, 121
        etiologies, 124
        gestational transient thyrotoxicosis, 124–125
        heart failure, 118
        maternal and fetal effects, 118–120
        maternal thyroid hormone levels, 123–124
        obstetrical complications, 119
        thyroxine binding globulin levels, 122
        TSH levels, 122
    systemic symptoms, 48–51
    thyroid examination, 51
Thyrotoxic phase, of PPT, 186
Thyroxine-binding globulin (TBG), thyroid hormone level regulation, 72, 73
Total iodide organification defects (TIOD), 93
Toxic adenoma (TA) treatment, 61
Toxic multinodular goiter (TMNG), 47
    treatment of, 60–61
Transient hypothyroxinemia of prematurity (THOP), 86

W
Wolff-Chaikoff effect, 7, 88

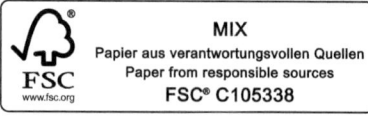

If you have any concerns about our products,
you can contact us on
ProductSafety@springernature.com

In case Publisher is established outside the EU,
the EU authorized representative is:
**Springer Nature Customer Service Center GmbH
Europaplatz 3, 69115 Heidelberg, Germany**

Printed by Libri Plureos GmbH
in Hamburg, Germany